GOING LONG

LEGENDS, ODDBALLS, COMEBACKS & ADVENTURES

THE **BEST STORIES** FROM

RUNNER'S WORLD®

EDITED BY DAVID WILLEY

RODALE

© 2010 by Rodale Inc.

Rodale books may be purchased for business or promotional use or for special sales. For information, please write to:

Special Markets Department, Rodale Inc., 733 Third Avenue, New York, NY 10017

Runner's World® is a registered trademark of Rodale Inc.

The essays in this book have appeared in *Runner's World®* magazine.

"Finding My Stride" reprinted from *Strides* by Benjamin Cheever. Copyright © 2007 by Benjamin Cheever. Permission granted by Rodale, Inc., Emmaus, PA 18098.

"Leading Men" reprinted from *Bowerman and the Men of Oregon* by Kenny Moore. Copyright © 2006 by Kenny Moore. Permission granted by Rodale, Inc., Emmaus, PA 18098.

"The Interval Workout" reprinted with the permission of Scribner, a Division of Simon & Schuster, Inc., from *Once a Runner* by John L. Parker. Copyright ©1978, 1990 by John L. Parker. All rights reserved.

"The Power and the Glory" reprinted by permission of International Creative Management, Inc. Copyright © 2008 by Michael Perry.

"Long Time Gone" excerpt from *Again to Carthage*, copyright © 2007 by John L. Parker Jr., published by permission of Breakaway Books, www.breakawaybooks.com.

Printed in the United States of America

Rodale Inc. makes every effort to use acid-free ♾, recycled paper ♲.

Book design by Christopher Rhoads

Library of Congress Cataloging-in-Publication Data

Going long : legends, oddballs, comebacks & adventures / edited by David Willey.
    p.   cm.
ISBN-13: 978-1-60529-533-6 paperback
ISBN-10: 1-60529-533-7 paperback
  1. Running—Miscellanea. I. Willey, David. II. Runner's world.
GV1061.G64 2010
796.42—dc22   2010005116

Distributed to the trade by Macmillan

  8 10 9

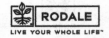

We inspire and enable people to improve their lives and the world around them

For more of our products visit rodalestore.com or call 800-848-4735

CONTENTS

THE RUNNER'S HIGH

ADVENTURES & INVESTIGATIONS

INTRODUCTION

OVER THE COURSE of his brilliant and prolific career writing about sports, the late George Plimpton developed his "Small Ball Theory," which he describes in the introduction to *The Norton Book of Sports*, an anthology he edited in 1992. Plimpton found a correlation between the quality of writing about a particular sport and the size of the ball used to play it: the smaller the ball, the better the writing. You might think that carrying this theory to its logical conclusion would place stories about running at the top of the podium—no ball at all! This would be especially true if you knew that Plimpton, well-known for taking readers inside "the most sacrosanct of worlds" (by, among other things, going three rounds with light heavyweight Archie Moore and playing quarterback for the Detroit Lions), claimed to have gotten his start as a participatory journalist by seeing what it would be like to "win" the 1947 Boston Marathon.

"I was prudent enough to enter the race a block and a half from the finish line," he said some years later in an interview. "There was one person ahead of me. I put on a desperate sprint but still lost, indicative of my speed. But I was exhilarated in a curious way."

Alas, Plimpton's appreciation for running, and for its literary potential, never really took off. Of the 70 fine pieces he collected in the 489-page Norton anthology, not one involved running. Nor is there a single running-related story among the 59 anthologized in *The Best American Sports Writing of the Century*, edited by David Halberstam and published in 1999. These two tomes explore baseball and football and golf—balls of all sizes—as well as boxing and horse racing and even frog jumping. But not one exemplary running story in 100 years? I know that runners have traditionally (and rather happily) trod around the periphery of the American mainstream, but something is wrong here. Even Red Smith, widely regarded as the greatest sportswriter who ever lived, wrote sparingly about running, explaining why in a 1981 *New York Times* column called "The Mile Is a Mockery." "If God had intended man to run," Smith wrote, "he would've given him four legs, or at least made him late for a bus. To be sure, speed afoot might have been useful to some of the young ladies pursued by Jack the Ripper, but unnecessary running is a crime against nature. This goes for the joggers who clutter our country roads and infest our parks, and young men like Sebastian Coe and Steve Ovett who perform publicly in their underwear."

A crime against nature. Okay, then.

At least some exceptional books from the past five decades have emerged, despite this strange sportswriting bias: Alan Sillitoe's *The Loneliness of the Long-Distance Runner;* Roger Bannister's classic *The Four-Minute Mile;* the cult novel *Once a Runner* by John L. Parker Jr.; Dr. George Sheehan's bestseller *Running and Being;* Jim Fixx's breakthrough call to arms, *The Complete Book of Running;* Bernd Heinrich's *Why We Run.* But when it comes to long-form magazine and newspaper writing, the storytelling promise of running seems to have eluded a couple generations of literary journalists.

This is especially odd considering that running is among the oldest sports known to man. The first Olympic Games, in 776 BC, featured just a single event: the *stadion,* a sprint from one end of the stadium in Olympia, Greece, to the other. And even though performance-enhancing drugs have tarnished running in recent years and cast many of its contemporary heroes into doubt, it remains a high-profile sport with sublime athletes and huge, world-class competitions. So all the elements are certainly in place for some good old-fashioned sportswriting.

But that's only the half of it, because we don't merely watch the elites run. We run ourselves, for all kinds of reasons. Running is often called "the people's sport," in part because it's such a short leap from our regular lives. At any given moment, the only thing separating us from a run is a quick change of clothes. We can go out alone or with a group, any time of day, wherever we are. We don't need lessons or formal training or fancy equipment. This doesn't mean that running is easy. It's not, but the effort always pays off, in ways seen and unseen. For all these reasons, running contains more humanity than any other sport, in every sense of the word—more people (tens of millions in America alone), more built-in joy and anguish, more depth, more soul. There's even compelling evidence that running actually made us human in the first place. It was our ancestors' ability to chase down their dinners over long distances on the African veldt, some scientists believe, that enabled them to survive and evolve. I say the following as a devout Red Sox fan and a former football player, but when was the last time you heard an evolutionary biologist postulate that hitting a curveball makes us human? Or throwing a nice, tight spiral? Or smacking a dimpled ball with a club before hopping in a motorized cart to race ahead and hit it again?

Here's something else that makes us human: telling stories. It's easy to imagine our ectomorphic ancestors sitting around a fire, telling their friends about finally running down that herd of wildebeest—or at least painting the scene on the wall of their cave. Like twin strands of DNA, running and storytelling are connected on a human, elemental level. Any run can be viewed as its own private drama with a beginning, a middle, and an end. For the vast majority of us, there is no stadium or crowd of cheering spectators. We generate our own progress according to our own definition of success. Time passes slowly, unless it's one of those blessed days when it flies by. We're left with our thoughts and our labor. This sounds a lot like writing. And reading.

The storytelling possibilities extend from there, to runners themselves (a remarkable lot, by and large), the places running takes them (both geographical and psychological), and the life-changing potential of putting one foot in front of the other again and again (beating cancer, kicking the bottle, taming your demons ...).

So that's *why* running lends itself to great writing and storytelling. This book is intended to demonstrate *how*—and to level the playing field on the anthology front. I originally hoped it would be a survey of the best long-form narratives, profiles, and essays from the magazine's beginning in 1966 to the present day, so I immersed myself anew in the *RW* archives, reading dozens of stories from the past four decades. But when the final selections were made, all but one of them had been published in the past seven years. To borrow a ball-sport metaphor, ambitious long-form feature writing just wasn't a club that *Runner's World* had had in its bag for 30 years, or at least it wasn't a club that had been swung with regularity.

We're taking bigger cuts now. Yes, runners still come to the magazine for instruction and advice. But they also want to be moved and inspired. So at a time when long-form narrative journalism is disappearing from many magazines and newspapers, *Runner's World* remains committed to telling great stories at the length they deserve, which often means 8,000 or 9,000 words. Those are the kinds of stories collected here. To land in these pages, they had to go long *and* deep, transcending running as mere sport in some way, connecting it to larger themes such as fame, faith, family, love, and even life and death.

Here's what this book isn't: a collection of the seminal moments in running history. With a few notable exceptions, these stories are about what happens out of competition, away from races and rivals. Because I decided at the outset not to include columns, some of the magazine's most prolific and iconic writers—Dr. George Sheehan and Joe Henderson to name two—are not represented here because they wrote primarily in column form. Also, I elected to leave out interesting snapshots of accomplished runners at a particular moment in time, unless the writing was simply too good to ignore. The profiles collected here are meant to feel timeless.

The 30 final selections are arranged into five chapters. "Inspirations" gathers profiles of people who have overcome seemingly impossible challenges—disease, amputation, the 9/11 attacks on the Twin Towers—through running or lived remarkable lives in relative obscurity. The runners profiled in "Legends" are more likely household names—phenomenal athletes whose stories reveal the beauty and soul of the sport. Because running doesn't only draw the earnest and the noble, and because I wanted the book to have a few laughs in it, "True Originals" gathers a handful of colorful characters who never took the road well-traveled. "The Runner's High" is a collection of personal essays (plus two pieces of fiction from John L. Parker Jr.) that explore the inner and often ineffable aspects of being a runner. And in "Adventures & Investigations," great writers set out on quests—some noble, some quixotic, some reportorial—all over the world in pursuit of running-related quarry.

I'm deeply grateful to all the writers whose work appears here and who make such a vital contribution to *Runner's World*. I also want to thank the editors, past and present, who brought such care and attention to the crafting of these stories: Amby Burfoot, Charlie Butler, Peter Flax, Tish Hamilton, and Jay Heinrichs; and also to Lori Adams, the keeper of the archives. Thanks also to the editors at Rodale Books who worked on this project: Courtney Conroy, Gena Smith, Karen Rinaldi, Colin Dickerman, and Zachary Greenwald.

Finally, thanks to our readers for *wanting* stories like these in their magazine every month, and for cluttering our roads, infesting our parks, and running around in their underwear, cynics and legendary sportswriters be damned.

David Willey
Editor-in-Chief
January 2010

INSPIRATIONS

16 MINUTES
FROM HOME

BY STEVE FRIEDMAN

[
As a father, husband, runner, and astronaut,
Willie McCool seemed to inspire everyone who knew him.
Even at the end. And even now.
]

DECEMBER 2005

MOST PEOPLE KNOW WHAT HAPPENED. That a piece of foam broke off *Columbia*'s external fuel tank and hit the shuttle's left wing. That NASA officials on the ground gravely underestimated the severity of the damage. That, in fact, the damage caused the shuttle to burn and break into pieces in the skies over Texas, just 16 minutes before its scheduled landing on a clear, bright Saturday morning in February of 2003. What everyone doesn't know is something NASA investigators learned when they sifted through and analyzed the wrecked vessel on the ground.

Among the shuttle parts that investigators recovered was a damaged but intact piece of equipment called the R-2 instrument panel. When they unfolded it, they saw a series of switches that, according to NASA investigator Jon Clark, appeared to have been engaged and manipulated in the final minutes of the doomed astronauts' lives by the person in the shuttle's right seat—the pilot. Although NASA's official report is inconclusive, one theory is that the pilot was making adjustments and maneuvers even as *Columbia* was pitching and spinning toward Earth. That even when death was certainly imminent and known to the crew, Willie McCool was still trying to save the shuttle. Clark, whose wife, Laurel, died along with McCool and five others in the crash, says that what McCool did in those final moments "was a big deal. A very big deal."

Willie McCool was 41 years old when he died, and his singular achievements are what the obituaries and eulogies focused on: Eagle Scout, exceptional runner, test pilot, astronaut. He died serving his country, was publicly mourned. Towns where he lived erected statues in his honor. He was a hero, in every conventional sense of the word, pronounced so at a memorial service by no less a person than the president of the United States. He lived a life deserving of the public recognition he has received.

But to really know Willie McCool is to explore a private world where the heroism is less obvious, but no less profound. Where the actions are human, but extraordinary. To understand Willie McCool you need to step back from the statues and take a closer look at the life.

THEY MET IN GUAM, where Willie's father, a Navy pilot, was stationed. Willie was blond, blue-eyed, and pasty-skinned, lean and sinewy. Atilana Vallelos had black hair and dark eyes and brown skin. He sat behind her in their high school speech class, and for months neither spoke to each other. She went by Lani. He had changed his name from Willy to Willie, because he idolized Willie Mays. "Which is cute," Lani says, "because he's so white."

When they finally spoke, they talked about sports. Lani Vallelos told Willie McCool that she was a sprinter. And that's when Willie, a swimmer, discovered running.

"Lani," he wrote to her, after he had joined the track team, after he had set records in the 1500- and 5000-meter races for Guam's John F. Kennedy High School track team, "of all the people to whom I owe thanks for getting me into track and influencing me to continue on, I think you deserve the most thanks. If it hadn't been for you ... I never would have joined track. Because of your efforts I have finally found something that I enjoy doing and that I do, in all modesty, fairly well.

"Lots of times in a race when my whole body aches, my lungs are burning, my stomach hurts, I feel like stopping and quitting, just saying, 'The hell with this.' But then I think to myself, *What would Lani think if I just stopped and quit? Finish the race for Lani!* Also lots of times, just to get my mind off the pain and off the race, I'll just kind of relax and 'run dream' about you and being together and of the times we had together in the past and the times I wish we could have in the future. Having you as my own sure makes my life an awful lot less painful (most of the time) and much more enjoyable."

He was 15 years old.

After his sophomore year Willie and his family moved to Lubbock, Texas, where Barent McCool had been transferred. Texas had many more, and swifter, teenagers than Guam did. Impressing people with his running wouldn't be easy. He found other ways.

Willie was in a gym, fooling around with a jump rope. His friend Dale Somers had told Willie that one minute of jumping rope expends the same amount of energy as running six minutes. So Willie jumped rope for five minutes. Then another five minutes. Dale yelled to him, Go another five and I'll buy you a Coke. Five minutes later, another high school pal joined in. Another five minutes, he yelled to Willie, and you're a quarter richer. Then one of the dads saw what was going on. Willie, the dad said, five more minutes and I'll buy you a steak dinner.

He jumped rope for 35 minutes.

Somers was on the Coronado High School basketball team, and in the summers he and Willie would play one-on-one. Willie wasn't very good, but when he lost, he would demand another game. And another. And another. Sometimes, the boys would still be playing—and Willie would still be losing—when day turned to Texas twilight.

While running and competing and earning grades good enough to get nominated for the United States Naval Academy, Willie was also a lovesick adolescent. He just wasn't a delusional one. He still wrote to Lani, and Lani wrote back. But after a while, what was there to say? Besides, Willie had developed a crush on a girl named Becky. It took him three months to ask her to lunch. That first date he spent most of it talking about his girlfriend on the island. But she wasn't his girlfriend anymore. How could she be, an ocean between them? Lani dated, got pregnant, and married, had two children.

Adolescent crushes are heady things, but they don't last.

"MY EARLIEST, VIVID MEMORY OF HIM?" Al Cantello asks. "I was screaming at him, something about a crappy workout. Now, most kids, they'd listen, then say, 'Yes, but, yes, but,' but not Willie. He just looked straight at me, with those big, steely blue eyes, taking it all in."

It was 1979, McCool's first, or plebe, year at the Naval Academy in Annapolis, Maryland, and Cantello's 15th year as coach there. He knew "hardly anything" about the runner from Texas. "Willie had a modest high school career. Which was fine by me. What we do here is we take an athlete, and we develop him." Here's how: "We're in a meeting," Cantello remembers, "and I say, 'Okay, Willie, what percent of you is devoted to running?' Willie says, 'I don't know, with graduation, service, maybe 20 percent?' And I say, 'Willie, you'll never be a friggin' runner!'"

Early in their relationship, Cantello told McCool that he was nothing but a baton. It's a standard Cantello trope, one in a series of fierce and ego-deflating lessons the coach imparts to virtually all his plebes. Maybe you won some high school races, maybe you're going to be a big-shot officer one day, he'd tell the boys. But really, you're nothing special. Don't forget it. When it comes down to it, "You're nothing but a baton, carrying DNA from one generation to the next."

McCool became the most disciplined, dedicated baton Cantello had ever seen. He listened to the coach's instructions about technique, and employed them. He listened to the coach's lessons about nutrition and rest, and followed them. He was in bed by 10, asleep by 11, every night of his college career. He listened to the coach's lectures about giving your all, and gave his all.

All that work made him a better runner, but not a great one. By the end of his Navy career, he had the 26th-fastest time ever, 24:27, by a midshipman on the Naval Academy's five-mile cross-country course. Which means his name isn't on the plaque in the glass case of the athletic department building. That's reserved for the 25 fastest. His greatest accomplishment as a Navy runner occurred when he medaled in the 10,000 meters in the league outdoor championships. Cantello can't remember much else.

Looking back, the coach wonders whether Willie could have been better had he been tougher, a bit more ruthless. "He was a little bit sheltered," Cantello says. "If someone stepped on his toes during a race, Willie would say,"—here Cantello affects a high-pitched whine—"'That's poor sportsmanship.' Meanwhile, a guy from New Jersey is running next to him, getting ready to throw an elbow, saying, 'I'm gonna put that jerk in lane three.'"

But Willie was other things. He was relentlessly cheerful, given to striding up and down the hallways of his dorm, exclaiming, "Five weeks till the meet. Beat Army!" He was elected captain of the cross-country team as a senior, the guy the team rallied around. "He was energetic, he was enthusiastic, he was smart," says Mark Donahue, the captain when McCool entered the Academy. "When I look back on it, the word that comes to mind is innocent." McCool was the brainy runner that Cantello asked to help his son with algebra one Saturday night. For a midshipman, a Saturday night is a precious thing, one of the only times he is allowed off the Academy grounds. McCool didn't hesitate.

When he graduated from the Academy in 1983, he was ranked second in his class. "He made more of himself in four years than anyone I can remember," Cantello says. Then the coach pauses. "But is he the most inspirational? You gotta remember. I've been here 43 years."

A COUPLE OF YEARS LATER, when he was studying for his masters in computer science at the University of Maryland, Willie made a point of taking care of Cantello's newest group of batons. He drove the plebes to meets. He joined them in practice. He filled up the team cooler with water. Every night before a meet, he invited them to his condominium in Crofton, eight miles west of Annapolis. He cooked them spaghetti. ("Willie knew as much about making spaghetti sauce as..." Cantello trails off mournfully. "He used carrots! That's a misdemeanor. That's a no-no.") But the batons were grateful.

"He protected all of us," Ron Harris, a plebe in 1983, says. The plebes called McCool's condominium the "Bat Cave" and treasured their time there. They didn't know what lay ahead for him, the greatness in store. They just knew the guy making funny spaghetti sauce. "The amazing thing," Harris remembers, "was that he had so much time for us. He had time for everything."

It was about this time that Willie heard from another Navy man that Lani was separated from her husband. Willie hadn't forgotten her. Sometimes when he ran with his Navy teammates he talked about the girl he had been in love with in the South Pacific, the one with the black hair who got him into running in the first place. He wrote to her and she wrote back. He flew out to see her in Tempe, Arizona, where she was finishing college, and they drove to a nearby football stadium. He handed her his watch, which she had used to time him while he ran quarter miles on Guam. She had always loved watching Willie run. She knew how happy it made him.

"Everything came back," Lani says. "The smells, the phone calls. It was like we had never been apart. My heart...it jumped. You know the saying about seeing a rainbow? I was seeing double rainbows."

After her divorce, Lani and Willie were married, in 1986. She knew how much he loved children and that he would be a wonderful father to her two boys; Sean was then 5, Christopher was 3. "I asked him if he wanted kids," Lani says. "And he said, 'I already have kids. We have kids.'" But another son, Cameron, was born on September 15, 1987. The next day McCool, by then a Navy pilot, left for a six-month tour of duty aboard an aircraft carrier.

Willie and Lani and the boys spent most of the next decade in Washington State, in the town of Anacortes, just a short drive from the naval base on Whidbey Island, where McCool flew the Prowler, a four-person aircraft used for jamming radar and other electronic warfare tactics. Once, at the Patuxent River Naval Air Station in Maryland, he pulled a Prowler out of a spiral, or a "death spin." No one had ever done it before. Today, every Prowler pilot and would-be pilot studies what McCool did that day; it's the official Navy procedure for pulling a Prowler out of a spiral.

His work meant Willie was gone from home a lot, but Lani had the children to take care of, and her passion for photography, and she played the harp that Willie had bought for her. Lani was a military man's daughter. So she knew the drill. When Willie was home they played chess together and went on backpacking trips with the kids. He wrote her poetry.

In 1996, NASA selected McCool for its space program. The family moved to Houston, where Willie joined 43 others in a group of future shuttle astronauts— they called themselves "the sardines" because there were so many. It was the largest group of shuttle astronauts since the 1978 class. By then McCool, the Navy pilot, had amassed more than 2,800 hours of flight experience in 24 aircraft and made more than 400 landings on aircraft carriers, which even among pilots is a very big deal.

But the other sardines were big deals, too. They had been selected from a pool of 2,400 applicants. McCool was surrounded by people just like him. There was a former circus gymnast who was also a fighter pilot and doctor. There was a flight surgeon who could name most birds—in Latin. Joining McCool on the shuttle *Columbia* would be an Israeli Air Force colonel, a son of Holocaust survivors, who flew on the mission that had destroyed Iraq's nascent nuclear reactors in 1981. Top guns all, oozing competitive juju.

Steve MacLean was one of the sardines. What struck him most about McCool wasn't his intelligence, or his skills, or his competitive zeal (though MacLean says all were extraordinary, even by NASA standards). What MacLean remembers is watching McCool run. "It was like he was on wheels," MacLean says. "It was a thing of beauty." What he remembers even more is how he treated others, especially children. At weekly soccer games involving astronauts and their families, a goal couldn't be scored until the smallest kid playing had touched the ball at least once—a rule McCool pushed for. As MacLean says, "When he was talking to somebody, no matter who it was, that person was very important."

ALMOST EVERY DAY, AT TWILIGHT, whether in Houston or in Anacortes, Willie would come home and find Lani cooking dinner for the kids. He loved his work, but he hated that he was gone so much. He would offer to help. Lani would decline. He'd insist. She'd tell him to go for a run. Sometimes, she'd watch him take off. "It looked like he ran on air," she says.

Half an hour or an hour later he would come in, dripping with sweat, and he would slam a knight to a new position on their chessboard in the living room, or write a line of poetry. And then he would lie on the living room floor and stretch, and Lani would play her harp as the dinner cooked. And Willie would move closer to Lani. And closer. Until finally, he was stretching his legs while he leaned against Lani.

"Our friends said we were the luckiest people in the world," Lani says. "And they were right."

One day, McCool asked Cameron to join him on a run. But his son, then 13, didn't want to. I have too much homework, he'd say. McCool promised to help him with the homework if he'd run. Well, then, I'm too sore. McCool promised he'd feel better after a run. He'd run, but the teenager would whine about it. For Willie's 41st birthday, a few months before the shuttle launch, Cameron gave his dad a card, promising 15 "complaint-free runs, to be used whenever you want."

Lani told her husband to entertain the boy, to make the running more fun. She told Willie to tell him stories, to take the boy's mind off how much he hurt.

But Willie was a natural listener, not a talker. Still, he tried. He began by retelling novels he thought a teenage boy would like. The first, told over weeks and weeks of running, was *The Worthing Saga*, by Orson Scott Card. By the end of the book, Cameron could talk and run without gasping. Then there were other novels—Cameron can't remember them all—and now that the boy could talk without gasping, they would discuss the works. They'd talk about "the philosophy behind the stories or just ideas in general," says Cameron.

Willie ran out of new novels. He started telling his own stories.

He talked about throwing berries at cars on Guam, getting in trouble. He talked about building model airplanes with his father. Those were fine, but Cameron wanted stories from the Academy. He wanted to hear about his father's life as a plebe, how he had to tuck his chin into his chest and recite dinner menus and jet parts while upperclassmen screamed at him. He wanted to hear about the ice-cream-eating contests his father participated in as a senior, how a plebe stood behind him and massaged his temples to prevent "freeze" headaches. Willie wouldn't just tell the stories, he would act them out—as the frightened plebe, the screaming midshipman, the ice-cream-gulping senior. By the time his father flew into space, Cameron had quit counting the poles. They were running three and a half miles from the gates of NASA. Three and a half miles out, three and a half miles back.

JUST A FEW WEEKS BEFORE McCool and the rest of the *Columbia* crew would head into space, in December 2002, he went for a run with a man named Andy Cline, whom he had met on a backpacking trip a year earlier.

The men ran in Anacortes, where the McCools planned to return full time after the *Columbia* mission. McCool wanted to show Cline a spot he had discovered. They ran through the Anacortes Forest Lands to Cranberry Lake. Cline told the astronaut how he wanted to run faster, how he would like, for once in his life, to break the three-hour mark in a marathon.

"And Willie said that was no problem, that he'd pace me and that he would help me get to that. And I believed him. When you were with him, you felt like you had his undivided attention. That life seemed pretty clear."

McCool and Cline always talked a lot on their runs, but on this run they talked even more than usual. "About God and faith, and what that looks like and the variability of that," Cline remembers. "He said that everyone of us has some sort of faith and the trick was in recognizing it, in seeing it.

"And I know it sounds odd to say this, but I couldn't help thinking as we talked. And what I thought was, This might be the last time I ever see Willie."

WE LIKE OUR HEROES' LIVES TO ADHERE to the simple and ascending trajectory we associate with great men. And in its public outlines, Willie McCool's life was all of that. A disciplined and strong-willed distance runner from an early age, a little boy who built and flew model airplanes, an honors student who loved chemistry and poetry equally well.

But his life wasn't quite so simple. No one's is. Willie's biological father was a heavy drinker known to have a bad temper and quick to take it out on his wife, Audrey, his son, and Kirstie, Willie's little sister. After his parents divorced, Willie took it upon himself to be Kirstie's protector when they went to visit their dad. Soon, the visits stopped altogether. Audrey was a dietitian then, in Southern California, working full time, doing her best to take care of her children and to keep her husband from finding them. "We had to grow up young and early," says Kirstie Chadwick.

Can a hero come only from a crucible of agony? Did McCool watch out for others because he had a tough childhood? Did he run because he had discovered a place where his life was not so painful? Did his biological father—by most accounts a highly intelligent man—pass on some of his best genetic material to his son? Did Barent McCool, Willie's adoptive father—a Navy pilot and by all accounts a loving if demanding and unsentimental teacher—mold the boy who became his son into such a perfectionist? Was it Audrey's drive and need that turned Willie into a man before he was even a teenager? There's a theory for every question. One sounds as good as another. None matters too much.

Just look closer at the life.

Lani McCool is gazing at a hawk in a tree, with his wings spread, drying. She has just hiked 20 minutes or so to Sares Bluff, a scenic outlook just a few minutes' drive from her home in Anacortes. It is cool, late summer in the Pacific Northwest and she is happy. She wishes more people would understand that joy is something Willie would have wanted.

"I'll be out somewhere, maybe at a function involving NASA, and I'll be throwing my head back laughing and people will stare and say, 'There's Willie McCool's widow.' What do people want? That we continue grieving forever?"

Late summer, two and a half years since the accident, and for the past two days she has been remembering the 24 years they knew each other, the 17 and a half years they were married. We have visited the naval station at Whidbey Island to pay respects at the memorial for Willie. There, engraved at the base of a replica of the Prowler, is CDR WILLIAM McCOOL STS-107 COLUMBIA 1 FEB 2003. Lani traces a heart in the concrete with her finger. We have poked around her house, looked at the chessboard where he used to slam pieces after his run, at the harp Lani played while Willie leaned against her legs. She has shown poetry he wrote to her, photographs she took of him.

The past two and a half years haven't been easy. His Navy and NASA files are in the garage. She managed to open one box, but couldn't open any more. She thinks about the trip to Switzerland he'd been promising since she saw double rainbows. She thinks about the darkroom he was going to build for her.

She's tried to go to church, but every time she got close, she started crying, "because the Eucharist is as close as we get to someone who's dead," and that's reminded her of the times she and Willie attended church together. Sometimes, because of terrible allergies, she couldn't walk to the front of the church to receive communion. So Willie would transfer part of the Eucharist to her, and people thought they were kissing and it scandalized the congregation, and it makes her laugh to think about it.

Soon she will drive Cameron to college in Seattle, and after she drops him off and returns home, she will pass a theater and see on the marquee the name of the film, *The Corpse Bride*, and she will break down sobbing.

She has five books on her bed, is reading all of them, but in the afternoon, overlooking the Pacific Ocean, she can't remember the name of a single one. Sometimes she looks at Willie's books. Books of Russian, which he was teaching himself. *The Odyssey. Macbeth.* Sometimes she leafs through them. In the margins of a biography of Einstein, she found something that made her smile. Willie's delighted scrawl: "Light Bends!!!"

Life hasn't been easy, but it has been ... life. It has been good. That was something Willie and Lani always agreed on. That it was good. That it should be good. "There are so many gifts," she says. The poems he wrote, the letters he sent. The memories she has of him. The future.

"I miss him horribly," she says. "It was a loss, but I realized it was okay, because we lived a good life. I have no regrets. I don't think I ever said he died too young. . . .

"People misinterpret it, because I'd give anything to have him back, but he's not here. I am okay. I miss Willie and I loved him. But I am okay."

She attended the launch on July 26 because she feels like her husband's death and the lessons NASA learned from it will help other astronauts. Still, she is much more at home in Birkenstocks and leggings than pearls and a dress. She says that all the memorials for the *Columbia* crew members were somewhat easier to take because "I love wearing black." In the hotel rooms afterward, she says, "I'd get a plate of chocolates and I'd take a bite out of each—I didn't have to worry about being good."

She knows that some other naval wives view her with something other than love. She knows that she doesn't quite fit the image of a military spouse. She says that Willie adored that about her. Some of his friends say the same thing. She shows me a poem that he read to her from space; it was the last time she heard his voice.

"He said, 'Hold on, I've got something here.' And then he read this: 'I've witnessed the beauty of Earth from space, far, far above. What a treasure it is to behold. But I would trade this view for your embrace, my sweet love, for only you enrapture my soul.'

"That was the last two minutes I heard him. So yeah," she says, "I feel lucky."

Look closer at the life.

Andy Cline is running. Some days it's in the Anacortes Forest Lands, some days it's somewhere else near his new home in the Pacific Northwest. He still wants to do a marathon in less than three hours, but he doesn't know if he'll be able to. Today, the running isn't easy. It doesn't feel good.

"And I'm dying," Cline says. "And then I'm thinking, 'If Willie were here, he'd kick it up a notch.' So that's what I do."

Look closer at the life.

Cameron stopped running as the launch date got closer, then his father went into quarantine, and then there was the *Columbia* accident. But after a while, he started again. As he ran, he says, "I was thinking in the back of my head that I was doing it for him, but always remembering that he had been doing it for me." Then Sean, his oldest brother, said he wanted to run, too. But he wasn't in the greatest shape. So Cameron set up a schedule. He encouraged his brother to tune out his pain. And he told him stories. "Like my dad did for me."

Look closer at the life.

Al Cantello is sitting in his office at the Naval Academy. On his wall is a framed sweatshirt that Willie wore. In Cantello's file cabinet are the size 10 and a half white Air Pegasus shoes that Lani mailed after the accident. In his drawer is a letter McCool wrote to the coach, inviting him to the launch: "Your coaching laid a foundation of discipline, drive, and passion that has carried me across the many milestones of my life. With boundless appreciation, Willie."

Willie McCool may have been heroic for all the conventional reasons—not least of which that he died while serving his country. But what made him extraordinary, even by heroes' standards, was something else entirely. Something rare. Something almost ineffable. The way he lived his life, every day, almost every moment. The way he touched others.

The coach, former world record holder of the javelin throw, still burly and vigorous at 74, leans forward across his desk. "Look," he says of the boy whose presence seems to fill his office, "he wasn't the Second Coming. He didn't network very well. He wasn't a very good correspondent. Too much sensitivity."

This is my second day visiting with Cantello. During that time, he has talked about the crushing demands of running at Navy, politics, coaching, life. He always returns to Willie McCool. To his naiveté. His love for Lani. His death.

"Afterwards," Cantello says, "there was the initial bereavement, in Houston, when the president spoke. Then, shortly after that, the vice president spoke here and some admirals, too, and a couple dozen busloads of congressmen. But it was perfunctory grieving.

"And then a year goes by and they have a ceremony at the National Air and Space Museum. Candles, subdued lighting, all the appointments and trappings were there. It's supposed to be a night of solemn closure. We're supposed to be in the cathedral of this nation's highest aspirations. I look around and who's there? Lockheed Martin, Boeing, Grumman." People who didn't know Willie. People who wanted to trade on his symbolism. More perfunctory grieving.

"Here. You want to understand Willie? You should listen to this." Then Cantello pulls something from one of his desk drawers and slides it into his computer. It's a CD labeled WILLIE MCCOOL WAKE UP MUSIC "IMAGINE" ABOARD SPACE SHUTTLE COLUMBIA FLIGHT DAY 15 JAN 29, 2003. It's from three days before the accident.

We sit and listen to the melancholy, aching strains of "Imagine." Then, a female voice: "Good Morning, Blue Team. The song 'Imagine,' by John Lennon, was for Willie this morning." A few more bars of the music, subtle hissing that hints at the distance from Mission Control to the orbiting craft.

Then, the voice of Willie McCool. Cheerful. Enthusiastic. Still innocent. "Good morning, Linda. That song makes us think that from our orbital vantage point we observe an Earth without borders, full of peace, beauty, and magnificence, and we pray that humanity as a whole can imagine a borderless world as we see it and strive to live as one, in peace . . ."

The coach is looking away from the computer, away from me. In the short time I have known him, it's the first time I've seen him speechless. His eyes well up.

"Okay, Willie and your team," says the voice from Houston, "we appreciate those words and we wish everyone down here could have the view you do."

13

Cantello leans forward, hits his keyboard, takes the CD from the computer. Then he leans back in his chair. "What's the right way to grieve?" he asks. "Do you go to a tree, rub some sand between your fingers? Hell, I don't know." More than a few cross-country runners have told me how hard Cantello took Willie's death. Not the coach, though. "How do you grieve?" he repeats. "I'm going to tell you how I'm going to do it."

He slides a letter across his desk to me. It's a memo, "Subj: CDR Willie McCool, USS Memorial at Navy XC Course." In the memo, Cantello proposes a stone marker on the cross-country course, "placed just to the left of the current tee shack [so it] would not impede golfers, runners, or golf-course management.

"This simple monument would serve to inspire generations of Navy runners, who, like Willie, endured the resolute pursuit of being a Navy runner...." Cantello sent the letter in July 2003. Still, no marker. "Man, for all practical purposes," he says, "is a son of a bitch."

Then the coach complains about golf courses, and golfers, and buildings on golf courses, and the nature of man, and about why petty-minded bureaucrats and penny pinchers are making it so damned hard to get a monument to the runner who wasn't the Second Coming but who made more of himself than anyone Cantello ever saw. Then he says that he doesn't care how long it takes, he's going to get a monument built to Willie McCool.

He and some of his runners walked off the distance on the cross-country course, factored in Willie's best time ever on the course, figured out Willie's pace. They want the monument to stand at the top of a grassy hill, a brief level stretch of the five-mile course, just before it descends to a narrow path through trees. It's 3.1 miles from the finish line. Willie would have covered the distance in 16 minutes.

Cantello's cross-country record at Navy is 236-64-1. He has coached three All-American runners, has been named the NCAA Mid-Atlantic Regional Coach of the Year three times. He had a 67-9-1 dual-meet record when he coached Navy's men's indoor and outdoor track teams. In 1997, the Academy Alumni Association awarded Cantello the Distinguished Athletic Leadership Award for a coach or faculty member who did the most for the physical development of the midshipmen. He has coached at the U.S. Naval Academy for 43 years.

This is how Cantello wants to be remembered: "My legacy," he says, "will be to preserve Willie's time in perpetuity for the five-mile course, so when I'm dead and gone, people will know where he was when he was 16 minutes from home.

"I'm just carrying Willie's baton."

A SECOND LIFE

BY CHARLES BUTLER

*Matt Long had life by the horns—until the day he
got crushed by a 20-ton bus. Though the once unstoppable
firefighter and Ironman suffered horrific injuries, he somehow survived.
Then he had to do something even harder: learn to live again.
So Long took on another impossible challenge.
He decided to run a marathon.*

MARCH 2009

THE SUN IS BARELY UP ON THIS NOVEMBER MORNING, but already Matt Long is in a rush. The career fireman knows the importance of moving fast: it can save a life. Today, however, he can't seem to move quick enough.

It took 10 stressful minutes to find the disabled-athlete starting area for the ING New York City Marathon. Until three years ago, he'd never have imagined lining up for a race alongside people who are blind or depend on crutches or sit in wheelchairs—and who will get a three-hour head start on the field. But those three years have been packed with humbling surprises.

Long is flanked by two longtime buddies, fellow fireman Frank Carino, and Noel Flynn, who works at a Manhattan hedge fund. Carino has done an 11-hour Ironman triathlon, while Flynn is on the cusp of a sub-three-hour marathon. Still, they've agreed to hang with their friend, step by step, for a very slow run through New York City. It could take eight or nine hours. Long's really not sure. All he knows is that until he finishes, his exhausting battle to restore his body, his identity, and his connections to loved ones won't be complete either.

Long wobbles over to a police barricade to stretch his legs. He adjusts his black skullcap. Then he gives his knee-high compression socks a final tug. He hopes they'll give his battered legs some extra support. Long's friends take note—and let him have it.

"Yo, Frank," says Flynn. "Check out Matty's legs."

"Very nice, Matty," says Carino. "Ya look like Paula Radcliffe."

For a while, Long joins in as the jokes fly, but he has other things on his mind. The fast-talking, hard-charging fireman is about to run the slowest race of his life, and even if he finishes, he's surely going to suffer. He paces around like his life depends on what happens over the next 26 miles. And maybe it does.

ON DECEMBER 22, 2005, NEW YORK CITY WOKE UP TO 28-DEGREE temperatures and day three of a transit strike. For 48 hours, the 33,000-person Transport Workers Union had violated a state law prohibiting city employees from staging a job action. Union and city negotiators kept bargaining, but no settlement was in sight. The strike forced New Yorkers to find new ways to get around.

Matt Long was among them. That morning around 5:30, the 12-year veteran of the New York City Fire Department left his apartment on East 48th Street on his road bike, wearing a ski mask and a red and silver jacket over a winter biking kit. He had a 20-minute ride ahead of him, to the Rock on Randall's Island.

The Rock is shorthand for the FDNY's training academy. It's where probationary officers go to see if they can make it in to the nation's largest firefighting department. The Rock resembles a Hollywood back lot, 22 acres dotted with faux walk-ups and high-rises. For six months, probies haul hoses up and down stairs with up to 100 pounds on their backs. They crawl through dark tunnels while breathing through oxygen masks. They do whatever they're told so they're ready when a fire alarm goes off.

It was the next-to-last day of Long's yearlong assignment with the academy's health and fitness squad. His job was to ensure probies were physically prepared to graduate and save lives. After the assignment, he was planning to take a week of vacation, then return to his permanent post at Engine Company 53, Ladder 43, in East Harlem.

Long, 39 at the time, fit in perfectly at the Rock. He was relentlessly upbeat and radiated strength. He came from blue-collar Bay Ridge, Brooklyn, and was one of nine siblings. He had two brothers in the FDNY. Long had worked amid the chaos at Ground Zero on 9/11. And he had a "save" to his credit. On Christmas Eve in 2000, his company responded to a fire in a tenement that was thought to be abandoned. But while putting out the fire, Long saw a stack of mail in front of one apartment. So, he entered the unit and found an elderly man unconscious on the floor. With another firefighter's help, he dragged the man to safety.

While at the Rock, Long worked himself into the best shape of his life. He had only been biking and running seriously for a year and a half; he got into the sports when he was having back pain and a doctor urged him to lose some of the 212 pounds he was carrying on his 5'11" frame. Within a few months, he was down 30 pounds, over the back pain, and suddenly addicted to triathlons. In fact, he competed in more than 20 events of various distances over an 18-month span. "The adrenaline rush—I loved it," he says. "It was like rushing to a fire. I was hooked."

So it was little surprise when Long attempted—and finished—his first Ironman triathlon, a 2.4-mile swim, 112-mile bike, and 26.2-mile run, in Lake Placid, New York, in July 2005. He finished in 11 hours and 18 minutes, placing in the top 20 percent for his age group and running the marathon leg in 3:44:38.

Next, Long set his sights on the 2005 New York City Marathon. But not just to run it. He wanted to go 3:15 and qualify for Boston. In August, Long began running workdays at 6 a.m. with three trainers at the Rock: Tommy Grimshaw, Shane McKeon, and Larry Parker. No day was a gimme. On Mondays and Wednesdays they ran 12 miles, pushing eight of those at a 6:15 clip. Tuesdays and Thursdays were easy eight-milers. And Friday was an 18-miler, with miles four to 12 at a six-minute pace. At first, Long couldn't keep up. "But after a month, Matty wasn't far behind us. Pretty soon he was sticking with us," says McKeon. "We pushed each other; our goal was for all of us to qualify for Boston."

As it turned out, all four made it. Long went 3:13:59, good enough to place fourth among the 201 New York firefighters who ran. They'd start ramping up for Boston right after New Year's. Today, on this frigid morning three days before Christmas, a light swim was in store. McKeon, Grimshaw, and Parker waited at the Rock as Matt Long started to cycle up Third Avenue.

"HEY, HOW DID WE DO WITH THAT FIRST MILE?"

"Around 17:30. That work for you, Matt?"

"Yeah, pretty close to what I expected."

By now Long, Carino, and Flynn are halfway across the Verrazano-Narrows Bridge. To their left, Manhattan's skyline is backlit in light blue. In front of them, there's nothing but the metal skyway. The other early starters are out of sight, having rushed off on crutches and in chairs.

When Long ran here in 2005, he did the first mile in an easy 7:40. Today he stutters across the span, his brawny shoulders listing and lurching side to side. As he pushes off his left leg, the one filled with titanium, the three grossly distorted hammer toes on his left foot jab into the ground. His right leg, two inches shorter than his left, follows in a contorted motion, barely bending as he forces his foot forward. Each step consumes inches, not feet.

THE BUS MOVED UP THIRD AVENUE, TWO LANES OVER from the shoulder where Matt Long and his bike were gaining speed. It wasn't a typical city bus. A brokerage firm, Bear Stearns, had hired the coach to transport employees to work during the transit strike. The driver was from Albany, so maybe he didn't know that making turns outside of the marked bus lane was prohibited by law. Or perhaps he just didn't see the biker. Whatever the reason, the bus started turning right onto 52nd Street—and right into Matt Long.

Later, one cop at the scene would wonder why the biker didn't ricochet backward on impact. That's what typically happens in a collision like this. But when Long crashed into the bus, he got vacuumed underneath. By the time the bus came to a stop, Long and his bike were twisted near the rear axle. The bike's handlebars were jammed into the coach's metal base and had speared Long, opening a fissure from his belly button to his rectum. Blood slid from under the vehicle and began pooling near the street corner.

A police officer happened to be nearby and called for backup. The NYPD's Emergency Service Unit arrived four minutes later. One detective, Charles King, went to work lifting the front of the bus with a hydraulic jack, while two others, Ralph Logan and Charlie Raz, crawled under. They heard Long moan, "so we knew he was alive," recalls Logan. They yelled out for a portable saw so they could cut the handlebars from the bus and Long's stomach. But because of the blood gushing from Long's midsection, "it was like an oil slick under there," Logan says. "I had to wedge my feet up on the bottom of the bus to keep from sliding." As the officers sawed, firefighters from a midtown station arrived. One of them, Donal Buckley, crawled under the bus to help. He grabbed the bike frame, steadying it as officers kept sawing.

After a couple of minutes, the officers had freed Long. They rolled him onto a backboard, pushed him from under the bus, and lifted him onto a gurney. Long was drifting in and out of consciousness, though he managed to mouth the word *forty*. Buckley looked at his face; it was pasty white but familiar. He remembered a fireman who used to park his car in front of his firehouse to run in nearby Central Park.

"Hey," Buckley blurted, "that's Matty Long, from Ladder 43."

AS LONG, CARINO, AND FLYNN STUTTER DOWN THE ramp off the Verrazano and start looping into Brooklyn, Long says, "I used to come out every year and watch this race. Never missed it." Bay Ridge is the first neighborhood runners hit after the bridge. Long's family moved there when he was a teenager.

In a few hours, locals will line Fourth Avenue, cheering on a sea of marathoners. But now, the street is practically empty, except for a clump of about 40 people waiting in front of Our Lady of Angels Church, near the three-mile mark. It's Long's family and friends. Matt told his mom and dad that he'd stop for exactly 90 seconds—enough time for them to snap a few pictures. The noise grows until Long shuffles to a stop in front of his parents and hugs them. His two sisters, Maureen and Eileen, hold their kids and cry. Some of his brothers and nephews hold signs that say Matty, We Love You and Matty, You Will.

The 90 seconds pass quickly. Long tells his family he has to go. A block later, he turns to his left. He's tearing up. "Hey, Frank."

"Yeah, Matt."

"The allergies, bro. They're starting to kick in."

"Take it slow, bro. Take it slow."

MOST MORNINGS, DR. SOUMITRA R. EACHEMPATI, a trauma surgeon at New York-Presbyterian Hospital on Manhattan's Upper East Side, walks to work from his nearby apartment. On this day, however, he walked a bit faster after getting a call from the ER about a biker who'd been carved open by a bus.

Orthopedic surgeon Dr. Dean Lorich had a trickier commute. He lives 20 blocks from the hospital. Because of the transit strike, police were restricting cars or taxis with fewer than four passengers. So to get to work that day, Lorich had to fill a cab with his pregnant wife and two young daughters.

Both doctors arrived to find Matt Long bleeding to death.

Jim Long was the first family member to get to the hospital; he's a year younger than Matt and works in the FDNY's public affairs office. When Jim arrived at the ER, a nurse told him that his brother was already in the operating room. "This is as bad as it gets," she said. "We're doing everything we can." Jim Long then looked to his left toward the emergency room, where puddles of red were everywhere. He asked the nurse if they came from his brother. She nodded. "My parents are coming very soon," he said to the nurse. "Can you please clean that up?"

Due to the heavy blood loss, Long's blood pressure was dangerously low by the time he reached the OR. His body was mangled, with a compound fracture of the left tibia and femur, a compound fracture of the left foot, a fractured right shoulder, a fractured right hip, perforated abdominal walls, a torn rectum, extensive pelvic nerve damage, and a crushed pelvis.

"His chances for living were five percent," Eachempati says. "Maybe even less than that."

The OR was a madhouse, as multiple teams of doctors, residents, anesthesiologists, and nurses scrambled to follow Eachempati and Lorich's orders. The two lead doctors went about separate, syncopated tasks to keep Long alive. Eachempati tried to stanch the bleeding, but as soon as he could control one perforated vessel, another would appear. Twice he had to abbreviate his work so radiologists could embolize bleeding that his fingers couldn't reach. All the while, the team kept transfusing pints and pints of blood into Long's body as he kept bleeding. "He lost an extraordinary amount," recalls Eachempati. "In 12 hours, he lost 48 units." That's six gallons—four times the amount of blood in a body Long's size.

Lorich worked to stabilize Long's broken pelvis. "All the big blood vessels are coming through the pelvis from the aorta and going down to your legs, so when he ripped everything, he tore all those arteries," says Lorich. "And it ripped through his anus and tore his rectum out, so he's pouring stool into the pelvis."

That night, the best physicians could tell Mike and Eileen Long and their eight kids was that Matt was still alive. Doctors also said that even if Long survived the blood loss, he could die of pneumonia or another infection or wind up in a vegetative state.

"That first day," recalls Lorich, "I think everybody other than Eachempati thought he would die." Lorich did a stint in Germany treating U.S. soldiers who'd been hurt in Iraq, and says that Long's abdominal and pelvic wounds exceeded the injuries of many soldiers who'd been hit by mortar fire.

Over the next few weeks, Long remained in a chemically induced coma as doctors continued to open and close Long up for follow-up surgeries. Finally, he came to on January 7. But he looked nothing like an Ironman. Long would lose nearly 50 pounds, most of it muscle, while in the hospital. "The first time I went to see him, I walked right past him," said Shane McKeon. "He looked like an 85-year-old dying of cancer."

So why didn't Long die? One theory, says Eachempati, is that "we actually got the blood loss controlled within eight to 10 hours." Just as critical, the doctor adds, Long was "obviously very fit, and that definitely contributed to his survivability. His body was resilient enough to withstand such a metabolic insult.

"Taking care of Matt reinforced some things that I'd already thought," he adds. "One is to never give up on anybody. Two, the human body can be trained to withstand severe insults. And three, never shortchange the will of the patient."

Matt Long certainly had a strong will. He'd qualified for Boston the first time he put his mind to it. He'd survived bouts with lots of burning buildings and the World Trade Center crumbling around him. But after five months and 22 surgeries, the man whom doctors had saved and rebuilt was no longer the same man who'd gone under that bus. Surviving that kind of trauma was one thing. Finding the will to live again would be another thing entirely.

THEY RUN THROUGH BROOKLYN SIDE-BY-SIDE, stopping to walk only when they come to a water stop or need a bathroom. They tell stories and jokes. Flynn offers one up about a Chinaman, an Irishman, and an Italian. Carino follows with one about a Pole, an Irishman, and an Italian. After that, Long says, "Enough," and they all laugh.

Next, Long riffs a bit about the nearby Catholic high school he attended and some of his favorite bars in the city. Then he tells a story about his younger brother Rob. "I got an e-mail from him last night just before I went to bed. He wrote me something he'd never told me before. I guess on Christmas Eve, just after the accident, my whole family was at the hospital. But around 6 o'clock, Rob left to go to an AA meeting—he's an alcoholic. And on the way back to the hospital, he passed this dirty, dingy bar. There were three old men in it, and he said it would have been a perfect spot to go in and just sit, and, you know, have a drink. He stood outside for, like, 20 minutes. And he kept thinking of going in. Finally, he said, 'No, Matty's dying up in that hospital. I can't be that selfish.' He said there was definitely a power higher than him, and it was me—I brought him back to the hospital and kept him from going in. And he's still sober today. He said me lying there in that bed inspired him."

Everyone runs in silence for a while after that.

HE WAS A FIREMAN, a bar owner, and a bachelor. He ran, biked, and played hoops, always hard. He traveled, drank beer and wine, and was the top cook at his firehouse. He had six brothers but called everybody bro. He teased, tweaked, and told a good story. He had hundreds of friends. He raised lots of money for charity. He liked country music even though he was from Brooklyn. He always made people laugh.

Long was popular with the ladies, too. He dated, often. There was the pretty brunette with whom he made eye contact as he was watching the marathon by his firehouse—a look that yielded a few dates with the young actress. (His firehouse pals like to remind him of the time they saw her in a commercial for a herpes remedy.) There was the girl from Bay Ridge, but that crumbled after they ran a marathon together. And there was the girl he was engaged to, but they never made it to the altar. As one friend said, "He was always looking for the right one."

"He had the whole works," says his brother Rob. "Good-looking guy, good personality. All the girls chased after him."

For months, when he was in the hospital, the party came to him. Every weekday, firefighters from all over the city brought meals to the Long family and everyone else who'd come by to see him. On Saturdays, the Asphalt Green Triathlon Club made lasagna, pot roast, chicken, you name it. "Matt was our teammate," says Allison Caccoma, who supervised the meals. "He used to host our parties at his bar. How could you not help?"

Of course, friends couldn't always see what Long had to endure. A titanium rod ran through his left leg, virtually from his hip to his ankle, supporting his shattered tibia and femur. Metal screws kept the bones of his left foot in place. The damage to his pelvis had made his right leg two inches shorter than it had been before the accident. His right abductors (the powerful buttock muscles that keep us erect and help propel us) were basically dead. He could raise his right shoulder no higher than 90 degrees. He had undergone several surgeries to try to heal his battered abdominal-wall muscles, and his stomach was sealed by processed cadaver skin. His internal injuries left him tethered to a colostomy bag. He had to relearn how to walk. Lorich warned him that it could take two years before Long could dispense with crutches or a cane, and to expect an early onset of arthritis.

Still, Lorich was stunned by how quickly he healed. On May 24, 2006, five months after getting run over by the bus, Long got the okay to go home. He held a press conference in the hospital lobby before leaving. Every major New York City TV station, radio station, and newspaper covered it. He came off an elevator in a wheelchair, then stood and walked to a podium on crutches. Flashbulbs blinked, and family, friends, and hospital staff in attendance applauded. He looked thin and unsteady behind the podium, and his voice sounded strained. But at points he sounded like the old Matt Long. "When I decided to become a fireman, someone said, 'You'll become bald and fat.' Well, I'm definitely bald," he said as he lifted off his baseball cap, "but I ain't fat." He also showed anger. He lashed out at Roger Toussaint, the transit union leader who had called the December 2005 strike. "It's against the law for civil servants to strike. If the Fire Department went on strike, and it was his neighbor's house or his house or someone's house, and we stood idly by watching that burn while you had to wait for firefighters from Jersey or somewhere else to come and put it out, how would you feel, Mr. Toussaint?"

He told reporters he still had hopes to do some of the things he once planned to do. Maybe, he said, he'd tackle another Ironman. Those dreams were for another day. "I can only say I wish this was the end," he said, "and I know it's not." And then he left the hospital and returned to his one-bedroom apartment.

AT MILE NINE, THEY LOOK BACK and see the elite women closing. Among them are Paula Radcliffe, the defending champion from England, and Kara Goucher, the American Olympian making her marathon debut. Finally, after a few hours, the guys are about to have some company. Long doesn't waste a second.

"Noel, listen. When they get closer, run up ahead and get a picture of them passing me. Got it, bro? And try to get me in a shot with Kara. I met her the other night."

"She's cute, Matty."

"Yeah, and she's also married. Just get the shot."

"Okay, here they come. Smile, Matty."

THE LETTER CAME FROM SOMEONE he didn't even know—a friend of a friend—while he was still in the hospital. She wrote, Don't worry. You'll run again. I can help. I work with disabled athletes. When he read *disabled*, the color returned to his face. He called his friend at once.

"What the fuck? What does she mean, *disabled?*"

"She means well."

"Well, this is the way it came across: she's telling me I am going to be crippled."

After a couple of weeks and then months back in his apartment, though, Long started to wonder if maybe the letter writer had been right. He did his rehab, 90 minutes every day: exercises on the treadmill to rekindle his walking muscles, upper-body weights to make that right shoulder more flexible. But any progress seemed marginal compared to his larger goals. How could he stroke through the water if he could barely lift his right arm above his shoulder? How could he ride his bike when it was uncomfortable just to sit? And how could he run if he couldn't even walk? Lorich had said that the abductor muscles in his right glute might never pick up neural signals again. Often, Long's right leg would uncontrollably flare out at a 45-degree angle.

Gimping around the city streets on crutches left him nervous about what might tip him over. And while he had no memory of that morning when his life changed, he still winced when a bus would come to a stop nearby. More and more, he came to realize how challenging his life was and would continue to be. "I have disappointment in my life, and mental struggles every day," he said one day nearly a year after he left the hospital. "How much do I have to pay for this? How much longer am I going to suffer before I can walk longer, before I can live longer? All I do now is therapy. I don't have much going on."

Others close to him saw the rising frustration. "His body was in shambles, his life was in shambles," his father says. "He was always a fast-moving guy—not only in sports but in everything. And now he hit a wall, and everything came to a real stop."

Long's poor mobility was only one part of his social paralysis. There was also that colostomy bag that never left his side. Forget about swimming or biking or running—try going to Thanksgiving dinner with all those relatives, or meeting his buddies for a beer at Third & Long (a Manhattan bar he owned with his brother Jim), or chatting up a pretty blonde with that smelly bag hanging around. He could cover it up with an extra-large shirt or a winter coat, but it wouldn't go away.

So Matt Long stayed away.

"We lost Matty," says Shane McKeon, his old running partner from the Rock. "For a year and a half, Matty wasn't the same guy. He wasn't returning phone calls; he was avoiding people."

Noel Flynn also felt a relationship changing. "Prior to the accident, we used to talk just about every day," he says. "Then there came a time where it would take a couple days before Matt would call back. You'd lob in a call, and it would go into voice mail. I think that was his 'why me' time. A lot of tears. You know?"

One day Long visited a psychiatrist and ran down what was playing in his head. He listed the things he'd wanted to do with his life: run more marathons, do more triathlons, maybe get married. He said he was the guy who made sure everyone enjoyed themselves, that their glasses were filled and they went home laughing. That was Matty Long. That's who he wanted back.

The doctor listened and then told him, "Matt, maybe instead of you trying to make everyone else feel good, you let someone make you feel good." It sounded logical, but that's not what Long wanted to hear. His first trip to the psychiatrist was his last.

The anguish came to a head one summer day in 2007. He met his parents for lunch at Turtle Bay Grill and Lounge, another bar he owned with Jim. Long had just been to a checkup and had learned that he might need the colostomy bag forever. He was distraught. His parents reassured him that it was just one more obstacle to overcome.

He snapped. "You know, you two are all happy because I'm alive. But I'm miserable because I'm alive," he yelled, starting to cry. "If I had died, at least it would have been short-term pain for you. But I got to live with this every day of my life."

Eileen Long held her breath for a moment, tears welling in her eyes. She looked over at her husband, damp-eyed, too. Then at her crying 40-year-old son. And then she let him have it. "If you want to miss family parties and sit around in your apartment feeling sorry for yourself, go ahead. But let me ask you, Do you want to be miserable all your life?"

"Maybe I do," Matt shouted back.

"Well, then be miserable, but let me tell you, you have a lot to offer people other than misery."

But Long couldn't see it that way. So much of his life had been taken away from him. He couldn't be a lifesaver, a stud triathlete, a ladies' man. He couldn't be the guy who made everyone else happy. He didn't have the bonding of the triathlon clubs, the antics with all his friends, the noble purpose, and fun at the firehouse. All he had was a one-bedroom apartment where he spent so much time thinking of what used to be and what was supposed to be. "It hurt to watch everyone around me continue with their lives," he says. "My friends were still racing and training, and one brother was having a baby and another was getting married. Their lives were moving forward and I was stuck." Stuck—and searching for a way to be Matty Long again.

WHEN THEY APPROACH THE QUEENSBORO BRIDGE, the dark, steel-grilled link between Queens and Manhattan near mile 15, the three runners slow down. Long had planned from the start to walk the bridge, hoping not to overtax his aerobic capacity. In training, his longest run was only 14 miles.

He's quiet for most of the walk across the bridge. Every few seconds, as people race by, a runner spots him and yells, "Great job, Matty" or "Way to go, bro," and Long yells back, "I hear ya, bro. We'll catch up to ya soon." Otherwise, he keeps to himself. Finally, at the 16-mile mark, as runners get set to descend a ramp into the canyons of Manhattan, he starts running again.

THE IDEA CAME IN A FLASH ONE NIGHT. It was as sudden as the alarm that would ring in his old firehouse, and he's still not sure what prompted it. Maybe it came from a lot of little things. Maybe it was the phone calls and e-mails from Shane McKeon, who got the idea that if he trained for an Ironman, and Long could coach him, then Matty might become Matty again. "I left him one message where I said, 'If you don't want to respond to any e-mails, don't, but on a daily basis, I'll tell you where I'm at with my training and what I'm doing," McKeon recalls. He soon got a whiff of the old Matty. "I'll tell you, within three days he was yelling at me, 'Where's my update?'"

Or maybe it was hearing his mom in his head, and recalling what she had already been through—watching her middle-aged son lie unconscious in a hospital, not knowing if he would live or die. Years earlier, she had waited by a hospital bed to see if her husband would survive being gunned down by a mafia member outside a Brooklyn bar. Then there was the car accident a few years later that nearly killed another son, Frank. And, of course, there was 9/11, the day her two firefighting sons, Matt and Jim, didn't call home until that night to let her know they were alive. Maybe she didn't need any more misery herself.

Or maybe it was that psychiatrist. Maybe he had a point. Maybe it was time to let others make him feel good.

Maybe it was all of that, or none of that. All Long knows is that one night he was at home with his brother Eddie, "moaning and crying about everything I had wanted to do. I wanted to break three hours in the marathon. I wanted to run Boston. I wanted to do the Ironman in Hawaii. And then, I just stopped. And I remember saying to Eddie, 'You know, a lot of people want stuff. People want this, people want that. People want to win the lottery. But just because you want something doesn't mean you're going to get it. You got to, you know, work for it.' So right there I just said, 'I will run. And I will run a marathon.'" And just like that, he started on the road back to being Matty Long.

But why a marathon? Months earlier, he'd told friends that if he were ever ready, he'd like to run with them around the Central Park loop they'd done so often. And if he could ever do those six miles, they'd go out for beer and pizza, and he'd be happy. Now, out of nowhere, six miles had mushroomed into 26, even though he still needed crutches to walk one block. Why? "Because that's what I had done before," he said shortly after that night. "To prove that I'm back as an athlete, that's what I have to do."

He knew that if he maintained his rehab schedule, his legs, eventually, would get stronger and more stable. Lorich had said so. The colostomy bag was more troublesome. To reverse the colostomy, he would need to return to New York-Presbyterian Hospital that October for surgery. That procedure turned out to be a wrenching 14-hour ordeal, followed by a two-week hospital stay. Ultimately, though, it served its purpose.

On December 22, 2007, after two years of rehabilitation and 40 surgeries, Long traded his crutches in for a cane. Within a few days, he did his first pool workout and booked November 2, 2008, to run the New York City Marathon. He had less than 11 months to learn how to run again.

AS IT IS ON EVERY MARATHON SUNDAY IN NEW YORK, First Avenue is lined three rows deep with people cheering and waving. Long, Carino, and Flynn aren't talking much right now, just listening. Finally, Carino says, "Can you believe this?"

"No way," says Flynn. "I don't think I ever heard it so loud."

"Incredible. And it seems like they're all cheering for Matty."

Long doesn't seem to hear them.

Around 65th Street, they're joined by some members of his triathlon club, who plan to run with Long the rest of the way. Then, a few blocks later, Tom Nohilly, a trainer he's been working with, hops in with a backpack. He trails behind, and sees that Long is laboring even more than normal. His feet are barely getting off the ground, his head keeps bobbing. "Matty, push off on your feet. Use your feet," Nohilly yells. "Pump your arms."

It's not easy. Each minute on the course equates to 160 footfalls. That means those three gnarly hammer toes curving into the bottom of his left foot have already sustained at least 21,000 poundings. They'll have to endure 16,000 more if he wants to finish.

At 99th Street, just past mile 18, Long pulls off to the side of the road and points to his left foot. "It's killing me," he says. Nohilly has him lean on Carino and Flynn and then stretches out both legs and flexes his foot. "You okay, you okay?" Nohilly asks. Long sort of nods. "Okay, then, hang in there. Try to keep your shoulders and head from getting so far ahead of you."

The group trudges on. For a while the mood is upbeat and relaxed. Heading through the Bronx, the runners talk about how many burgers they'll devour later. As they swing back into Manhattan, in Harlem, a group of five or six teenagers are rapping on a street corner, trying to recharge the runners. Long breaks into a funky dance routine, and the others just break up laughing.

The fun evaporates near mile 22. This is where most marathoners start to wonder if they have enough left to finish, if they've prepared enough. The point when the head hurts as much as the quads. But Long isn't like the runners around him. He couldn't prepare enough. He only began running in March. His longest training run was 14 miles. And already, today, he's run for more than six hours, twice as long as the people passing him, on a contorted left foot that's killing him. It's attached to a leg filled with titanium that has been working double-time today because his right leg has abductor muscles that don't work. People around him are suffering, but not like him. They didn't get hit by a bus.

Flynn and Carino sense something, and they move closer to Long, making sure passing runners can't knock him over. As they enter Central Park, a wisecrack from someone gets little response from Long. With less than three miles to go, he finally barks, "No more jokes." The only noise that breaks the silence is Long grunting every few seconds.

IN FEBRUARY 2008, LONG FLEW TO Tempe, Arizona. He'd wanted to escape New York City for a while, to "someplace where people didn't know me as the guy who got hit by a bus." He'd found a rehab center that seemed suited to "getting me running."

The two trainers he worked with, Mark D'Aloisio and Kyle Herrig, use an approach that relies less on isolating individual muscles and more on getting muscle groups to work in sync. Their clients range from members of the Arizona Diamondbacks to senior citizens recovering from hip surgery. For three months the trainers put Long through daily 90-minute sessions geared at firing up dormant muscles and building strength. He also swam and lifted weights at a nearby gym. The work paid off quickly. After about six weeks, he wasn't using the cane as much, and he was putting more weight on his right leg. "His confidence was getting better," says Herrig, "and that's when we decided that we'd go out and do a little jog."

Around noon on March 14, along a canal path in Phoenix, Long, with D'Aloisio and Herrig at his side, ran his first mile in two years. It took him 17 minutes, 24 seconds. "I can look at it two ways," he wrote in an e-mail. "It's 17:24 faster than any mile in the last two years or 1:30 slower than my best 5-K. Either way I'm running!"

A few weeks later, he returned to New York and saw Jim Wharton, a sports physiologist known for his flexibility techniques. Long wanted to be taken on as a patient. On his application, where it asked for his medical condition, he simply wrote, "Fucked." When Wharton saw that, he chuckled; the two hit it right off. Long shared his plan to run the marathon that fall. That's when Wharton knew the guy was serious. "It is rare to see someone with such challenges to the body come back and try the marathon. But Matt has a great attitude," Wharton said last summer. "That makes it easy. He was an athlete before he came here, and he still is."

Over the next six months, Wharton and his staff spent hour-long sessions working with Long to improve his strength and range of motion. They concentrated on his right abductors, seeing if they could get them firing again. Wharton made no promises. In case the muscles didn't respond, they made sure muscles like Long's hamstring and quads were ready to compensate. Wharton also devised a 16-week running schedule that would gradually rebuild his cardio capacity.

It began at the Rock on July 1. Long returned to active duty with the FDNY that day after two and a half years of disability leave. While hoping that he could one day get back to his old firehouse, Long was happy to be with his training buddies and shouting orders at the probies. That afternoon, he took his lunch break at a nearby track. He asked Tommy Grimshaw to join him, and the two set out for six laps. Long, who wore a new raised shoe that compensated for his shorter right leg, gimped more than he ran, but after 24 minutes he had finished the first one and a half miles of his marathon plan. As they walked from the track, Grimshaw laughed and said, "Matty, I can taste the Guinness we'll be drinking after the marathon."

"I hear ya, bro."

The days he didn't run, Long swam, used the elliptical, and lifted weights. His upper body became stronger and bigger than before the accident. "Hey, I'm going to be out there a long time on marathon day," he said while training one afternoon. "My arms are going to have a lot of work, too." He gradually increased his running miles. By mid-August, he hit the five-mile mark. Carino and Flynn started to join him for his longer runs. In mid-September he did nine, and then a couple of weeks later, 14. But then, on October 3, during a scheduled 16-miler in Central Park, he felt a sharp pain in his right hip. He stopped after 11 miles, and his two friends assisted him to a cab. It turned out that he'd torn his right labrum, a ring of cartilage around the hip socket, probably due to the position of his pelvis. He iced it, treated it with herbal remedies, and cut back on the long runs, as Wharton suggested.

That wasn't the only concession he made. When he first had decided to do the marathon, he expected to be with the other 38,000 runners at the start, maybe even with his firefighter buddies. But three weeks before the race, he called Dick Traum, CEO of the Achilles Track Club, which supports disabled runners. He told Traum his story, and about his injuries and his desire to run— and his wish to run with other disabled athletes. Later, he recalled the letter he had received while in the hospital, the one from the lady saying she could help him become a disabled runner. "I was pissed then," he said days before the race. "But, you know, I've come to accept that I am disabled. I'm a challenged athlete. I can't do things that I used to do. So, yes, I'm a challenged athlete." He paused. "But if I finish the race on Sunday, I'll be an athlete again."

That meant much more than running 26 miles. It meant that he'd be back among people with whom, for so long, he shared life and its pleasures. People who ran and biked and swam for hours each day, not because they expected to win marathons or Ironmans, but simply because they loved to compete, participate, work hard—and laugh, too. Friends whom he could talk to about training plans and nutrition strategies and who didn't bug him about his various pains or his limp or his psyche. Connections from around the city and from different professions whom he could tap to help him launch his "I Will" foundation, a program he hoped would help sick or severely injured people accomplish goals they never thought achievable. Most of all, it meant he'd be back among people who saw him as a fitness junkie and not as the guy who got run over by a bus. He'd be Matty Long again.

LONG AND CARINO AND FLYNN and the friends who've been with them since First Avenue come out of the park onto Central Park South—there's just a half mile to go. Long is that close to saying he's an athlete again. And when that happens, perhaps he'll call someone in Boston and plead his case to let him run their race. It was on this stretch, nearly three years ago to the day, when he made his final push to qualify for Boston.

Today, he goes about 100 more yards, and suddenly stops. Flynn and Carino look at him. "You okay, Matt?" Carino asks.

For so many months, ever since that frigid December morning, people had been asking him how he was doing. Was he okay? And for a long time he hadn't wanted to answer them. Then he decided to run a marathon to prove to everyone—especially himself—that he was okay. No, running a marathon wouldn't make him whole again. His first step out of bed each morning would still be excruciating, as if he were "stepping on broken glass." And he would still come home each night to stacks of hospital and doctor bills, and wonder how long it might take before the outstanding lawsuits (against the bus company, the driver, and Bear Stearns) might give him some relief. No, things would never be like they were before the morning he had decided to bike to work. They would be different. And that was okay, too. If he could just make it another half mile.

"Yeah, yeah, it's the foot," he tells Carino and Flynn. His toes can't take it anymore. "Let's just walk a bit."

Walk? Now? Practically everybody who has helped Matt Long fulfill this crazy dream is either running beside him or waiting at the finish. They're here to pay back the man who was always the go-to guy for everyone else. His mom and dad are there, and all his brothers and sisters, nieces and nephews. They've been tracking him all day; they want this thing done. Dean Lorich is there, too. He's brought along his wife and children—now numbering three daughters—just like he did the morning when he had to hail a cab to get to the hospital to save Long's life. Many of the top FDNY brass are waiting there, too; they want to see their latest hero come in safely.

They'll have to wait a little bit longer, because Matt Long is walking. Flynn and Carino and the others follow his lead, for how long no one knows. He takes five, six, seven steps, until finally, like an old engine sputtering to life, he pushes off his left foot, and starts running. Everyone follows. They run the rest of Central Park South. They run through Columbus Circle. They run back into the park. There's no Boston qualifier to race for, just a finish line to reach, 0.2 miles away. They run tighter together; they run, it seems, a little faster. They run with smiles on their faces, closer and closer to the finish. With just yards to go, a random runner gets too close. Long shoves him aside. There won't be a collision today. With Carino on his right and Flynn on his left, he crosses the line—in 7:21:22—and hits the ground.

He reels off 10 push-ups, lifts himself up, and starts searching for all the people who helped him get back on his feet.

It doesn't take him long. There, gathered near the finish line, they're waiting for him to join them.

TEAM HOYT
STARTS AGAIN

BY JOHN BRANT

On April 17, 2006, Dick and Rick Hoyt, the most inspiring father-son team in sports, took their hallowed place at the Boston Marathon for the 25th time. A series of setbacks threatened to make it their toughest one yet. But, as usual, they found a way to keep on rolling.

MAY 2006

RICK HOYT LIES AWAKE but unmoving, watching clear winter sunlight spill into his bedroom. He often spends whole days watching light move across a room, or along the course of a road race—the pale April sunshine filtering through the bare trees along Route 135 in the early miles of the Boston Marathon, for instance, or the tropical sun lancing the clouds that shroud Mauna Loa volcano at the Hawaii Ironman.

He lies on his belly, his head turned to the right, alone in the apartment, in exactly the position that Naomi, his personal care attendant, left him at 10 o'clock the night before. You would think that Rick's nights would seem endless, but the medication he takes to relax his chronically clenched muscles allows him to sleep soundly for 12 hours at a stretch. Unable to voluntarily move any part of his body but his head, and that just barely, Rick lies calmly studying the morning light. By its slant and texture he reckons the time to be around 10.

The sunlight keeps filling the bedroom, like April in January. It must be warm out on the streets. The women would have shed their heavy coats. From the vantage point of his wheelchair, Rick regards women from an arresting, navel-level angle. His two brothers give him a hard time about that. They call it a perk of cerebral palsy.

He hears the key in the lock, and then a step in the hallway, then, "Good morning, Rick!"

AT 8 A.M. ON THIS SATURDAY MORNING, Dick Hoyt swings his van onto the Mass Pike, heading east toward Boston, 75 miles away. He lowers the visor against the rising sun and turns the car radio to an all-news station. "I've driven this route so often all I gotta do is sort of point the van and it finds the apartment on its own," Dick jokes.

He yawns behind the wheel. It's been a crazy week. On Tuesday, he was in Florida to give a motivational speech to business executives. On Wednesday, he was in Texas giving another one. Thursday night he and Rick were honored at a dinner in Hopkinton, where the Boston Marathon starts every April. Now, on to Boston. He makes this 90-minute drive to Rick's apartment, in the Brighton section, almost every Saturday morning. He'll pick up Rick, bathe and shave and feed him, and then they'll drive back together to Dick's house in Holland, a village on the Connecticut border. Most Sundays they'll rise at 5 a.m. to prepare for whatever 5-K, 10-K, marathon, or triathlon is coming up. They race 40 times a year, in a manner that, over the past quarter century, has become no less miraculous as it has become familiar: a short-legged, barrel-chested, 65-year-old man with a rocklike jaw, running at an 8:30-per-mile pace pushing a slight 44-year-old quadriplegic in a 27-pound wheelchair.

Seven miles into his drive Dick pulls off the Pike to make his ritual Starbucks stop. "I shoulda bought stock in this place 10 years ago," he says with a grin. The barista starts Dick's drink the moment he steps in the door—a venti chai tea, extra hot. He has been careful with his diet ever since his heart attack three years ago. The scare caught the extremely fit Dick by total surprise, as have several other setbacks the Hoyts have faced of late. In December, a gale raked New England, sending a tree through Dick's roof and into his living room. Days later, the lift on Rick's specially designed van broke down, necessitating the purchase of a new rig. Then, just before Christmas, Dick needed arthroscopic surgery on his left knee to repair cartilage damage, the first serious injury of his 29-year running career. The knee is still healing and has kept Dick from running for a month, his longest inactive stretch ever. The Boston Marathon is only three months away.

Dick's tea is ready, but just before he turns to head to the door, he spots the Starbucks' manager and asks him if the store might contribute to the Easter Seals fund-raising drive he has launched in conjunction with the Boston Marathon. "We want to raise a million dollars," Dick tells him. The manager pledges his support. Smiling, Dick heads out the door, back to his van, and back on the Pike.

He's drinking his tea and talking about races and running while changing lanes frequently and making great time getting to Boston. By 10 a.m. he's steering off the expressway and threading through the streets near Boston University. He parks near Rick's building, takes an elevator up five floors, and moves down a long corridor to Rick's apartment. He puts a key in the lock and turns. He opens the door and steps into the hallway.

"Good morning, Rick!"

THE ATHLETIC PHENOMENON that is known as Team Hoyt began one spring day in 1977. Rick was 15 at the time and came home from school asking his dad if they could run a five-mile road race together in their town of West-field, Massachusetts, to benefit a local college athlete who'd been paralyzed in an auto accident. It was a strange request, considering Rick's situation.

Cerebral palsy is a debilitating condition often caused by complications during pregnancy or at birth. In Rick's case, the umbilical cord got tangled around his neck, cutting off the oxygen supply to his brain and causing irreparable damage. Aside from his head, the only other parts of his body he can voluntarily move even slightly are his knees. His muscles chronically contract, hence the need for muscle relaxants. He can't control his arms, which jerk and wave spasmodically. He has a "reverse tongue," meaning he drools and reflexively expels food and drink, so he can't eat on his own. His head is usually tilted, his smile lopsided, but genuine, accompanied by a mischievous glint. He can't speak at all, but because he can move his head, he can communicate with the help of a specially designed computer. As a cursor moves across a screen filled with rows of letters, Rick highlights which letter he wants by pressing his head against a narrow metal bar attached to the right side of the wheelchair. When he completes a word and then a thought—a tediously slow process—a voice synthesizer verbally produces it.

At the time Rick asked to run that race, Dick was a 40-year-old nonrunner. When he and Rick got to the event, organizers saw the wheelchair, the disabled son, and the middle-aged dad and gave them a look that said, "You two won't make it past the first corner." They didn't know Dick. It wasn't in his nature to quit a job he'd started. And besides, by that first corner, Rick was having too much fun. They ran the entire five miles, and didn't finish last. Afterward, a wild grin lit up Rick's face. Later he tapped out: "Dad, when I'm running, it feels like I'm not handicapped."

Dick had a slightly different reaction. "After that race I felt disabled—I was pissing blood for a week," he says. "But we knew we were onto something. Making Rick happy was the greatest feeling in the world."

Running made Dick happy, too. A career Army guy, he felt like he was back in basic training again, breezing through a forced march while the other guys struggled and bitched. And, like the military, running was structured. If you followed the program, you got faster. Dick bought a pair of running shoes and researched a training schedule. Judy, Rick's mother, located an engineer in New Hampshire to build a wheelchair modified for running, with three bicycle wheels and a foam seat molded to Rick's body. The Hoyts' first running chair was produced for $35, and its basic design forms the template for all the racing chairs the men have subsequently used.

Since 1977, Rick and Dick Hoyt have completed more than 900 endurance events around the world, including 64 marathons and eight Ironman triathlons. They've run their hometown Boston Marathon 25 times. With a marathon PR of 2:40:47 and a 13:30 personal best for the Hawaii Ironman World Championship, they are the furthest thing from a charity case imaginable. Just consider how they managed the 1999 Hawaii Ironman. After completing the 2.4-mile swim (for triathlons, Rick lies in an eight-foot Zodiac raft, Dick pulling him with a strap fastened around his waist), their brakes froze with 30 miles left in the 112-mile bike leg, and, lacking a replacement part, they had to wait more than an hour for the mechanic's truck. When the repair was finally completed, Dick asked the wind-blasted and sun-burnt Rick if he wanted to continue. (Rick rides on a specially constructed seat that fits on the bike's handlebars.) Rick instantly nodded yes. So they soldiered through the bike phase in last place, and then transitioned into the marathon, their strongest event. There seemed little hope of completing the run by midnight, the deadline for official finishers. But feeling stronger as the night wore on, Rick and Dick passed dozens of runners and powered across the finish line with 45 minutes to spare. They had run the notoriously difficult marathon leg in a remarkable 3:30.

Over the course of their quarter-century-long career, the Hoyts' incredible athletic achievements have made them, arguably, the most famous distance runners in America. They've met Ronald Reagan and Rudolph Giuliani, appeared on *Oprah*, and been the subject of a full-length documentary. In 1996, during the Boston Marathon's centennial celebration, the Hoyts ranked tenth in a poll of the most influential runners in marathon history—a list that included such legends as Bill Rodgers and Joan Samuelson. Dick has become a sought-after motivational speaker, making 50 appearances a year before corporate groups. Inevitably, after such speeches, Dick will hear the same well-meaning questions: How do you and Rick communicate during a race? What happens if Rick has to go to the bathroom? And, of course, How much longer can you do this? When the questions come up, he replies readily and cheerfully. "We feel real good . . . we love what we're doing . . . we've got no plans for quitting." But the questions, and the implication that Team Hoyt's run has to end at some point, still rankle.

The fact is, Dick Hoyt can expect to keep hearing the questions, especially after the heart attack, the knee surgery, the missed training. All that, and Dick turns 66 in June. How many more Bostons are really likely?

People can keep asking that question, but if they do, Dick insists, it means they don't know what drives the distance runner.

A FEW MINUTES after arriving at Rick's apartment, Dick lifts his naked, 110-pound son off his bed as if he weighed no more than a case of beer and sits him on the toilet. Dick is built like a catcher, his position as a star high school baseball player (he had a tryout with the Yankees, who rejected him, ironically, because he was too slow a runner), with a stocky frame and heavy legs featuring such exceptional muscular definition that his physical therapist jokes that he ought to model for an anatomy class.

Rick has trained himself to use the bathroom just twice a day, upon rising and retiring, a boon to his father and personal care attendants (similarly, Rick doesn't ingest fluids during marathons or shorter road races; during triathlons, he drinks only at the transition areas). Lifting Rick again, Dick places him in the steaming water of the bathtub, where he bathes and shaves him. The water feels good. Rick gives a crooked smile of pleasure. Although he looks childlike sitting in the tub, his shoulders are surprisingly broad. Dick explains that the chronic contractions caused by Rick's spastic condition, along with the stress and stimulation of his athletic career, have given him excellent muscle tone. Paradoxically, Rick emanates an air of health and well-being.

"The human performance lab at Boston Children's Hospital wants to study Rick," Dick says. "His life expectancy is the same as any other man his age."

As he works, Dick talks quietly about the weather, last night's Celtics game, and his recent visit to the physical therapist for a checkup on his knee. "Jackie says I'm ahead of schedule," he says, toweling Rick's close-cropped, gray-flecked hair.

Dick originally injured his left knee in San Diego last November. The two were running with students from an elementary school through a bumpy field when Dick twisted the knee, tearing cartilage. Then, a few weeks later, when the Hoyts were in Florida for a race, their hotel's fire alarm sounded in the middle of the night. It was almost certainly a false alarm and another man—even another father—might have turned over in bed and gone back to sleep. But Dick didn't have that luxury. He got Rick into his wheelchair and humped down a narrow fire escape. While making one of the tight turns, Dick again twisted his knee. There was no denying this injury and, three days before Christmas, he underwent surgery. Thus the doctors' orders not to run for a month.

Dick lifts Rick into his wheelchair and guides him to the kitchen table. The walls are covered with running memorabilia, including a quilt stitched out of T-shirts from 1980s-vintage road races, and a photo of Rick and Dick being greeted by then President Reagan. Dick pours orange juice into a tumbler and, for the next 20 minutes, feeds it sip by sip to Rick, palpitating his jaw and neck with a milking-like motion to assure the juice stays down. Each moment ministering to Rick requires exacting effort, but his father never seems to lose patience.

"I was never angry or resentful about the hand we were dealt," Dick says. "People assume that I work out my rage through running, but that's not the case."

RICK HOYT IS ONE of an estimated 760,000 Americans who suffer from cerebral palsy. Unlike that for such crippling conditions as spinal cord injuries or Parkinson's disease, cerebral palsy research currently offers little hope of a cure. Through technology, physical therapy, counseling, and prodigious work, however, the condition can be managed. Perhaps the best indicator that Rick has successfully dealt with his condition is that in 1993 he completed a special education degree from Boston University, though it was an arduous process. A personal care attendant had to sit with him through every class, taking notes, and then reading assignments aloud to him. He had to communicate with professors through the voice synthesizer. With such impediments, he could only take two classes a semester and he needed nine years to complete the degree.

Still, a college degree was hardly what Judy and Dick Hoyt expected from their firstborn when he arrived in January 1962. One pediatrician told the couple that their new son, his condition classified as nonverbal spastic quadriplegia, would be a vegetable for the rest of his short and miserable life; place him in an institution, the doctor recommended, and, in effect, forget him. Judy and Dick adamantly refused, though the first weeks and months with their severely disabled boy were unquestionably hard ones.

Judy and Dick had met in high school in North Reading, a community 15 miles north of downtown Boston. She was a cheerleader and he was captain of the football team. The sixth of ten children, Dick was always a demon for work. At the age of 8 he was earning money at odd jobs, and at 16 he was running a crop farm. He taught himself masonry and other construction skills. After high school he joined the National Guard. He loved basic training—the order, the challenge, the physical rigor—and decided to make the military his career. The Army placed him in the Nike missile program, assigning him to posts around New England.

When Rick was on his way, two years after they had been married, the couple looked forward to having a boy who would grow up to play catcher like his old man and go fishing with his grandfather. Instead, when he arrived, he couldn't manage a newborn's cry. Judy was crushed, and fell into a deep depression. "I hated Dick, and I hated all the mothers in the hospital and all my friends who were mothers of babies that were not handicapped," Judy says in the Hoyts' biography, *It's Only a Mountain.* "My feelings kept seesawing from hate to denial for months.... Rick couldn't suck, he couldn't even open his little clenched fists. He was tight, tight, tight. We had to force him to eat every two hours just to keep him alive. We would wake him up by pinching the bottom of his feet."

Judy soon recovered from the depressive bout and insisted, along with Dick, on raising Rick at home. She started to fight for her son's rights and those of other disabled individuals. After earning a degree in special education, she helped establish a summer camp for children with disabilities, and she battled endlessly to keep Rick in Westfield's public schools. While an estimated two-thirds of people with cerebral palsy suffer some degree of mental retardation, Judy says she could tell just by looking at Rick's eyes as a baby that he had an active mind. "His eyes would follow me around the room. My son was intelligent. He was alive inside."

As Judy worked this front, Dick was busy with his military career, rising through the enlisted ranks to attend officer candidate school and eventually attain a rank of lieutenant colonel. Nights and weekends, to pay for Rick's wheelchairs and other necessities, he moonlighted on masonry jobs. But for all their varied activities, Judy and Dick tried to maintain a typical family life. Rick's two younger brothers, Rob and Russ, both healthy, were taught to treat their older brother as normal as possible. Rick played goalie in neighborhood hockey games. Dick or the brothers would tie the goalie stick to the boy, then steer him in his wheelchair as he tried to block shots in the crease. Rick would go wild with each blocked shot. There would also be family hiking trips. Dick would drape Rick over his shoulders and carry him up mountains.

Then came that race in Westfield in 1977, and the family's life changed forever. The epiphany of that first race fed a desire to do other races around New England. But just because the Hoyts wanted to run more didn't mean they were necessarily welcomed by the running community. At a 10-K in Springfield, Massachusetts, Dick remembers getting snubbed by the other athletes. "They shied away from us as if they thought they were going to catch a disease," Dick recalls. The race officials were even less hospitable. "The officials said they didn't fit because Dick was pushing him," Judy remembers in the Hoyts' biography. "Dick did it 'differently' than all the other runners. The wheelchair athletes didn't want them because Rick wasn't powering his own chair, and the able-bodied runners said, 'You're just going to get in the way. Why do you want to push this kid of yours who doesn't talk and just sits in the wheelchair?'"

Judy was there to watch the two at all their races, strongly supporting them through the early stages of their running career, even when some people questioned Dick's motives. "I got maybe 20 or 25 letters," Dick says. "Parents with disabled kids saw the stories about us, and they assumed that running was my idea, not Rick's. They thought I was using him to get publicity for myself."

Four years after their first race, Dick and Rick sought to run the 1981 Boston Marathon, but again met resistance. They were told that they needed to meet a qualifying time, just like any other runner officially entered in the race. There would be no exceptions, even for a guy pushing his kid in a wheelchair. "The Hoyts were proposing a nontraditional form of participation and, at the time, any change at Boston was a big deal," says Jack Fleming, spokesman for the Boston Athletic Association, organizers of the marathon. Fleming, who was not with the BAA in 1981, adds, "It wasn't just Rick and Dick; the same thing had happened with women running for the first time, and then professionals."

Team Hoyt decided to run the 1981 race unofficially, as bandits, and clocked a remarkable debut marathon time of 3:18. They ran unofficially again in 1982, going under three hours for the first time (2:59), and then shaved another minute off in 1983. Still, no waiver came from the BAA. Finally, in October 1983, they went to Washington, D.C., to run the Marine Corps Marathon, looking to clock a 2:50, the time Boston required for runners in Rick's 20 to 29 age group (even though Dick, who was doing all the running, was 43 and would have qualified with a 3:10). On a cold, rainy morning, they ran 2:45:30. They officially raced the Boston Marathon the following spring and have run all but one since, becoming one of the event's most popular participants. "They personify the race as much as the elite athletes do," says Fleming. "Besides being inspirational role models, they are also quintessential New England guys. The crowds love them."

In those early years, Judy proudly watched as Rick and Dick's celebrity grew with each Boston or with their first Hawaii Ironman in 1989. Her pride, though, faded as Dick began assuming more responsibilities for their son and, over time, supplanted Judy as Rick's primary caregiver. Rob, the Hoyt's middle son, says he can understand how Judy must have hurt. "I think my mother had a hard time with all the attention that my father got through running," says Rob, 42, who lives in Holyoke, Massachusetts. "The accolades seemed to come much thicker and faster for him than they had with her. She had been everything for Rick. My mother got a nonspeaking spastic quadriplegic through high school and then through college, and now that role was taken by my father, and in a much more public manner."

Judy's frustration and alienation culminated in 1992, when Dick and Rick completed a 45-day, 3,753-mile bike-and-run trek across the United States. Her men's interest in running had morphed into a time-consuming obsession. After 34 years of marriage, she and Dick divorced in 1994.

After so many years, Dick tries not to dwell on what happened to the couple's marriage. "I know that Rick's and my involvement in running and racing was hard on Judy," he says. "First, because of all the attention that got put on me, and second, because, for all the time she spent around the sport, she never understood distance running—why Rick would want to spend all that time on the road, and why I would insist on going to bed at 9 o'clock on a Saturday evening so I would be fresh to race the next morning."

Today, Judy lives in Union, Connecticut, just a few miles from Dick's house, but she avoids contact with him. She visits Rick once every three months or so, but no longer attends Dick and Rick's races. Her animosity toward Dick is still fresh. "I fear that Dick is going to drop dead some day in the middle of a marathon, and I just pray that Rick doesn't go down with him," she says one afternoon while sitting in her kitchen. "Why should Rick suffer more, and put himself at risk, just to please his father?"

IT'S JUST ABOUT NOON as Dick pushes Rick through the parking garage of his apartment building and over to Rick's new van. Dick had shopped carefully and found the slightly used vehicle, with a working lift, at a dealer near his house. Dick lowers the lift, eases Rick onto it, and then works the lever. Staring into a private middle distance, Rick rises into the van. Dick snaps the chair's wheels into the locks on the van floor and fastens the shoulder belts so that Rick will ride securely.

Still not totally familiar with how the van maneuvers, Dick spends the next several minutes hassling it out of the garage; the customized raised roof clears the ceiling only by a few inches. He must back up and pull forward repeatedly to get past a car that is parked illegally in the exit lane. Once out of the garage, he retraces his route to the Mass Pike and points the van west, back toward Holland. In the back Rick listens to NBA scores on the radio.

As they get close to home, Dick stops at a Greek pizza joint to pick up a couple of oven-baked grinders. The shop owner is a friend of Dick's, and with the sandwiches he sends along a flagon of homemade ouzo.

Once inside the house and settled in the kitchen, Dick sets the ouzo aside. He purees Rick's grinder in a food processor and then spoons it into his mouth. In between spoonfuls, Dick takes bites out of his own sandwich, and talks about what's planned for the year ahead. After the Boston Marathon, he explains, he'll begin serious training for the Hawaii Ironman in October. He and Rick are both eager to vindicate themselves after what happened in the 2003 race, when they wiped out at the 85-mile mark of the bike leg.

"The last thing I remember, we were gliding into a water stop," Dick says. "I still don't know what happened. Most likely we skidded on an empty water bottle. Anyway, when I came to, we were both on the road, and blood was gushing from Rick's forehead. An ambulance took him to the emergency room. The doctors there were concerned because of all the blood and the fact that Rick was a quadriplegic. I kept telling them he was okay, but they insisted on taking 52 X-rays. Later, I got a bill from the hospital for $6,000. I refused to pay it, of course."

Hawaii, though, is still nine months away. As always at this time of year, the two are focusing on Boston. Rick and Dick prepare for the marathon by running several half-marathons from January through March. Because Dick trains solo during the week, typically running about eight miles a day, he relies on the half-marathons for building upper-body strength and adjusting to pushing Rick and the wheelchair. He frets over the missed training.

"I've put on seven pounds since my knee operation," Dick says. "I'm heavier now than I've been in years, although the weight should come off pretty quickly once I start running again." He frowns at his grinder. Watching what he eats isn't always easy, as much as he has tried since the heart attack.

It was in the winter of 2003. Midway through a half-marathon, as he and Rick prepared for that year's Boston, Dick felt an unfamiliar tickling sensation in his throat, along with an unusual buildup of saliva. The sensation passed, and they finished the race without difficulty. But the phenomena recurred at races over the next few weeks. Dick consulted his doctor, who administered an EKG.

"A day later I'm driving to my gym when my cell phone rings," Dick recalls. "It's my doctor. She asks me, 'Where you going?' I tell her, 'I'm going to work out.' She says, 'No you're not. You're coming straight to the hospital for a stress test. The EKG showed that you had a heart attack.' My problem is strictly hereditary—high cholesterol. She said that if I wasn't in such good shape, I'd probably be dead by now." The stress test indicated he needed an angioplasty.

That procedure was done just days before the Boston Marathon, which meant Team Hoyt would miss the race for the first time in 22 years.

While Dick tells the story, Rick listens intently. His eyes flicker and his right arm jerks in a slow, almost graceful fashion.

Word got out about Dick's heart attack, and then he began getting calls from around the country from people offering to push Rick in his place. One running club offered to bring in 26 people, and each would push the chair for a mile. "They said they would consider it an honor," Dick says. "I left the decision up to Rick. He said no. Team Hoyt was exactly that, a team. We would run, or not run, together."

Rick's decision echoed one his father had made many times before. Shortly after the pair began running—as soon as Dick's vast latent talent for the sport manifested—people suggested that he should launch a concurrent solo career. If Dick ran so fast pushing a 140-pound load, the reasoning went, imagine what he could do unencumbered. But Dick declined to compete without his son. "The only reason I race is Rick," he says. "I've got no desire to do this on my own."

Dave McGillivray, the race director of the Boston Marathon and a close friend of the Hoyts, thought that if Dick had competed solo, he could have become a world-class age-group runner. In fact, it was McGillivray who first suggested that Dick try triathlons. "Maybe Dick has been fooling us all these years," McGillivray says. "Maybe Rick has been his big advantage, and not his handicap. Look at Dick's stride when he's pushing the chair—it's amazingly clean, he's doing a minimum of pounding, and with both hands on the chair he's always well balanced. He's always leaning forward, even when he's climbing a hill. Of course, he's also pushing 140 pounds. If there were a real competitive advantage, you'd see hundreds of guys in marathons pushing baby joggers. But you don't see that. In fact, after 25 years, and all the publicity, only a few have ever tried."

And that's okay, because watching the Hoyts roll down Commonwealth Avenue in the final mile of the Boston Marathon can be a near mystical experience. The roars of the spectators reverberate off the brick buildings and swell behind the two men like a following wind. Dick bears down and begins to sprint. Rick writhes and jerks ecstatically, the screams of his fans shooting through him.

The event in Hopkinton earlier in the week demonstrated the intense emotional bond that the Hoyts have forged with their fans. A local newspaper had gotten wind of their recent difficulties—Dick's knee surgery, the tree coming through the roof, Rick's van breaking down—and ran a story that seemed to suggest that the two had fallen on hard times. The Hopkinton Athletic Association started a funding drive and hundreds of people from around the country sent in checks—a poor old lady didn't buy a Christmas tree so she could send a few dollars, and an anonymous wealthy donor contributed $50,000.

When Dick learned about the size of the gift, his first impulse was to refuse it or funnel it into his Easter Seals drive. But ultimately, given the need for a new van and other things for Rick, he accepted the association's check for $90,000 and the accolades that came with it. He and Rick had sat quietly on the stage of the school auditorium and patiently listened to a series of speakers. There were tears and testimonials. The Hoyts were made honorary citizens of Hopkinton. A state senator read a proclamation. Bob Lobel, a popular Boston sportscaster, called Dick and Rick the greatest athletes in Boston over the past 30 years, greater than any of the Red Sox, Celtics, Patriots, or Bruins. "Rick and Dick are originals," Lobel told the crowd. "We will never see their likes again."

How many more Bostons are really likely?

"I can understand why people always wonder when I'm going to quit," Dick says, finally willing to offer more on this subject. "It's a natural question to ask a man my age. But I can honestly say that stopping never crossed my mind. And I know Rick feels the same way. What keeps us going is that we see how much good we're doing, and not just for disabled peopled. We have inspired a lot of able-bodied people to start running or try some other kind of exercise."

Like the Austin insurance executive who heard Dick speak at a company sales meeting. She was inspired not only by his message of overcoming obstacles, whether physical or mental, but by Dick himself to fight through a long marathon training run. "I've been sitting here brainstorming the past week and trying to come up with a way to show how much your presentation meant to all of us, not only in our professional lives, but personally," she later wrote Dick. "When I was running my longest prerace run, 22 miles, Saturday after the meeting, I kept picturing your face, and it truly helped keep me going." There are other stories like this, too many to count.

After finishing lunch, Dick wheels Rick into the living room and places him in his favorite spot by the bay window, where he can look out over the sloping lawn to the edge of Hamilton Reservoir. His father hooks him up to the computer and headpiece equipped with a mouse that rests just behind his right temple. Now it's Rick's turn to answer questions.

Letters appear on a small screen at Rick's eye level. He twitches his head to move the cursor through the letters, double-twitching when he wants to select one. Each twitch requires a concentrated effort. As he works, his arm waves spasmodically, occasionally getting caught in the computer wires.

He is asked, "Do you ever have a bad race?"

Rick considers for several moments, then sets to work. He scans down the letters, each twitch of his head accompanied by a small electronic beep, like a bird chirping. Y, he types. Then, three minutes later, E, and finally, after a similar interval, S.

The next question comes, but Rick isn't finished with the first one. W ... three minutes ... H ... three minutes ... E ... three minutes, and so on for a half hour. Rick communicates no sense of frustration or impatience. "Yes, when the weather is too cold ..." finally appears on the screen. The reply is read aloud, but Rick still isn't finished. The twitches and chirps continue. And then the full reply sounds through the voice synthesizer. "Yes," the disembodied electronic voice says after several more long minutes, "when the weather is too cold and the women are too covered up."

Rick laughs, his face twisting into a grin, his shoulders shaking. Forty-five minutes after the first question, the next one comes.

"Do you ever regard running as an unhealthy obsession? Do you ever think you should stop or cut back?"

"No. By running we are actually educating the public."

"Do you think that not being able to speak gives you a special insight into other people?"

"Yes. I understand them not in terms of running, but as far as general life."

"What do you do when you feel down or depressed?"

"I just think about the poor people in the world."

The final, two-part question comes as dusk falls and Rick's father quietly enters the room to turn on a lamp. Three hours have passed since the Q&A started, roughly the time it takes Team Hoyt to run a marathon.

"Was fate at work at the time of your birth, and on that day nearly 30 years ago when you told your parents that you wanted to run? And do you think fate chose you to live such a confined life but also one so free?"

Rick doesn't need the computer to answer this one. His face lights up. His whole body says yes.

DOGGED

BY STEVE FRIEDMAN

> As one of the world's best endurance runners,
> Danelle Ballengee was always up for a challenge.
> But when she got severely injured and
> stranded in the desert, she prepared to give up.
> Fortunately, she brought a friend along.

JULY 2007

HE WAS A BAD DOG. That was an awful thing for the runner to think as she lay dying. He had curled next to her that first night in the hidden canyon, after the accident. He had put his snout on her belly, and licked her face as she stared up at more shooting stars than she had ever dreamed. And that first morning—could it have been just the day before?—when it was so cold she had to crack the ice on top of the miraculous puddle, he had played with a stick, run in little circles, and barked with what she thought was happiness, and he was such a good dog then. He made her think that maybe things weren't so bad. She saw an eagle glide overhead that morning. It was beautiful. It was a beautiful morning. She was in a beautiful spot. Red rock and sandy soil and a juniper tree and the soft sighing of the high desert wind, and to lope through it would have been a wonder for a runner whose body wasn't broken and bleeding inside.

All she had was the puddle, and her dog. And then she didn't have the dog, because when she was screaming, when it took her two hours to reach behind her head to fill a water bottle from the puddle, the dog ran away. She couldn't stop screaming. She screamed because she hurt, and because she needed help, and because she was afraid that help might not come in time. The dog came back, but he wouldn't lie down next to her that second night. It was just last night, but it seemed so long ago. There were no shooting stars the second night. The second night, she saw things in the sky that made no sense, and heard a strange voice from the dark, and it made no sense, either.

Today, the third day, the dog was gone. Then he was back. Then he was gone again. Maybe she was hallucinating. Even though she was well known for enduring things others could not, for persevering through heat and cold and all manner of punishing climate and topography—even though she was one of the most accomplished endurance runners in the world—she still had her limits. On the third day, in the hidden canyon, her body broken, she discovered them.

And then the dog was back, and now he was coming closer, and now he was lapping at the puddle, her only water source, and she couldn't help it, she yelled at him. It was the only water she could reach. Couldn't he find another puddle? Bad dog!

No one knew where she was. It would be dark again, and cold. No one could hear her scream. No one was coming. Today, her third day on the rock by the puddle, she allowed herself to see the truth.

She had won the Pikes Peak Marathon four times. She had raced up all 54 of Colorado's 14,000-foot peaks in less than 15 days, faster than any woman in history. She had competed in 441 endurance events (races that took from an hour to 10 days to finish) since 1995 and finished in the top three in 390 of them. Three times she was part of a four-person team that won one of the most punishing endurance events in the world, Primal Quest, a 400-mile trek over land and water, mountain and desert terrain. She had earned six U.S. Athlete of the Year titles in four different endurance sports. She had kept going when others had told her she had to stop. Now, she couldn't move.

It was midafternoon on a Friday. She had degrees in biology and kinesiology, and as much as she had invested, personally and professionally, in the awesome power of the human spirit, she also possessed grim knowledge regarding the limits of flesh and bone. It was 10 days before Christmas. That's when Danelle Ballengee, just 35 years old, prepared to die. That's when the runner who never gave up, gave up. It really was a beautiful spot. She felt peace. And then she heard another sound. And it didn't make sense, either.

TWO DAYS EARLIER, ON WEDNESDAY, DECEMBER 13, Ballengee had spent the early part of the morning e-mailing with sponsors, writing articles, answering questions from clients who had hired her as a personal trainer. She left her house on Cliffview Drive in Moab, Utah, at 10 a.m. She had landlord duties to attend to, too. She owned three rental properties in Colorado, and she rented out space in her Moab house, and one of her tenant's friends had stolen some money, so she had to go to the bank to file a fraud report. Only then could she begin the highlight of her morning—the run.

With her dog, Taz, a 3-year-old reddish-brown mutt with a long jaw and a broad chest, she climbed in her white Ford Ranger truck, her kayak on top of the roof. She stopped at a Burger King for a chicken sandwich and French fries and a large coffee, because she had forgotten to eat breakfast. The dog got a bite, because the dog always got a bite. She had spoiled him since the day she got him from the pound, when he was just a few weeks old.

It was a good day for a run, cloudy but not too cold. She listened to "Beautiful Day," by U2. She thought about the guy she had met a few weeks earlier at a race in Leadville, Colorado, and smiled because she thought there was potential. When she got to the parking area at the Amasa Back Trail, five miles out of town, she kept driving, continued a quarter mile north on the road to a turnoff near a cliff. She did it because she wanted to shave a quarter mile off her run. The endurance runner was feeling lazy.

She put on a pair of cheap orange sunglasses, grabbed her MP3 player, a large plastic bottle filled with water, and a raspberry-flavored energy gel. She wore running pants, a fleece hat, silk long underwear, a polypropylene shirt, and a thin fleece jacket. The temperature was in the 40s, but she wanted to be prepared. She invested as much in preparation as she did in the power of positive thinking. Just before she locked her wallet and cell phone in the car, she spotted a fanny pack in the backseat. She had forgotten it was there. She grabbed it, stuck her water bottle in, and took off.

Her plan was to run and hike an eight-mile loop. She would start on the Amasa Back Trail, popular among bikers and hikers, especially in spring and fall. But she would veer off of it after just a few miles, just before the top of a mesa, where she would follow a seldom-used jeep trail known to the locals as the Mine Sweeper and into a hidden canyon, then she would scramble up the rocks of that canyon, toward Hurrah Pass, onto another seldom-used jeep trail, through another canyon, up some more rocks, and she would eventually land back on another jeep trail that would take her back to a road that led to her truck. Taz ran alongside her, panting happily. An hour in, she had covered five miles. She had drunk half her water bottle. She was scrambling up the rocks in the first hidden canyon, Taz just behind her. It really was a beautiful day.

If you stopped to think about the things that could kill you, you could drive yourself crazy. Another second in an intersection. Another inch on a highway. One misstep on some ice-covered slickrock. Or maybe it was just slippery lichen.

One second she was one of the best endurance runners in the world, out for a late-autumn loop in the high desert, breathing in the soft, juniper-scented air, barely paying attention to the low, grayish clouds scudding by. One second she was a world champion out for a light workout.

And then the second was gone. Now she was sliding, like a kid down a giant water slide. That's what she thought at the time, that it felt like a water slide. Past lichen, past rocks, past sand. She slid on her butt, hit "a little bump," then "another little bump." Then she came to "a little ledge."

People hear Primal Quest and they think of adrenaline junkies. People read about Danelle Ballengee and they think risk seeker. But in her kayak, she steered clear of white water. On skis, she descended carefully, avoided steep, out-of-bounds areas. She had no interest in bungee jumping. Other adventure racers yipped with glee at sections that demanded hanging from ropes. That was the point in the race when Ballengee frowned and gritted her teeth.

She kept picking up speed. According to a newspaper account published a week after the accident, she flew off a cliff and plummeted the equivalent of two stories, landing on her feet. The reality was messier, and more plain. She ended up halfway down the hill, prone. She caught her breath. She had once survived eight sun-baked days in the Morocco Eco-Challenge, a race equally fearsome as Primal Quest. A leech had attached itself to her eyelid in another race, given her a corneal ulcer, blinded her for three days. That was punishing. This was just a nasty tumble. But she was smart, and careful. She had her two degrees from the University of Colorado. She would be methodical. She put her right hand on her right leg, her left hand on her left leg. *Whew.* That was the word she thought. *Whew.* She wasn't paralyzed. This was her next thought: *Man, it's gonna be a long walk out of here.* A moment later she realized she couldn't stand up.

She would crawl 30 feet to the bottom of the canyon. She would drag herself over rocks and through scrub. Then she would crawl the three miles to the Amasa Back Trail and hope that someone would see her. It was noon when she started.

Her left leg wouldn't move. She scooted forward on her right knee, balanced, then reached back with both hands and pulled her left leg forward. She knew things were broken. She knew she was in trouble. When she reached the bottom of the canyon, she looked in her fanny pack to see if there might be something to help. She found another pack of raspberry energy gel, a shower cap, and two ibuprofen. She swallowed the pills, kept crawling. She crawled through sand and brush and some snow—the canyon floor was not just sand—and by the time she arrived at a flat rock, and a sinkhole filled with water, the air was getting cold and shadows in the canyon were lengthening. It was 5 p.m. She had crawled a quarter of a mile, and it had taken five hours.

She lay down on her back, drank the remaining half of her water bottle, put her hands between her legs because they were so cold. She decided she would refill the water bottle from the sinkhole—she didn't care about parasites. But it hurt too much to turn over. So she reached backward over her right shoulder and filled the water bottle without looking.

She did crunches with her head and neck to keep warm. Her knees were bent, and she tapped her feet on the rock. She rubbed her hands together. She reached for the shower cap in the fanny pack, but she couldn't find it. Taz curled up next to her. He put his chin on her stomach and looked at her. The temperature dipped into the 20s. She lay on her back, freezing, exhausted, and looked at the moonless sky. She saw the Milky Way and shooting stars. She had never in her life seen so many shooting stars.

She wondered what the guy in Leadville was doing. She wondered if someone would see that her truck was missing from her house. Then she realized how dumb that was. She loved working with others in the endurance challenges, but she hadn't told anyone where she was going. And what she was most famous for was enduring. Why would anyone worry about her?

It was so cold. She didn't want to die. She couldn't die. There were friends and family she wasn't ready to leave. She continued her crunches, her feet-tapping, her finger-curling.

At first light, she saw Taz playing with a stick. That cheered her. She ate one of the energy gels. She tried to refill her water bottle, but the water in the sinkhole had frozen. She reached over her shoulder and broke through it with the cap of the bottle.

She decided that today she would crawl out of the canyon. She tried to roll over, to get on her hands and knees, and she screamed. She felt pain radiating down her legs, up her back. Taz licked her face and she lay back down, on her back, to gather her strength. And she screamed for help, in case anyone could hear her, and when she looked up, Taz had gone.

Then it was three o'clock and he was back. She wasn't sure how so much time had passed, but it had. The temperature had risen into the 40s, and that felt good, but it would be dark again soon, and the cold would come. She screamed for help, even though she knew no one was coming. That's when she saw the shower cap—it was just a couple feet away. It was too far. She raised her head, lowered her voice. She looked at Taz.

"I'm hurt," she said. He looked at her and tilted his head, first to the left, then to the right. She knew it was ridiculous, but it looked like he understood.

"Taz," she said, "you know, maybe you could go and get some help for me."

He tilted his head again, didn't move. She told herself not to be stupid, that he was a dog. Just a dog. And then Taz ran away again, down the hidden canyon.

Now it was four o'clock. She had to get the shower cap. She would need it for the night, to keep what meager body heat she still had. Two feet. It took an hour to get it.

And now the sun had left the hidden little canyon, and it was getting colder again, and she felt a swelling in her midsection, a lump the size of a water bottle, and she knew she was broken inside. Then Taz was back, which was comforting, but it meant that he wasn't magic, he didn't understand English, he was a good dog, but he was just a dog. No one would be coming down the hidden canyon to rescue her.

She started the crunches again, the feet-tapping, the hand-rubbing. Taz refused to curl up next to her. Was it an animal's instinctive recoiling at imminent death? Did he want softer ground? It made no sense to her. Every so often, though, he would place a paw on her chest, lick her face. "Good dog," she would say.

It got colder, and colder, and darker. She gazed up, looking for shooting stars, for the Milky Way, for evidence that the world hadn't ended. That she hadn't ended. She saw only stripes. Long, white stripes slicing through the black night sky. She knew her body was shutting down, her brain malfunctioning. She was seeing things. She cried. She cried for her family and her friends and the nascent romance with the guy from Leadville that would never go anywhere. She is not religious, and she did not pray. What she did was plead.

"Please," she pleaded. "Please, somebody, notice that I'm gone."

DOROTHY ROSSIGNOL IS 76 YEARS OLD, a "nosy neighbor" by her own account. Others in Moab call her a "piece of work," a "little old lady," and "the busybody of the neighborhood." She is childless, a widow since 1990. She loves mining, and if there is a town in the American West that ever produced a significant amount of any valuable mineral, whether gold, silver, or lead, she can name the town, along with its mineral. Chances are she lived there with her husband, Robert, who mined it. "My husband would rather mine than eat," she says. They first came through Moab in 1957, a young bride and her husband, a miner looking for work during the uranium boom. They returned in 1969 and settled there for good. Moab was something in the boom years. "Parties you wouldn't believe," she says, ". . . dancing girls from Spain."

Life is slower now, nights quieter, days longer. She volunteers at the Dan O'Laurie Museum, eats lunch four days a week at the Moab senior center ("I'd eat there five days, but they're closed on Thursdays"), tends to the five peachcot trees (peach trees with apricot fruit grafted on) in her yard. Rossignol liked the young woman who moved next door five years ago, which is saying a lot. "I don't rush over to meet new neighbors right away," she says, "because you don't know what kind of people they are."

But the young woman seemed nice, and quiet, and she bought a puppy who jumped over the little metal fence separating the yards so often and scratched at the widow's door so relentlessly that she finally gave up and bought a bag of dog biscuits. Every day Taz would come over, and every day Rossignol would give the mutt two biscuits. He'd eat one there and take the other one home. Ballengee was gone a lot—"training for one of those adventure things"—so Rossignol fetched her mail, made sure her pipes didn't freeze in the winter when she was traveling.

They would do yard work together and chat "about everything in general and nothing in particular." As nice as Ballengee was, she wasn't so great on following leash laws. "So when I see the police or the dog catcher," Rossignol says, "I tie him up."

Taz didn't come to visit on Wednesday, December 13, and that night Rossignol looked outside and saw that Ballengee's truck wasn't there. She also saw that Ballengee had left her drapes open, her lights on. She saw Ballengee's laptop computer on. She knew that Ballengee was a free spirit, that when she wasn't training or visiting her parents in Evergreen, Colorado, she sometimes left to visit friends. She knew that Ballengee sometimes didn't tell anyone where she was going. The widow didn't exactly approve of all that gallivanting. On the other hand, she had to admit, she admired it. They weren't all that different, the endurance runner and the miner's widow. Self-sufficient women in a man's world. Rossignol might have been a nosy neighbor, but she wasn't a scaredy-cat. She would feel foolish calling the police if her young neighbor was out just having fun. She went to bed.

On Thursday afternoon, Rossignol looked again and saw the open drapes, the blazing lights, the computer. That's when she called Gary and Peggy Ballengee, in Evergreen, Colorado. She told Danelle's parents she was worried.

SHE WAS SO TIRED. And cold. What was the point of tapping her feet? No one was coming down the hidden canyon. She stopped tapping. Then she heard a strange voice, commanding her. She knew she was alone. She knew there was no one telling her anything. She didn't believe in God. She knew there couldn't be a voice. But there was. And it wouldn't shut up. Keep tapping, the voice said. She kept tapping.

WORD HAD SPREAD THROUGH TOWN, along with rumors, and someone from the bicycle shop called someone else who called the guy from Leadville. "I promise," the guy told Ballengee's parents over the phone. "I did not take your daughter to Mexico. I don't know where she is."

Police spent three hours inside Ballengee's house that Thursday. When they arrived, Rossignol was waiting. She told them her neighbor was in trouble, that they should be looking for her truck, and her dog. She told them she would show them where things were inside the house, where to find important clues. When they refused her entry, she stood on the sidewalk outside. She stood on the sidewalk for three hours.

One of the police officers was a woman. She listened to the widow's requests and suggestions and urgent entreaties. Then the officer gave her a card. It was dark now. If Rossignol heard anything, the cop said, feel free to call. Then the cops left.

THE STRANGE VOICE HAD STOPPED. The stripes were gone. It was light and she was alive. But the water in the puddle was frozen again and Taz was gone. She broke through, filled her bottle. She ate the other raspberry energy gel, the last one. No one was coming. She estimated she couldn't make it more than a few feet an hour, and wondered if it was worse to die trying or to die next to her little puddle. She started crawling.

She dragged herself off the rock, and her pants came off, because she couldn't lift her pelvis off the ground. She found herself in a shallow depression. She was stuck. She saw the stupidity of her decision and crawled back onto the rock. A round trip of four feet. It took two hours. Now she was hyperventilating. Now she felt the ball of clotted blood and swollen flesh moving inside her. And now it was 1:30 p.m. She would never leave this hidden canyon. Why had she wasted hours, and time, and precious energy to go four feet? Why hadn't she told someone where she was going? Why hadn't she told more people she loved them? And where the hell was Taz? What was wrong with that dog?

CRAIG SHUMWAY GREW UP IN MOAB, dug in its soil for uranium during the last years of the boom. He loves the high desert, the wide-open spaces. He has been in law enforcement for 17 years, a Moab detective for four. On Friday morning, December 15, he was sitting in his office at the police department on East Center Street when Sergeant Mike Wiler walked in and sat down.

Wiler told Shumway there had been a missing-person report the previous night. He said it looked like someone had left a house unsecured. He said he had given the information to the Grand County Sheriff's Department and that they would be checking trailheads to see if the truck might be there. In the meantime, Moab police had put out an Attempt to Locate (ATL). In Moab, a magnet for the young, the adventurous, and the risk-seeking, an ATL is not exactly a red alert. "You just don't jump out and go look for every one of 'em," Shumway says.

Shumway nodded, plowed through some paperwork, then decided, before lunch, he would take a drive. No one was too alarmed about the missing woman—people took off for days without telling anyone all the time in Moab, and she was a world-class athlete. And it wasn't his job. It wasn't his jurisdiction, either. But he knew how big the desert was, how many trails crisscrossed the canyons and rivers of southern Utah. First he stopped at Ballengee's house, took a quick look. Then he drove 10 miles north to the Sovereign Trail and checked the trailhead, and found nothing.

Law enforcement officers often talk about intuition and gut feelings and how important it is to recognize them. On the way back to Moab, though, Shumway felt something unfamiliar.

He drove down Kane Creek Road, to the parking lot of the Amasa Back Trail. He's not sure why, but he passed it, kept going, to the top of the hill, to the little spot near the cliff. That's where he saw the white Ford Ranger. He wanted to document things, in case there had been a crime. He pulled out his eight-megapixel Canon digital camera and took pictures. Later, he would look at the receipt that the runner had left inside the car. It was from Burger King, for a chicken sandwich and large fries and a large coffee. It was dated Wednesday, December 13, at 11 a.m. Now it was 1:30 in the afternoon, two days and two cold nights later. Shumway had another feeling, a bad one.

IT WAS THE EFFORT SHE HAD EXPENDED CRAWLING into and out of the little depression. It was her body shutting down. It was fear. She knew she needed to stop hyperventilating. She forced herself to breathe more slowly, and it worked. She breathed. She didn't know where her dog was, and soon it would be cold and dark, and she was broken and bleeding inside, and no one was coming, but at least she was breathing. So she breathed. She breathed and she waited to die.

BY MIDAFTERNOON, when the Grand County Search and Rescue team gathered at the Amasa Back trailhead, they knew who they were looking for. John

Marshall, the officer in charge of the team that day, had met Ballengee once before, when he worked as a volunteer at the 2006 Primal Quest in Utah. When he had first seen her then, she had just finished a 46-mile trek across the desert. The temperature had been 105 degrees. She had been without water for the past four hours. Her feet were more blisters than flesh. Marshall suggested an IV drip that day. Ballengee declined. She was in a hurry.

And now she had disappeared. "I'm thinking," Marshall says, "this was a world-class, I-eat-nails-for-breakfast person we're looking for. I'm thinking she's been out there for two nights.

"I'm thinking she didn't twist an ankle. I'm thinking there's something very, very serious going on."

As soon as Marshall and the others got near Ballengee's truck, they saw the dog. It was running in circles, "going a million miles an hour." Marshall suspected it was the runner's dog.

"Most dogs won't leave their master as long as their master has a pulse," he told a newspaper reporter. "To see that dog was a truly saddening sight."

He called Taz, tried to coax him over. But Taz wouldn't come. The dog circled Marshall and the others, then dashed toward town. Marshall thought they should try to grab him, but no one could. Then the dog stopped, looked back over its shoulder. Then the dog was gone.

Marshall sent Melissa Fletcher, a team member who works as a backcountry mountain bike guide, running up Jackson's Trail, a narrow, steep, single track, because it was the most difficult and she was the most fit member of the team. He stayed near the truck to coordinate the search. Though he wasn't a Search and Rescue team member, Craig Shumway, after calling his discovery in, had gone home, changed into hiking clothes, and trekked up the Cable Arch Trail to make sure Ballengee wasn't there. She wasn't. Marshall sent two men and a woman up the Amasa Back Trail in ATVs. Riding the second ATV were Mike Coronella and Barb Fincham. In the first ATV was a 60-year-old commercial heating and refrigeration installer named Bego Gerhart.

Gerhart is 5'8", weighs 180 pounds. He has a full gray beard and piercing blue eyes and a potbelly. He looks like he'd be more at home in front of a cheeseburger than driving an ATV through the backcountry, looking for a woman about to die. He hitchhiked to Moab in 1970, a onetime California Eagle Scout with no particular direction. A Moab cop asked him for identification, and Gerhart asked if the cop knew anyone looking for work. That's how he ended up as a trucker, "with guys who had 200-word vocabularies, and 100 of 'em were obscene."

Gerhart has volunteered for the Grand County Search and Rescue squad for 11 years. He rigged ropes in New Zealand for filmmakers shooting *Vertical Limit* in 1999. He served as a consultant to a television show called *I Shouldn't Be Alive* in 2006. In 2003, he was on the team that hiked into Blue John Canyon to winch a boulder and retrieve the hand of Aron Ralston, who had hacked it off in order to free himself. Others might have broader shoulders and younger legs, but of the 91 calls that went out to the Grand County Search and Rescue team in 2006, Gerhart responded to 88 of them, more than anyone else.

A lot of men and women who run (and hike and bike) in wilderness-rich areas like Moab speak of the majesty of the outdoors, the intoxicating consequences of fresh air. Many submit that the majestic sweep of the sky and the exquisite desolation of the desert serve as prima facie evidence of a loving spirit. But those tend to be the younger, leaner runners. Gerhart sees things a little differently.

"What happened to someone like Danelle is pretty good evidence against the existence of a benevolent God," he says. Regarding the secret to survival, he says, "It's all about knowing how to suffer."

Gerhart was a mile down the Amasa Back Trail, puttering along in his ATV, when his two-way radio sputtered to life.

"The dog! The dog!" It was Marshall. Taz had come back. He had sprinted up the trail, passing Coronella and Fincham's ATV. Fincham had gotten out of his ATV to follow the dog on foot, and the dog had promptly disappeared.

The dog dashed by Gerhart's ATV, and it stopped. It looked at Gerhart, then it dashed off the trail, up to a little mesa. Gerhart clambered out of the ATV, walked up the mesa, where the dog was waiting. Gerhart stared at the dog. The dog stared at Gerhart. And the dog was gone again.

People journey into the desert without enough water or the proper clothing every year, and people die. People slip, and they never rise. People get lost, and they stay lost. Search and Rescue team members do their best, but when someone is gone for three days and two nights, on the fringe of winter, help often consists of a recovery mission. It often includes a body bag. Less than a month earlier two men had died near Moab. They had frozen to death. Both were wearing heavier clothes than Ballengee. Gerhart knew all that. But he had a feeling. Gerhart is not a sentimental man, nor prone to a lot of religio-mystical mumbo jumbo. This is about as close as he gets: "My mind said, Follow the dog."

But the dog was gone. So Gerhart backtracked to where he had first spotted Taz. A few years earlier, he had taken a tracking course from U.S. Marshals, and now he studied the ground. He looked for dog tracks next to footprints of a woman runner. When he saw them, he followed them, away from the main road, down a little spur, toward a hidden canyon. He saw that the trail got rockier and more and more rugged. He hopped into his ATV, and he drove toward the hidden canyon, the sounds of his engine echoed off the red-rock walls. And he drove, and drove some more. And then he stopped. He thought he had heard something.

THE DOG HAD BEEN DISAPPEARING all day. This time when he got back, he ran straight to the puddle and he started drinking. And he drank and drank. And as much as the runner loved the dog, as inured to pain and loss as she was, she was still human. Bad dog! She yelled at Taz, "Can't you drink out of another pothole?"

And there they lay, less than a week before the shortest day of the year, a woman broken and bleeding inside, a dog lapping up her precious water. She cried. She thought again of the people to whom she hadn't said, "I love you." And then something shifted. It wasn't the dog's fault. It wasn't anyone's. Is this what acceptance felt like? She wasn't angry anymore. Now, she was ready to die. Now, she was at peace. And then she heard a sound that didn't make sense.

LATER, A LOT OF PEOPLE WOULD INVOKE DIVINE mysteries, seek answers in the supernatural. Shumway would reflect on the strange feelings that led him to search for the missing truck, the inexplicable and powerful urges that guided him up the Kane Creek Road and to the little patch of dirt on top of the hill, near the cliff. "You can call it whatever you want," he says. "Call it coincidence, or fate, or whatever. I'm a God-fearing person and I can't explain it. It was a sense of urgency. I had never felt it before." Marshall would ask out loud how someone with virtually no body fat could possibly live through two cold nights in the high desert, "how her internal metabolism defied the laws of physics." People referred to the entire episode as a "Christmas miracle." When it came to myth-making, though, no one beat the dog lovers. In the news accounts and stories of the accident, Taz morphed into a furry genius, a four-legged phantasm, a kind of barking, galloping Gandalf. Some Search and Rescue team members talked about how, in hindsight, it looked like Taz had planned the rescue the whole time. "It was like he was trying to get us to pay attention to him, so when he showed up later, he could lead us to her," Marshall says. (Marshall is a dog lover.) Even academics sang the praises of the wonderdog. Marc Bekoff, a biology professor at the University of Colorado and author of *The Emotional Lives of Animals*, says there's a good chance Taz knew what he was doing. "I don't know what his doggy brain was saying, but it was probably something like, 'There's something novel, there's something new here.' I bet you that dog was just going, 'This is new, this is different, I gotta do something.' There's no doubt that [Ballengee's] scent was changing. At some point, he was picking that up. At some point, I'm sure the dog realized there was some opportunity to save her. I know people will laugh at me, but I don't care. I believe that."

But that was all later.

First, Gerhart had to drive toward the sound. That's when he saw them. There, on a rock, in the little hidden canyon, was a woman on her back. And there, lying next to her, with his snout on her chest, the mutt.

"I'm so glad to see you," Ballengee cried, weeping.

"I'm glad you're glad to see me, and that you can say so," Gerhart replied. At least that's the way he tells the story. The way he remembers, she was lucid, but emotional. He was amazed she was so articulate, but he was concerned about keeping her core temperature from falling, so he fetched from his ATV a heavy sleeping bag with Velcro straps, what Search and Rescue team members call Doctor Down. The way he remembers it, he kept her talking, even as he was radioing for help, scanning the landscape for a place where a rescue helicopter might safely land, shoving her hands into heavy gloves. All of that, according to Ballengee, is accurate, but incomplete. The way she remembers it, Gerhart was weeping, too.

Taz ran to Gerhart and licked him. Then the commercial heating and refrigeration installer said something to the runner that people have said to other people as long as there have been pets. "You got one heck of a dog," Gerhart said.

SHE DIDN'T SLEEP WELL LAST NIGHT. Every time she shut her eyes, she was tumbling down the slickrock, picking up speed. Every time she opened them, she was on her back, halfway down the steep wall, cold and alone, broken and bleeding inside. And if she did sleep, then what? She was afraid of the nightmares. She didn't want to find herself back in the hidden canyon, cold and alone and dying.

It was midafternoon, January 23, almost six weeks after she fell, and she was tired, and she hurt, and though she was lying on the couch in the basement of her parents' house in Evergreen, and they were upstairs, and she was safe, and though Taz was lying on the floor next to her, and even though she and her dog had been on the *Today* show, even though she and Taz had ascended in the popular consciousness to Christmas Miracle and Wonderdog status, the reality was messier, more difficult.

She didn't have complete control of her left hand. She wasn't sure if she ever would. Her feet felt as if she were standing in an icy stream. She wasn't sure if they would ever feel differently. Both were consequences of frostbite.

She was taking six Neurontin pills a day to help reduce the pain. She was taking three 600-milligram tablets of ibuprofen for inflammation, four 30-milligram iron pills to help increase her red-blood-cell count, and Percocet for more pain. And anti-anxiety pills, for the nights she had trouble sleeping, like last night. And stool softener. Until a few days ago, her father had been injecting her every day, in her stomach, with a drug to lessen the chances of her blood clotting. After she complained about the pain, her doctor finally relented. Now she was taking 325 milligrams of aspirin daily.

She is almost 5'5" tall, and weighed 120 pounds before the accident. Now she weighed 100. She has dirty-blond hair, blue eyes, and anyone who has spent any time around her comments on her impishness and how she can't stay still. Today, she was squinting with pain and exhaustion. Her pelvis had broken in four places. At one spot, it splintered into too many pieces for doctors to count. She cracked three vertebrae. She lost a third of her blood. Doctors at Denver Health medical center had operated on her for six hours, inserting a titanium plate in her pelvis.

When the *Today* show called afterward, she wasn't all that interested. Of course she was grateful to be alive, but in the hospital, she hurt, and she was tired, and hungry and—truth be told—scared about what the injuries would mean. Then the *Today* show people said they wanted Taz on the air, too. She hadn't seen the dog since the Search and Rescue helicopter had lifted her into the sky, right after she scratched him behind the ears and said, "It'll be okay, boy," and Taz had gone home with John Marshall, who couldn't have lived with himself if he'd let animal control take the dog. If agreeing to be interviewed by the Today show meant she'd be able to see Taz, she was on board.

Now she was talking about how after the shooting for the *Today* show was done, and after Taz had gone home with Ballengee's sister, Michelle, to her home in Denver, a quarter mile from the hospital, the dog had escaped, and her sister knew where he was going, so she walked to the hospital, and there was Taz.

She was a miracle, and Taz was a hero. Cards came from all over. One day, a box filled with dry ice arrived. It was from a woman in Michigan who had seen the *Today* show. Inside were five pounds of hormone-free aged rib steaks and a red-and-white Christmas stocking with a stuffed Santa inside. On the top, embroidered in green, was the name of the intended recipient—Taz.

Ballengee had visitors—including the guy from Leadville—and heard from friends and relatives and strangers. She wouldn't make the same mistake again—this time, she told everyone how much she loved them. There were a lot of them. And love was great, and maybe she was a Christmas miracle, but she was still human, and this was life.

She couldn't walk. She stayed in the hospital for 15 days, and the first week, her biggest accomplishment was forcing herself to sit up in bed without passing out. Ten seconds was a good day. Just a week ago, she tried to get out of bed to use a portable commode that was just a few feet away, and fainted. Now she could make it to the bathroom, using a wheelchair, by herself. That was a big deal. She couldn't afford all the medical bills. At the moment, the bill from Grand Junction, where she had been taken by the helicopter, totaled $45,000, and the insurance policy that had sounded so good when she bought it turned out to be not so good, and she hadn't even received her bill for surgery or her Denver hospital stay yet. She had managed a lap and a half around a West Denver mall in her wheelchair yesterday, and that had felt great, "just to get the blood flowing," and runners and endurance athletes she had competed with were holding fund-raising events for her, and that was great, too, but she knew she wouldn't be able to walk for at least two months, and after that, it would be another few months before she could run, and then it would be "how to run fast, then how to run aggressively. On trails and up and down mountains. Whether I'll be able to do it at the levels I used to—I'm gonna try. But if I can run again at all, I'll be so happy."

She works hard at planning to be happy. But she is scared, too, and she has nightmares.

She talks about those nightmares, and about Bego Gerhart (whose name, when she first heard it in the canyon, she thought was Bagel, "probably because I was so hungry"). She talks about Dorothy Rossignol, who, unbeknownst to Ballengee, has promised that when the runner moves back to Moab, she will be watched with special vigilance—even for a nosy neighbor—and nagged about where she's going, "even when it's just a trip to the mailbox." She talks about how much she misses being outside, "just being with Taz, running through the woods."

She talks a lot about Taz, how people ask if he gets extra treats now, or extra attention. He doesn't. "He's always been spoiled," she says. "I treated him pretty well before."

Mostly, she talks about her days in the hidden canyon, and the cold, and how she was sure she was going to die, and about the way she saw the white stripes in the sky, and heard the strange voice that commanded her to keep tapping her feet.

Daniel Smith, author of *Muses, Madmen, and Prophets*, a book on auditory hallucination, says the strange sounds Ballengee experienced were likely caused by "the abuse the body takes and the exhaustion. [They] often occur in that twilight moment between sleep and wakefulness."

Ballengee knows that. She earned degrees in biology and kinesiology, after all, not philosophy and religion. But she's not sure. "As far as I'm concerned," she says, "I'm going to be the best person I can. . . . I'm okay without an answer."

She has been watching movies at night. She recently watched *Touching the Void*, the story of a man who had to crawl his way off a mountain in the Peruvian Andes and through a crevasse with a broken leg, and *Eight Below*, the tale of eight sled dogs who face death by freezing in Antarctica. A visitor suggests a few comedies, considering the nightmares.

Then Taz starts barking. He sees a squirrel outside. Ballengee's father walks down the steps when he hears the barking and tells his daughter he'll take her mutt for a walk.

"He's kind of dumb," Gary Ballengee says, patting Taz on the head. "Brilliant at saving lives, but he'll chase that squirrel all day. He's just kind of dumb."

Her father and her dog are behind her, and it's not easy to turn her head, but that's what Danelle Ballengee does. She's done more difficult things. She turns and looks first at her father, who doesn't notice, then at her dog, who tilts his head and looks back at her. He tilts his head first to the left, then to the right, side to side, just like he did that terrible afternoon when Danelle Ballengee lay dying. And then the runner smiles at her dog and she puts her head back on her pillow, and she rests.

LIFE AND LIMB

BY BRUCE BARCOTT

[
How far would you go to preserve your life as a runner?
Would you cut off your own left leg? That's exactly
what Tom White did. This is his story.
]

OCTOBER 2008

ON THE DAY HE DECIDED to pay a man to cut off his leg with a power saw Tom White woke up with a powerful yearning to run. It was October, early morning. The girls were still asleep. White rolled over and found an empty bed. His wife, Tammy, had already pulled on her shoes and set off on a five-mile run on the streets of Buena Vista, Colorado. Without him. Again.

The Whites are well known in Buena Vista, a farm town on the sunny central Colorado plain between the Arkansas River and the 14,000-foot Collegiate Peaks. Tom, a 47-year-old country doctor, has delivered many of the kids in town. He's a trim, compact fellow with an unflaggingly sunny outlook—kind of a one-man optimists' club. It's not uncommon for a woman to stop him in the produce section of the City Market, put his hand on her pregnant belly, and ask, "Is that a contraction?" Tammy, 46, is a physical therapist whose patients sometimes drop by the family's house on Main Street for treatment right there in the living room.

The sight of Tom and Tammy running together was a part of daily life in Buena Vista. Tom was a nationally ranked cross-country runner in college, and Tammy completed a marathon about once a month. For ten years they'd paced each other along the river trails and up the high ridges outside of town. But by early 2007, the townsfolk didn't see Dr. Tom running so much anymore. A degenerative condition in his left leg, the result of a motorcycle accident in his 20s, was giving him pain. That summer the pain worsened. By autumn, Tammy was running alone. For Tom, the injury was more than a disappointment. It was maddening. Running was an integral part of his life, his identity; it was how he moved when he felt most completely himself. And it had been taken away from him once before, after the crash. He'd spent years teaching himself how to run on a badly wounded leg. Now he was losing it all over again.

It was a school day, so he had to get the show on the road. He showered, dressed, and woke the girls. Eight-year-old Whitney and her 4-year-old sister, Jasmine, both wearing Hannah Montana T-shirts, picked their way through matching bowls of Kix cereal. "Jassy, you want some oatmeal?" Tom asked. She made a face and shook her head. He mixed some Spanish coffee—hot milk, instant coffee, two teaspoons of sugar—and handed Tammy a mug as she came in the back door, flushed and damp with sweat.

Tammy drove Jasmine to preschool, and Tom walked Whitney a mile down the road to Avery-Parsons Elementary. This was their morning custom. Whitney kicked a soccer ball as she and her dad chatted about possible Halloween costumes. Tom quietly endured the pain shooting through his leg. On the walk home, he wrestled with his frustrations.

The previous weekend he'd taken the Buena Vista Demons to the state cross-country championships. In their spare time, Tom and Tammy coached the high school girls' cross-country team, and it was a tradition for them to join the runners on a 5-K warmup. But last weekend, the pain was too much to bear.

"Coach!" the girls called. "You running with us?"

Tom's heart sank. "I can't," he said. "You go on without me."

He watched his squad head off. Next year, he thought, I'm going to be telling my own daughters I can't walk to school with them.

Over the years he'd joked about getting his gimpy leg cut off. "When this thing doesn't serve me anymore," he'd tell Tammy, "I'm going to get it amputated. Get a prosthesis."

Now it didn't seem like such a joke. Three years earlier, at the New York City Marathon, he heard about the Achilles Track Club's Freedom Team, a group of disabled Iraq and Afghanistan war veterans racing on prostheses. Also at that race, he met Sarah Reinertsen, a triathlete who runs on a hydraulic knee and a Flex-Run foot, a variation of the carbon-fiber Cheetah foot used by Paralympic athletes. Reinertsen had lost a leg to a congenital condition and still outpaced many able-bodied runners.

Back at home, White slipped into the garage to get his bike. He walked past a corkboard pinned with finishing medals and a rack of running shoes custom-designed for his unorthodox gait. Because it didn't pound his leg, bicycling was one activity he could still enjoy without pain. He rode the mile to his office, where Rhoda Boucher, his nurse, handed him a full schedule of patients. Tom saw a little bit of everything at Mountain Medical Clinic, the practice he ran with two partners: broken bones, newborn checkups, injured river guides, obese patients with heart failure. His oldest patient was 95, his youngest, born last night.

The work took his mind off his own decision for a few hours. As a medical procedure, amputation goes back 2,500 years, but the human fear of limb loss hearkens back even farther, to something primal. It's a horror-movie cliché, and for good reason. The psychological toll—the self ripped apart, the disfigurement, the revulsion in the eyes of others—arguably dwarfs the pain. Amputation has always been an act forced upon a body. It's the last resort, the corner where gangrene traps the limb.

For Tom White it was a different story. The choice he faced wasn't life or death. It was life or better life. With his natural leg, he faced a future without running or hiking—the pursuits that animated his physical self. He felt fully alive, he was who he was, when his heart was pumping and his lungs were bellowing. Now he was considering cutting off a part of himself to retain that core identity. For Tom, amputation didn't look like a loss. It looked like a life regained—if everything went well.

That afternoon, he went through a stack of charts, dealt with prescription refills, and locked up the office. As he rode home, he recalled hitting a rut a few days earlier, and how it made his shin creak. Now a dull, familiar pain crept up his leg. Aw, man, he thought. Even the bike's giving me trouble now.

That night, lying in bed next to Tammy, he let his thoughts slip across the pillow. "You know," he said, "I think it's time to amputate my left foot."

Tammy's eyes shot open. Holy cow! I can't believe he's telling me this right when we're falling asleep, she thought. "Cool!" she said.

Her reaction surprised him. She missed him as a running partner. But more than that, Tammy wanted to grow old with Tom—*with* him. So much of their joy in life came from running and hiking. Vicarious pleasure sucked. She wanted Tom to feel the endorphin rush, too.

The next morning she chased Tom around the kitchen with a date book. "Let's schedule it next month," she said.

"Whoa!" he said. Second thoughts kicked in. He was still talking theory. She was pressing for fact.

Hours later, the 2007 *Runner's World* Heroes of Running issue came in the mail. Tammy flipped open a piece on Amy Palmiero-Winters. She'd run a 3:04 in the Chicago Marathon on a prosthesis. "Tom!" Tammy called. "Do you believe in fate? Look at her."

She held out a photo of Palmiero-Winters, looking powerful and confident on her mechanical setup. Tom took a good long gaze. He didn't see a disabled person. He saw an elite marathoner pushing to qualify for the Olympic Trials. He smiled.

"That's it," he told Tammy. "That's what I want."

TOM WHITE DECIDED TO CUT OFF HIS LEG at a time when there had never been a better time to be an amputee. In the few years prior, a profound change had swept through American society and the global sports culture. Seemingly overnight, amputees had morphed from pity magnets to competitors. What once was handicapped had become bionic. A generation ago, disabled activists fought to pass the Americans with Disabilities Act. Today, the International Association of Athletics Federations (IAAF), track and field's world governing body, wrestles with the implications of South African sprinter Oscar Pistorius, who uses prosthetic legs, beating able-bodied runners in elite competition.

New technology has certainly made an impact. Devices like the Cheetah foot and the C-leg (a biomechanical prosthesis that uses a computer chip to run a hydraulic knee) allow amputees a more natural range of motion. But the gear—which has been widely available for nearly a decade—is only part of the story.

The real change has come in public awareness and attitude. It has something to do with Iraq War amputees proudly wearing prostheses emblazoned with Harley-Davidson logos and American flags. It has something to do with athletes like Pistorius making a leap from Paralympic champion to Olympic hopeful. It has something to do with amputees like Reinertsen flashing her high-tech leg in glossy ads for Lincoln sedans. These athletes raise the visibility of prostheses at a time when the melding of man and machine seems not only possible but inevitable. Tech fanatics are talking about mobile-phone implants. Skin-deep microchips help owners locate lost pets. Pistorius and Reinertsen are no longer human tragedies. They're the future. And they look damn cool.

In fact, the perception of athletes using prosthetic limbs has changed so quickly that some are now howling about the perceived advantage of prosthesis users. Lawyers spent much of the year prior dueling over Pistorius's right to run in the Beijing Olympics. (When Pistorius failed to post a qualifying time, he ended the controversy over Beijing. But the issue—whether prostheses give him an unfair advantage—is far from settled.)

As the issue of prosthetics in sports made headlines around the world, Tom White chose to undergo one of the most radical transformations any runner will ever face: from two-legged to one. Tom's choice raised profound questions about identity, athletics, and the human body. How far would you go to sustain your running life? Would you sacrifice money, career opportunities, relationships? Would you give up your left leg?

I followed Tom through the entire process, from decision, to surgery, and on through months of grueling rehabilitation. Though Oscar Pistorius and Sarah Reinertsen make it look easy, running on a prosthetic limb—heck, walking on one—is hardly easy. It's a struggle. It takes grit and determination. When you lose a leg, it's a long, hard road back to running.

A WEEK AFTER MAKING HIS DECISION, Tom sat in the exam room of Dr. David Hahn, a Denver orthopedic surgeon. Dr. Hahn, 59, had seen a lot of legs in his career. White's was a piece of medical history. Twenty-five years earlier a motorcycle accident had nearly severed the limb four inches above the ankle. Reattachment surgery, pioneering for its time, saved the lower leg and foot. It was heroic work back then, but the bone had never fully healed. Now it was cracked beyond repair. For 25 years, Tom had run on the human equivalent of a patched tire. He'd finally worn it out.

"You know, my first job is usually to tell people all the ways they can keep their leg," Dr. Hahn told Tom. "But it looks like you've already done that."

Three weeks later, on November 27, Tom and Tammy and the girls made the two-hour drive from Buena Vista to Denver's Presbyterian/St. Luke's Medical Center. Along the way they tallied mountains Tom's foot had climbed. "Mount Princeton! Mount Yale!" A few days earlier, Tom and Tammy had told the girls what was going to happen. "My foot hurts me, and once the doctors take it off, it won't hurt me anymore," Tom said.

Whitney began to cry. Tammy wondered if the amputation scared her. But that wasn't it. "I'm sad because Daddy was hurting and we didn't know," Whitney said.

That afternoon, Tom sat in a hospital gown on a gurney, prepped for surgery. A saline drip line draped from his right arm. For a man about to lose a limb, he looked calm. "I don't have any fear about the surgery," he said. "I'm excited to get this going." Asked what he planned to do with the foot, he answered, "You know, it would make great practical joke material." He laughed. "Tammy wants it cremated and spread someplace. But no. I think I'll just let them toss it out as medical waste."

Tom understood the risks. He'd seen men his age die in routine surgery. Things can happen—bleeding, infection, embolisms, hospital screwups. You didn't have to tell him that doctors and nurses were human. He also knew there was no guarantee he'd run again. If the amputated leg got infected, they'd have to cut again, above the knee. And who knew how he'd take to a mechanical leg? Chris Jones, the prosthetics expert he'd be working with, had warned him: "These things don't walk themselves."

He took those risks and fears and stuffed them in a locker in a far corner of his mind. If he was going to get through this, he had to stay up, focus on the positive. "I just need to get through rehab, and then I'll be good," he said.

Late in the afternoon, a nurse wheeled him to the operating room. Tammy held his hand, told him she loved him, then let go. She turned and walked away. Once she was out of Tom's sight, she let herself wipe away a tear.

The anesthesiologist poked an epidural catheter into his spine. For years, Tom had advised pregnant patients not to fear the epidural. "It's just a little sting, like having blood drawn," he told them. But he never knew for sure. Now, as he nodded out, his last thought was this: I'm happy I was telling them the truth . . .

It took 22 minutes to lose the lower leg. Working behind a plastic face shield, Dr. Hahn used a scalpel to peel away muscle and tissue, exposing Tom's tibia (shinbone) and fibula, the beam-and-stud of the lower leg. The bones were small and thin, like the remnants of an order of pork ribs. A nurse handed Dr. Hahn a small reciprocating power saw, the kind of thing you'd use for small jobs around the house. Zip—tibia gone. Zip—fibula gone. Or rather, almost gone. In a maneuver known as an Ertl procedure, Dr. Hahn used a leftover bit of the fibula to form a bridge between the two bones, locking them in place with screws. The bridge would allow Tom to put more weight on the residual limb below the knee. With the bones secured, the surgeon clamped off Tom's blood vessels with tiny metal clips, then used flaps of skin hanging below the bone bridge to wrap the stump. (*Residual limb* is the medical term; *stump* is the word many amputees use.) Dr. Hahn sewed the works closed with surgical thread.

Then it was over. A nurse dressed the stump in bandages and wheeled Tom to a recovery room to let the anesthesia wear off.

THE NEXT MORNING, TOM SAT UP and stared at a spot 10 inches below his bandaged stump. "Phantom pain is real," he told Tammy. "It feels like my left heel is sitting on the bed, like someone is pressing down on it. And there's a slight pain in my arch." There was, of course, no heel, no arch. Ninety percent of recent amputees get phantom sensations (not always pain) that are triggered by brain neurons wired to receive signals from nerves in the amputated limb. Over time those neurons reprogram themselves to respond to adjacent body regions, and the sensations subside.

A nurse overheard him and stopped by. She had experience with fresh amputees. "That's nothing," she said. "Wait till your toes start itching."

Tom was in an ebullient mood, helped along by drugs that kept both his legs numb. Friends and family kept the phone jangling. "Listen dude, I just dropped five pounds in surgery, and I'm back at my college weight," Tom told one caller. "I'm going to be kicking your butt soon enough." He hung up. "That was Tim Terrill," he said. "He's an old Vigilante. They put an item about my amputation up on the green line, and now all the old runners are calling me."

The green line was an e-mail list connecting alumni of the cross-country team at Adams State College, a small liberal arts school in Alamosa, Colorado, about 50 miles north of the New Mexico border. They called themselves Vigilantes (the *g* is pronounced like an *h*) after their legendary coach Joe Vigil. Vigil is to cross-country running what John Wooden is to basketball. During his stint at Adams State, from 1965 to 1993, Vigil's teams won 15 national titles. He produced 425 All-Americans and 89 individual champions in various running disciplines. Since then, he has coached Deena Kastor, Meb Keflezighi, and other elites.

News of Tom's amputation set the green line abuzz. Of course, over the years Vigil had produced runners who were faster than the Buena Vista doctor, but none more beloved. The tales told about White were passed down from generation to generation at Adams State, part of a storied program's cultural lore. They were tales of promise and misfortune, courage and fortitude. They were stories of the time he lost his left leg—the first time.

As a teenager, Tom ran along lonely ribbons of road outside Albuquerque. A poster of Steve Prefontaine hung on his bedroom wall. He was the only white kid on his high school cross-country team. "We were half Navajo, half Hispanic, and me," he once recalled. The legacy of that team lives on in his hard-to-place accent. When he speaks, what escapes his throat is the ghost of a studious white boy navigating between the barrio and the rez.

Coach Vigil recruited him after Tom won the New Mexico cross-country state championship in 1977. Despite Adams State's small size and remote location, Vigil built a powerhouse program by combining effective motivational techniques—the man has world-class charm and magnetism—with cutting-edge scientific training methods. "We ran a bold style," said Tom. "We went out hard, got to the front, and stayed there. And if another team had a strong runner, Coach Vigil would specifically assign a couple of our guys to key on him. Didn't matter where they finished in the race; they just had to beat their man."

His first year at Adams State, the team finished third at the NAIA national championships. Tom took fifth in the individual race. The next two years, Tom and his squad claimed the team title. By the spring of his junior year, Tom had run a 4:02 mile and looked to vie for the individual title in the national cross-country championships the next fall.

Then came the accident. The summer before his senior season, Tom and two teammates, Randy Cooper and Pat Porter, found work as beekeepers in Rifle, Colorado, about 180 miles west of Denver. They lived in a tree house to save money. Porter would go on to dominate the U.S. cross-country scene in the 1980s, competing in two Olympics and posting a record eight straight national titles, but at that point he and Cooper and Tom were just three college kids trying to raise cash for tuition.

One night when Tom was making his way back to the tree house from Rifle, a drunk driver in a pickup swerved in front of Tom, who was riding a motorcycle. The truck's bumper caught Tom's left foot and tore it almost completely off his leg. He went down, skidded on the road, and came to a stop on his back. He lifted his left leg and watched his foot droop like a grotesque flag. All that kept it attached were his Achilles tendon and a flap of skin.

Thinking quickly, Tom applied his own tourniquet and then asked a passerby to compress a pressure point in his groin area, which prevented him from bleeding to death. A helicopter flew him to St. Mary's Hospital in Grand Junction, Colorado. When a doctor there saw him, Tom, still conscious, begged him not to amputate. "Doc, I'm a runner!" he said. "Save my foot. Please save my foot!"

As it happened, Dr. Richard Janson had just arrived at St. Mary's. Only two weeks before White's accident, Dr. Janson and a nurse wrote the hospital's first protocols for transporting amputated extremities. By coincidence, that nurse was on the chopper that flew Tom to St. Mary's. Dr. Janson hadn't been on call that day, but staffers called him anyway to see if he could help.

Dr. Janson reattached Tom's foot, but he didn't have enough skin to work with. After a temporary graft was performed by Dr. Janson five days later, White was flown to an Albuquerque hospital for a far more complex—and torturous—graft. Surgeons there peeled a patch from Tom's thigh and grafted it onto his lower leg. The skin wasn't just lifted and planted like a piece of sod. White's legs were pinned in a way that forced him to sit completely still for three weeks with his left leg bent cross-legged so it met his right thigh. Skin from the thigh was peeled back slowly, like the lid of a sardine tin, and grafted bit by bit to the left leg—while the skin was still attached to the right thigh. "You could tell he was in pain," recalled Vigil, who visited White often in the hospital. "His leg had atrophied to just skin and bones."

Though Dr. Janson saved Tom's foot, his racing days were over. He joined Vigil's staff as an assistant to finish his senior year, but all the rehab in the world couldn't bring back a 4:02 mile. For two years he lived on crutches. When he finally set them down and walked again, the crutches bowed like wishbones.

For seven years, there was no running. Then Tom met Tammy. They fell in love and married. Tom went to the University of California–Davis for med school. There in Davis, Tammy joined a running club called the Buffalo Chips. She'd leave on Saturday mornings and return with tales of runs through redwood groves, up the crest of the Sierra, or down to the Pacific. Tom felt like a hungry man hearing his wife describe a banquet.

He felt himself jonesing for a run. One day after watching Tammy finish a half-marathon, Tom acted on the impulse.

"Tammy, let's run to the car!" he said.

"What?"

"I want to run to the car!"

They ran to the car. "You couldn't really call it running," she later recalled. "It was a sorry sight. He looked like Quasimodo."

The next morning, Tom began teaching himself to run again. He made his way in a sort of stumble-hop around the block. The next morning he did a block and a half. Then two blocks. "It was ugly, but every day I went a little farther," he said. It took him a while to figure out how to adapt his gait. But eventually he started joining Tammy on her runs. His pronation was so extreme that he destroyed a new pair of running shoes every couple of months, until finally he found a custom shoemaker who designed an angled sole built to withstand his distinct pounding.

He started to enter races but encountered a unique problem. His limp was so pronounced that race officials would jump onto the course and pull him off. They thought he'd broken his leg. "Hey!" he'd shout. "I'm not done yet!"

The pain never went away. Every step hurt. But Tom trained himself to ignore it, to make it white noise. He built up his distance. One year he ran a marathon. Then a 50-K. He posted a 3:45 in the London Marathon. He tried the Leadville Trail 100 five times. He ran 50 miles several years, once making it to mile 72.

The race that made White a legend at Adams State wasn't a 100-miler, though. Every year a group of alumni return to Alamosa to challenge the current team in a five-mile race. It's not a typical, take-it-easy-on-the-old-guys match. Though the Grizzlies are perennial national championship contenders, the alums often include Olympic-caliber talent. In 1991, 10 years after Tom's motorcycle accident, Tammy called up Joe Vigil. "Coach," she said, "don't tell anyone, but Tom's coming to run the alumni meet." Pat Porter won the race, but Tom White won the day. "He hobbled through the entire five miles," recalled Vigil. "People were lined up and down the last mile just to watch Tommy finish the race. Everybody was cheering like crazy and crying."

Context is everything. When doctors warned him about the tough rehab and psychological adjustments he'd face after amputation, White just smiled. "Usually an amputation is a trauma," he said. "But I went through that trauma 26 years ago."

He was more concerned with the difficulties his daughters might face in seeing a stump-legged father. "For children, a missing limb is the most traumatic thing," he said. "You can't see diabetes or a heart attack, but this you can see. It's a jarring sight."

But when Whitney and Jasmine visited him the day after surgery, they seemed more spooked by the strangers in the hospital room than by their dad's missing limb.

"My operation went real well," said Tom. "I don't hurt at all."

"Yay!" said Whitney.

"What did they do with the other part?" Jasmine asked.

"I told 'em to just get rid of it," Tom said. "I'm done with it."

The girls were also there a few days later when Dr. Hahn arrived to unveil his handiwork. "Okay, girls, you know, it might look a little different, but it's really okay," Tom said. When Dr. Hahn removed the cast, he revealed what looked like a rounded slab of bacon—a stump marbled white and red with skin and blood. Dr. Hahn liked what he saw. When he left the room, Whitney and Jasmine brought out a treat they'd saved for their father: gingerbread-man cookies. The girls bit the left legs off their cookies and held them up. "Daddy cookies!" they said.

WHEN A LIMB IS SEVERED FROM THE BODY, the vertebrates of the world—creatures with spinal columns—face one of two fates. If they are salamanders, their bodies will grow new limbs. For everyone else, it's stumpville. Scientists are studying limb regeneration in salamanders, but until they come up with a way to transfer the amphibian's unique ability to other species, humans and others will have to be satisfied with a less-miraculous form of healing. After amputation, the sewed-up skin starts to form scar tissue to seal itself up. Broken capillaries near the amputation site leak blood and serum into surrounding tissue, causing the leg to swell. And in Tom's case, the ends of the tibia and fibula would begin to grow new bone tissue that connected to the Ertl bridge, turning the saw-and-screw job into an organic structure.

For that biological process to happen, though, Tom White had to do one thing: rest. That was tough.

"I'm planning to head back to work on Tuesday," he told Dr. Hahn a few days after surgery. "I'll start slow, just a half day."

Dr. Hahn's eyes narrowed. He urged Tom to rest. "You know how easily a half day can turn into a full day," the surgeon said.

Back in Buena Vista, Tom quickly slipped into a routine. He worked half days at Mountain Medical, using crutches to move between exam rooms. His patients were happy to see him back. But at night, he had trouble sleeping. The phantom pain kept him up. Sometimes it was like getting hit with a charley horse. Other times his missing foot ached or burned. Sometimes it itched, or felt squeezed, or seemed like electric shocks were running through it. "One time I felt my left toes dragging on the floor, clear as day," he said. "I felt them move."

Tammy worried about Tom's schedule. "You're working too much," she told him.

He brushed her off. "Ahh, you don't know what you're talking about." He was a doctor. He could read his body's signals. Everything was a go. Tom felt so good, he made a pact with Andrew Miller, a bike-racing friend. They'd do the Leadville Trail 100 Race Across the Sky, a 100-mile mountain-bike race, later that summer. It seemed like a reasonable goal.

One month after the amputation, though, Dr. Hahn told White to knock it off. "You're working too much," he said, and it was affecting the recovery. Before Tom could get fitted for a prosthetic leg, the swelling in his stump had to subside. That wouldn't happen until he stopped hopping around the clinic every day.

So Tom cut back to three half-days a week. After lunch he'd come home and catch up on paperwork, or sit in a recliner and page through a prosthetics catalog, daydreaming about his shiny new leg. Through the living-room window he saw the snow pile up, and guiltily watched his wife deal with it. Tammy hated clearing snow. That was usually Tom's job. And, of course, this winter had to be the one with record dumps. "You stay in that chair and rest, mister," Tammy told him. "The faster you recover and get your new leg, the sooner you can get out there and shovel."

ON A FREEZING JANUARY MORNING, two months after the amputation, White crutched his way into the clinic of Denver prosthetist Christopher Jones. It was time for his first leg fitting, and Tom was psyched. He wore running shorts and a Vigilantes T-shirt. He didn't really think he was going to tear into a 10-K that afternoon, but if it happened, he was damn sure going to be ready.

A prosthetist acts as a kind of pharmacist and physical therapist for amputees, designing and fabricating the right artificial limb, and then helping train patients to use the device. Jones was one of the best. His most famous patient, Capt. David Rozelle, has become a powerful symbol of the Iraq War amputee. In 2003, Rozelle lost his right foot and lower leg to an antitank mine. Working with Jones, Rozelle got himself back up and running within months. Less than two years after his injury, Rozelle returned to active duty in Iraq, becoming the first amputee in recent military history to resume command in a combat zone.

Tom unwrapped his residual limb. "Looks like it's healed well," Jones said.

"Yeah, the swelling's gone and now it's atrophied," Tom said. "My left thigh is half the size of my right."

Jones wrapped the stump with a silicone liner, then layered wet, plastered bandages on it to form a cast. From the cast, Jones would be able to make a socket for the prosthetic leg.

While the model hardened, Tom and Tammy wandered around Jones's office, which is part clinic, part woodworking shop, part museum. Today's new prostheses are high-tech wonders (with fancy price tags, between $15,000 and $35,000), but when it comes to the socket that binds them to the stump, there's old-fashioned drilling, grinding, filing, and sandpapering involved.

"Tom, did you see this?" Tammy said. She pointed to Jones's collection of antique prosthetic legs. They progressed from a wooden hand-whittled job worn by a Civil War veteran, through World War I models, 1950s-era legs, to today's cutting edge: the C-leg, a prosthesis for above-the-knee amputees that uses computer-controlled hydraulics to mimic the actions of a biological knee.

Until recently, prosthetics was largely a mom-and-pop industry. Innovations usually came from amputees who were so frustrated with old equipment that they went into their garage and created something better. But in the past 20 years, prosthetics has become a booming business. It's not because of war wounds. Too many Americans are fat, out of shape, and smoking—and it's costing them their limbs. About 3,500 amputations are performed in the United States every week. A little more than half result from vascular disease (usually caused by diabetes or smoking). Trauma and cancer account for 46 percent of amputations. The population of U.S. veterans of Iraq and Afghanistan requiring amputations makes up a small fraction of the nation's estimated 1.7 million amputees. Analysts say the market for prosthetic legs has been growing about four percent annually, and industry officials expect Americans' unhealthy lifestyles to double the amputee population by 2050. "It's the baby boom generation," says Jones. "As they age, vascular disease, diabetes, and smoking will lead to limb loss."

It's not just a demographic game, though. The increased visibility of Iraq War amputees has helped normalize the use of prostheses, and marketing has played a role. For nearly a century, the German company Otto Bock, founded to serve World War I amputees, dominated the market. Bock was a staid, established institution with little competition. Then in the late 1990s Ossur, an Icelandic upstart, began buying the mom-and-pop shops (including the company that made the Cheetah) and ginned up an aggressive marketing campaign. The company sponsored athletes like Oscar Pistorius, Sarah Reinertsen, Brian Frasure, and Casey Tibbs on "Team Ossur," picturing them in ads as bold risk-takers who embodied Ossur's motto, "Life without limitations." Ossur wanted to make prosthetics cool—and it did. Today's prosthetics industry is highly competitive, but it's still dominated by two players, with Ossur playing Pepsi to Otto Bock's Coke.

"Let's give this a try," said Jones. He appeared from a back room holding Tom's new foot, an Ossur carbon-fiber model called the Talux. Attaching the hardware to the limb has always been tricky with prostheses. Thirty years ago, an artificial leg was strapped on with buckles; today's designs use a ratcheting coupling, suspension sleeves, and various suction systems. Jones rolled a silicone-based sleeve, with a nonskid surface that felt like neoprene, over Tom's stump. Jones handed Tom the prosthesis. "Okay, now slowly fit yourself into the socket," Jones said.

Tom pushed his leg into the Talux. For the first time in months, he looked nervous.

"You hear that click?" said Jones. "That means you're connected. But you can get it tighter. If you can get to five or six clicks, you're solid. That's what you want."

Tom pushed harder. Four, five clicks. "That's it," Tom said.

"Take a few steps," said Jones.

Steps? Tom thought. Heck, it's amazing to just stand up. Instantly, he gained an inch of height. All those years of limping had induced a stoop. The new leg gave him perfect posture. For the first time in his life, he stood and looked at his wife eye to eye.

Tammy stepped back to give him space to move. Tom took three tentative steps across the room, turned, and walked back. His face drew into a rictus of concern and fear. This isn't exactly the glove of comfort, he thought. It was all wrong. He didn't feel like marathoner Sarah Reinertsen. He didn't feel like sprinter Oscar Pistorius. He felt like a man with a clunky hunk of metal on his leg. A hunk of metal that pinched and hurt. His head was aboil with misgiving. Uh-oh, he thought. This may not go as planned.

"Everything's going to feel heavy at first," Jones said. "Remember, you've been moving around for two months without any weight on that leg, and it used to have a five-pound foot attached to it." This prosthesis, a sort of training leg, weighed two and a half pounds. His final leg would weigh a little bit less.

"Yeah," Tom said. "Okay." He tried to put on a good face. He couldn't. His expression was that of a man whose doctor just told him he had cancer. "Let's adjust it, and I'll walk a little more."

Tom described where it pinched. Jones took the foot into his shop, where he used a router to grind away the socket. "Yeah, that's a little better," Tom said as he ambled, slowly, down the hall. Still, it wasn't great. He expected it to feel like his stump was hitting a cushy sofa. Instead he got a wooden chair.

For the better part of an hour, he worked with Tammy and the prosthetist, breaking down the mechanics of his new gait. He had to figure out the right hip motion and stride length. He had to learn how to strike the ground with his new carbon-fiber heel, roll and flex and push off without ankle muscles and tendons there to do the pushing. He had to find optimal mechanical efficiency in his gait, and he had to find it now. Any bad habits formed this early would be hard to break, and a slight flaw in his mechanics would waste huge amounts of energy. Researchers have found that below-the-knee amputees like Tom White require 20 to 25 percent more energy than nonamputees just to walk around. (Above-the-knee amputees use up to 60 percent more.) As a distance runner, Tom was used to training his body to move with exquisite efficiency, to think like a machine that turned calories into endurance and speed. Now he had to apply such thinking to every moment of his waking life.

THE NEXT DAY, TOM AND TAMMY drove back to Buena Vista with Tom's new leg. They went straight to their daughter Whitney's elementary school, where the teacher was expecting them. Whitney gave Tom a big hug, and the kids buzzed around his new leg. They made him take it off, put it on, take it off again. They passed it around, felt it, banged it on a desk, tried it on themselves.

"Is it made of titanium?" one boy asked.

"Yes," Tom said proudly. "Yes, it is."

By the end of the school day, word had spread through the playground grapevine. Whitney's dad had a robot leg. It wasn't weird or scary. It was cool.

He couldn't wear it all the time at first. He walked on the new leg in the mornings, then took it off in the afternoon and got around on crutches. His stump was sensitive, and putting pressure on it made it ache and swell a little. Every few days he'd call and check in with his old coach, Joe Vigil. They'd talk about life and running, coaching techniques, and Tom's progress.

"I had knee replacement, Tom, and I can tell you this: It's really going to affect your gait," Vigil told him.

"I know, Coach," Tom said. "It's like I'm learning to walk for the third time in my life. First as a baby, then after the accident, and now this. I'm going to get it right this time."

That was easier said than done. He worked at it, on his own and with Tammy. Had to perfect his leg swing. Get his hips balanced. Sometimes he'd walk past a store window on Main Street and watch what his right leg was doing, and then mimic the motion with his left. Tammy gave him feedback, but sometimes she bit her tongue. "It's great to live with a physical therapist," Tom said, laughing, "but sometimes it's hard, too. They're always watching how you walk, and the professional in them wants to correct it."

For three months he worked on getting used to the leg. It was never easy. Sometimes the prosthesis pinched or his stump ached. One day at work, he had to take off the leg and use crutches. While standing in the hall between an elderly couple using walkers, looking at himself on crutches, he thought, Oh my God. I'm in the lunch line at the nursing home. Back in November, he'd set a goal. He wanted to be running on his prosthetic leg six months after surgery. Now that looked like a pipe dream. He couldn't imagine the carbon-fiber contraption ever feeling like a natural part of his body. "I don't see how I'm ever going to run on this," he told Tammy. The idea of riding the Leadville 100 seemed ludicrous. He had to call up his friend Andrew and back out of the race.

In the midst of his discouragement, he talked to Amy Palmiero-Winters. She knew what Tom was going through. Eleven years earlier, at age 24, she lost her lower left leg due to injuries she suffered in a motorcycle accident that had occurred three years earlier. Now, at 35, she lived the life of an elite athlete. PowerBar featured her in magazine ads. She had nearly broken three hours in the marathon on a prosthetic leg. Tom wanted to know if she was doing all that while suffering as much as he was. Maybe he just had to suck it up and get used to the pain.

"Amy, is your leg uncomfortable?" he asked. "Does it hurt at all?"

"No," she said. "It's comfortable. I wear it all day long."

"How long was it before it started to feel comfortable?"

Palmiero-Winters couldn't remember. Tom took that as a good sign. "At least it wasn't a horrible period that was burned into her memory," he said. She passed on a few tricks: Detach the leg when you're sitting down to take a little pressure off. Don't bend your knee all the way or the socket puts pressure behind your knee.

Not long after that, he achieved a tiny bit of success. Christopher Jones cast a new socket for him. Tom's muscles had atrophied so much that the old one made his stump feel like a clapper in a bell. Then one day a stranger stopped him in a hallway. "Are you an amputee?" the man asked. Yes, said Tom, who was wearing pants. "I saw you earlier today, and I didn't even notice," said the stranger.

Yes! thought Tom. Finally he was walking well enough to fool somebody.

DESPITE THE INCREASED VISIBILITY of amputees, a certain amount of social stigma still comes with the territory. Even for Tom, who treated bodily deformities every day, it wasn't easy to endure the stares of strangers. Or the imagined stares. "Oh, get over it," Tammy told him. "Nobody's looking. Nobody cares." Easy for her to say, Tom thought. She wasn't the one shocking people every time she hiked up her pant leg.

Then Tom went to Boston and got schooled in the art of getting over it.

He and Tammy flew there in April for the marathon and the women's Olympic Marathon Trials. Tammy planned to run in Monday's marathon, and daughter Whitney came to compete in the Newton Heartbreak Hill International Youth Race, a kids' fun run up the course's notorious rise. For Tom, it was a running reunion. He kept bumping into Adams State friends, including Coach Vigil.

At the race expo the evening before the Olympic Trials, Tom finally met Amy Palmiero-Winters in person. Officials at USA Track & Field had told her she could run in the Olympic Trials if she posted a qualifying time, but her personal best of 3:04 came up 22 minutes short. She came to the race anyway to cheer on the hopeful Olympians.

She was walking around on her Flex-Run foot, a drink in one hand and a spare leg in the other.

"Wow, look at your leg!" Tom exclaimed.

"Have a look yourself," Palmiero-Winters said. She snapped the leg off, handed it to Tom, and stood on her remaining limb, perfectly balanced. "I give her back the leg," Tom said later in describing the scene, "and she just goes click-click and she's in. I'm cracking a sweat just putting my liner on!"

She analyzed Tom's setup like a NASCAR mechanic working over an engine. "The first thing you need to do," she told him, "is get yourself a knee brace and pull it over the socket. There's a CVS around the corner. They're probably open late. Go."

Tom smiled and mumbled something about picking up the brace in the morning.

"No," she said. "Go now."

So he did. When he pulled the brace over his knee, the contraption seemed to pull together. His walking improved at once. "Holy Toledo!" he told Tammy. "I had no idea!"

The next day, Palmiero-Winters joined Tom, Tammy, and Whitney to watch the Olympic Trials. Unlike the point-to-point Boston Marathon course, the Trials layout featured a loop that the runners lapped four times. Tom's gang found a spot where they could watch Deena Kastor, Magdalena Lewy Boulet, and other frontrunners pass by on one side of the course. Then, if they hustled, they could cross the Charles River and watch the runners pass on the other side of the loop. It was hot, sweaty work. Tom did his best to keep up, walking and jogging in a kind of gimpy hop. By the halfway point, sweat had turned his prosthetic liner into a sopping wet mess. His leg began to slip.

"You're not walking so well," observed Palmiero-Winters. "What's going on?"

"I sweat through my liner," he said. "I need to take it off and let it dry."

"Go ahead," she said.

Tom nervously eyed the crowd. Tens of thousands of people lined the course that day. "I'll wait until the crowd moves on, then I'll do it discreetly," he said. "A little bit of privacy, you know."

Tammy watched the whole thing go down. She often fought this battle with Tom and often lost. But Palmiero-Winters didn't back down. She'd been there, done that. If Tom was too shy to change his socket liner in public, at some point he would hurt himself—if not today, somewhere down the line. "Do it now," she told him.

Tom held firm. "I don't want to do it in front of all these people."

"Oh my God, just change it," she said. "Suck it up and do it!" She stood in front of him, hands on her hips, resolute. She wasn't going to let him off the hook.

"Arrgh!" Tom parked his butt on the grass and snapped off his leg. He unrolled the wet liners, let them dry, and then put them back on. Nobody in the crowd gave him a second glance. They were busy watching Kastor overtake Boulet for the lead.

At that moment, White realized that living with the leg was going to demand different kinds of courage. There was the courage to get up and walk on the thing—and eventually, maybe, run. And then there was the courage to snap it off at a party in a room full of strangers.

"Amy has this attitude like, 'Nothing wrong with me. I'm just gonna do my thing,'" he later said. "She taught me plenty of technical stuff, but nothing so important as that attitude. I don't have her command or her presence yet. But I'm working on it."

THE END OF SPRING drew closer, and with it Tom's realization that nearly six months had passed since his amputation, and he still seemed miles away from his two main goals. He hadn't yet walked Whitney to school, and he still couldn't run. His frustration mounted.

"Well, of course you're not running on that thing!" Palmiero-Winters told him in Boston. White was still walking on his training leg, which wasn't really built for the pounding of roadwork. She pointed out her custom-made model, which had a socket that flared up higher near her knee to give her much better stability. So when he got back home to Colorado, Tom met with Chris Jones and designed a new leg based on Palmiero-Winters's model.

By the middle of May, the Colorado snowpack was fast disappearing. Sandbags were stacked around Buena Vista, ready to stave off the meltwater floods. Tom checked the mail every day, and then finally it arrived—his new leg, boxed and packed in Styrofoam peanuts. He threw off his old model and started snapping on the new one. He felt some trepidation. What if this one wasn't any better? But ohh, it felt good. Stable. Snug. He walked out the door, and the new leg felt better with every step.

The next day he walked Whitney to school. The whole family went, and they walked all the way: one mile to school, one mile back. Tom and Tammy talked about the upcoming cross-country season. They'd been trying to talk a friend into coaching a sixth-grade girls' team. In the off-season Tom and Tammy organized a fitness and running club for elementary school kids, the Speed Demons, and recently Tom had begun coaching some local masters runners who met at the high school track Wednesday mornings at 5 a.m. The Whites were doing in Buena Vista what Joe Vigil had done at Adams State: building a running culture from the ground up. "Start them early, get them excited about it," Tom said. "The main thing is to get them out there doing some physical activity they enjoy." As a doctor, the toughest patients for Tom, emotionally, were those with heart disease, diabetes, obesity, or other ailments that stemmed from inactivity. "That's part of the reason I'm doing this," he said. "So I can say to my patients, 'Hey look at me, I've only got one good leg and I'm out there running, biking, staying active. You can do this.'"

"How's your leg feel?" Tammy asked on the way back home.

"Good," Tom said. "Like a combination stilt and pogo stick. It feels like I'm mastering a new sport. I have good steps and bad steps."

That Saturday, he tried something new. In between his daughters' soccer games, he snuck off to a quiet corner of the park, and he ran. Just for two minutes. But it wasn't walking. And it didn't hurt. And he couldn't keep the words from racing through his head: I can run!

He kept on running. He started at two minutes and added 30 seconds every day. "I'm realizing I need to get my ultrarunner's step back," he said. "It's kind of a slow shuffling gait, no high knees, stay low, conserve energy while moving forward." After several months of struggle, the path ahead was beginning to open up. Somewhere in the future he could see himself doing 10-Ks with his daughters, maybe even running a marathon with Tammy.

He smiled. "I feel like my third running life is just getting started."

THE MAJOR ADVANCES IN prosthetics have almost always been made by amputees themselves. Van Phillips, the engineer who created the Flex-Foot, lost his lower left leg in a waterskiing accident at age 21. Hugh Herr, director of bio-mechatronics at MIT's Media Lab, is pushing prosthetics into the bionics age with joints that use microprocessors, integrated sensors, and advanced actuators to mimic natural motion. He lost both legs below the knee at age 17 after being trapped in a blizzard on Mount Washington.

There's a reason for this: it's almost impossible to know how a prosthesis works—or doesn't work—until you wear one yourself. As a doctor, Tom looked to medical professionals for advice in the early months of his recovery. After a while, he discovered that the best information often came from the amputee grapevine. Amy Palmiero-Winters showed him how to brace his knee. A technician in Chris Jones's practice, an amputee himself, gave Tom crucial advice on cleaning his liner and minimizing sweat. ("Roll a little antiperspirant on your stump," the guy said—and he was right.) At a marathon in San Diego, Tom spent an hour talking with Sarah Reinertsen. She told him to give himself a break. "You've only been on your leg for a few months," she said. "It takes about a year before you really realize what you can do."

By mid-June, Tom was running for 14 minutes at a stretch. Then, almost overnight, his stump lost a huge amount of sensitivity—as if his nerves had been set to volume 8, then turned down to 3. The hard wooden chair wasn't so hard anymore.

When Tom, Tammy, and the girls flew to France at the end of that month, Tom kept a secret notion in the back of his head. They were going over to watch

Tammy run in the Marathon du Mont-Blanc, a spectacular race held in the streets of Chamonix and the foothills of the French Alps. When they arrived, Tom signed up for a 10-K held the day before the marathon. "I'll take it easy, see how far I can get," he told Tammy. "Run a kilometer, then walk, run, walk. See how it goes."

At the starting line, his leg caused no commotion at all. The other runners were preoccupied with their own prerace rituals. Anxiety crept into Tom's head just before the gun went off. Man, maybe I should have signed up for the 5-K, he thought.

A 12-minute-mile pace put him at the back of the pack. At 2 kilometers, he felt good. Maybe he'd stop at 5 kilometers and take a rest. But then things started humming. He picked up the pace. Passed a few people. Then a few more. The course turned onto a hiking path and snaked into the hills. That worked to his advantage—Tom could really crank on the leg when he motored uphill. At the 5-kilometer water stop, he didn't pause. Just kept on running.

By 7 kilometers, sweat was soaking his liner. He could feel his stump sloshing. The voice of Amy Palmiero-Winters came into his head. *Do it now.* White stopped, snapped off his leg, wrung the sweat out of the liner, rolled it back on, and snapped on his leg. Right there in front of God and the Alps and the nation of France.

He continued on. His ears became his coach. When he tired, his footfall made a sliding sound. Since he couldn't feel his foot strike the ground, Tom had to listen for the sound. For the last three kilometers, he concentrated on making good strikes, good sounds. And that's when he felt it—a little bit of that old rhythm. When he was a kid, before the motorcycle accident, the rhythm of running was his biological clock. Back in those days, if he ran long enough, with the proper mindset and respect, he could slip into the rhythm and transform his body's movement into a mystical experience. It was like a scent from childhood, a sense-memory of which he caught just a trace up there among the edelweiss. That's what he missed the most, all those years. That's what he gave his left leg to get back again.

And then the finish was upon him. Tammy, Whitney, and Jasmine screamed his name. The girls dashed onto the course and ran the final 50 yards alongside him.

He hugged the girls and felt them crinkle his race bib. Around him, runners caught their breath and checked their times. Tammy offered a smile. He savored the world opening up around him and the feeling, once again, of being whole.

A MOMENT OF SILENCE

BY STEVE FRIEDMAN

[
At 4:15 most mornings, John Moylan knew exactly where he'd be—
on a run, doing the roadwork that would get him through
the day ahead. Then came 9/11, and suddenly his routine stopped.
Reviving it would become his toughest battle.
]

SEPTEMBER 2006

HE WILL WAKE AT 4 A.M., as he does every weekday except Monday. He'll wear shorts and a T-shirt, even in the rain, unless it's winter, when he might pull on a Gore-Tex jacket and pants. When it snows and the snow is heavy enough, he'll stretch thin rubber sandals with metal spikes over his running shoes. He'll grab a small canister of pepper spray. Three seasons out of the year, he'll lace up one of his six pairs of "active" size 13 Sauconys that he keeps in a closet underneath his 100 hanging T-shirts, and in the winter he'll wear one of his half dozen pairs of active Nikes from the same closet, because the layer of air in them doesn't seem to compress in cold weather as much as the foam in the Sauconys. He'll be out his front door at 4:15, back inside at 5:05. Then he'll shower, eat a bowl of instant oatmeal, make himself a lunch of a peanut-butter-and-jelly sandwich or pack a cup of yogurt, and leave his house in Warwick, New York, at 6:10 to drive to the train station in Harriman for the 6:42 train to Hoboken, New Jersey. The trip will take a little over an hour, and in Hoboken he'll board a 7:55 underground train bound for Manhattan. Once there, he'll walk 15 minutes to his office at an insurance company at Madison Avenue and 36th Street.

John Moylan is a man of habit and routine and caution, and for much of his life attention to detail has served him well. Some mornings, when he's feeling adventurous or wild, he'll make a little extra noise between 4 a.m. and 4:15 a.m., just to see if his wife of 30 years, Holly, will wake up. She hasn't yet.

His running route starts outside his front door and it hasn't varied for six years, since he and Holly and their two daughters moved from Crystal Lake, Illinois, when his then employer, Kemper Insurance, transferred him to New York City. Down Kings Highway, through the small village, up a small hill, and by the time he passes the Mobil gasoline station at the end of the first mile, he'll know if the run will be easy or hard, and if it's hard, he'll remind himself to eat healthier that day, to make sure to get to sleep by 9 p.m. At one and a half miles, he might pass a gaggle of geese that like to waddle near the black granite memorial to the seven people from Warwick who died on September 11, 2001. He'll run past one dairy farm and its herd of cows, and he'll make mooing sounds and wonder why they never moo back. Later, he'll pass another dairy farm and moo at those cows, who always moo back. One of life's mysteries. He'll run past what's really no more than a giant puddle next to the road that he thinks of as the turtle pond, because he once saw a turtle waddling across the concrete toward the water. He'll run four to five miles, 10 or 12 on Saturday, and on Sunday anywhere from 10 to 16. Mondays, he rests.

Moylan is by nature conservative, by profession cautious. He has been in the insurance business for 33 years and has spent much of his life calculating risk, calibrating the costs of bad planning and devastating whim. Men who worry about the future can guard against the worst sorts of accidents. Men who look ahead can avoid life's greatest dangers. Even when running, even during the time of his life that is devoted to release and escape from daily tallies and concerns, he can't quite escape the principles that have guided him for so long.

"What do I think about?" he says. "God, just about everything. Am I on target for my marathon goal? How am I going to pay my daughters' college tuition? Do I have good retirement plans?"

Some days—one of life's mysteries—he thinks of that terrible morning in 2001.

THE SIMPLE THINGS

HE AND ONE OF HIS COWORKERS, Jill Steidel, had just arrived at their office on the 36th floor of the north tower at the World Trade Center in downtown Manhattan. They were carrying coffee they had picked up from the Starbucks in the building's atrium. He had his usual—a grande-size cup of the breakfast blend, black. It was 8:46 a.m., and Moylan was standing at his window, looking west, gazing at the ferries on the Hudson River. It was one of his great pleasures, what he called "one of the simple things in life." That's when he felt the building shake and heard a loud

81

thwaaang. He had heard longtime employees talk about the 1993 bombing in the building's parking garage, and now he thought the building might be collapsing as a result of residual structural damage. Then he heard screaming. He was one of the fire marshals on his floor, so he rounded up his employees—there were about 25 of them—and herded them to the stairs. A longtime runner, he reflexively checked his watch as the group entered the stairwell. It was 8:48 a.m.

The stairwell was packed, but orderly. He remembers two "nice, neat rows" of people, scared but polite. He remembers many breathing hard and sweating, wide-eyed. He remembers thinking that his experience as a runner helped him stay calm. "What was it?" someone asked. "It wasn't a bomb," someone else said.

The people in front of his group would sometimes stop suddenly, which made his group stop. That didn't make sense. Neither did the smell. Moylan had been in the Air Force as a young man, and it was a familiar odor. "I thought, What the hell is jet fuel doing here?"

It took 28 minutes to get to the ground floor. Moylan left the building at 9:16 a.m. He turned to his right and looked east, just as two bodies hit the ground. He saw other bodies on the ground, realized that's why firefighters had kept people from exiting the doors in a constant flow. He saw greasy puddles of blazing jet fuel, huge chunks of twisted metal. He saw more bodies falling. (It's estimated that of the more than 2,500 people who died in the twin towers, 200 had jumped.)

He and the others were marshaled to the overpass that stretched over the West Side Highway and to the marina next to the Hudson River. At the marina, he looked back. People on the higher floors were waving pieces of clothing and curtains from the windows. There were helicopters—he thought there were eight or 10—circling. He could see that the helicopters couldn't get through the fire and smoke, and he knew that the people in the windows could see it, too. He was used to synthesizing facts quickly, and it didn't take long to comprehend the horrible calculus confronting the people in the windows: be burned alive or jump. He wondered what he would have done.

Thousands of people were on the marina. Some stared upwards. Others walked north, toward Midtown. The Kemper employees for whom Moylan was responsible had all gotten out safely; now Moylan needed to get home. The subway was shut down, as was the underground train to New Jersey, so he boarded a ferry to Hoboken. When he got to Hoboken, at 9:59, he looked back, and as he did so, the south tower, which had been hit at 9:02 a.m., crumbled. The north tower, his tower, would fall at 10:28 a.m.

In Hoboken he boarded a train for home, but first he tried to call Holly and his daughters, Meredith and Erin. He had left his cell phone in his office, so he borrowed one, but it wasn't working. Neither, he remembers, were the landlines.

He remembers the hour-long train ride to Harriman, and from there the drive to Warwick. He remembers with absolute clarity walking through his door at 4 p.m., covered in soot, smelling of fire and death. Five years later, the memory still troubles him.

"The home office had called, looking for me, which just scared my wife even more. My suit was ruined. I was reeking. I scared the living daylights out of them. My daughters especially were emotionally ruined, or disturbed.... When your family thinks you're dead and you walk in your house and surprise them ..."

He stayed up all night, watching television. In the morning, he knew what he had to do. He rose from the bed where he had failed to sleep. "I wanted desperately to go out running," he says. He just couldn't get his shoes on.

Accidents Happen

MOYLAN KNOWS BETTER than most men how accidents can shape a life. He had been working in the East Norwich, Long Island, post office in the summer of 1970 when he learned he had drawn the 11th spot in one of this country's last drafts. He had always thought about how neat it would be to fly planes, so he enrolled in the U.S. Air Force. And that's how he got to Iceland.

There he was, in the summer of 1971, a cop's son from East Norwich, playing softball at midnight, soaking afterward in thermal hot springs, gorging on fresh salmon, drinking beer with pretty girls who spoke another language. Forget planning. He couldn't have dreamed that summer—"one of the best years of my life." Pure chance. Then another one of life's mysteries. Late one night, in April of 1972, there was a knock on his barracks' door. It was the chaplain. Moylan's father had died; he was only 46. After the funeral, Moylan asked his mother how she was going to hold onto the house. She told him not to worry, but he pressed. Did she need his help?

The Air Force gave him an honorable hardship discharge, and he went back to the post office. He might still be there if his mother hadn't insisted that he go talk to one of the leaders of the church she attended. He was an insurance executive, and he was always looking for bright young men.

So in 1973, Moylan became a company man, a trainee for Crum & Forster, a salaried student of chance and fate. Every morning, he waited for the 7 a.m. Manhattan-bound train from the station in Syosset, Long Island, and every morning he stood in the same spot and walked through the same door and sat in the same seat. And every afternoon, he did the same thing at Pennsylvania Station, when the 5:06 eastbound train pulled in. Then one afternoon, the train stopped 20 feet short of its usual spot and people pushed and shoved and Moylan's seat was taken and he had no choice, there was only one empty seat left. He found himself sitting next to a pretty blond dress designer from Huntington. Her name was Holly.

Accidents happen, and it's one of life's mysteries the effect they'll have, and all you can do is try to control what's controllable. And that's how a young, married company man started running. It was 1979, and Moylan had gone from a lean, 180-pound military man to a 220-pound, 28-year-old, pudgy, listless suit. He needed to do something. He had read an article about Bill Rodgers, and the New York City Marathon, and he decided that running sounded like fun.

Moylan is not a man to make a big deal out of things, and he doesn't make a big deal about that decision. But two years later, in the spring of 1981, he ran the Long Island Marathon. He ran it in just under four hours. In the fall, he ran the New York City Marathon, and did even better, finishing in 3:51.

He cut out junk food, started eating lean meats. He woke early, ran before the sun rose. He experimented with equipment and distance and learned "to not let my mind get in front of my body. I learned that patience is a virtue."

He wore his running shoes when he walked from the train to his office building, and he wore them when he took his midday 45-minute walks around Manhattan. He always worried that people thought he looked funny.

By 2001, by the time he was 50, he had run 14 marathons, many half-marathons, countless 10-Ks and 5-Ks. Running helped him reduce his blood pressure from 120/90 to 110/60, helped him reduce his weight from 220 to anywhere from 180 to 195, depending on where he was in his training cycle. His resting pulse is 50 now, and when he gives blood, Red Cross officials routinely question him to make sure he's not a fainter. Running helped him cope when his mother died in 1985, at age 59, with the birth of his daughters in 1982 and 1985, with the demands of being a middle-aged father and husband and provider and company man. He ran because he didn't want to die young, as his parents had, and because it relaxed him and was part of his life. Accidents would happen, and there were some things a man couldn't do anything about, terrible things. But with discipline and attention and will, a man could carve out a safe place, a part of life that was predictable, calming in its sameness. Half an hour or so in the early morning stillness could help a man deal with almost anything.

It was a Tuesday, in 2001, the week after Labor Day, and warm for that time of year, in that part of the country. A morning like this was rare and precious. It would be a good run. It felt like it would be a good day. At the Mobil station, Moylan picked up his pace.

He ran past the cows and the geese and the turtle pond. He thought about his retirement fund, even though he had many years to go before he'd need it. He worried about his daughters' college tuition, even though he had been saving for years. He wondered if he would run as swiftly as he wanted to in the New York City Marathon, even though it was still two months away. He was back at home at 5:05 a.m., he showered and had his instant oatmeal and caught his train and met Jill Steidel at Starbucks, and they rode the elevator up to the 36th floor, and less than a minute later, he felt the building shake. And the next day, he couldn't get his running shoes on. He couldn't put them on the next day, either. He woke at four each day, got out of bed, thought about running, got his shoes out of the closet, then put them back. Then he would sit on the couch and watch television and his mind would drift. He thought about a framed photograph he had left on his office desk. Holly had taken it, and it showed Moylan and Meredith and Erin at a Yankees game in July. It was cap day, and they were all wearing Yankees caps. He doubted he could ever find the negative. Then he thought about all the people who didn't get to say goodbye to their families.

Friday, September 14, was his 26th wedding anniversary, and on that morning he got dressed and he laced up his Sauconys, and he opened up his front door. He looked outside, into the darkness. Then he closed the door and went back inside.

THE FUNNY SENSE

IT IS LATE SPRING, nearly five years later, and he is looking at the space where the World Trade Center once stood. It is the first time he has been back here. He says he's surprised that the footprints of the two towers aren't more clearly marked. He's disappointed that the twisted cross of metal that became the focus of so many Christians is no longer on the site.

He gazes into the sky.

"When I came out," he says, "it was on this level. I had a view—right in this area, the bodies were already falling. I could look up and see the people hanging out the windows. The news footage, you just saw smoke. From down here, it was like looking up from the bottom of a grill. I remember seeing how ungodly hot it was—there was an orange glow."

Moylan is a handsome man, square-jawed, gray-haired, hazel-eyed. He is 6 feet tall, a solid 190, on his way, he says, back to 180. He wears a blue suit and a pin of the Twin Towers and an American flag, and he looks like a soap-opera actor or the Air Force pilot he might have been. If this were a different place, he might appear to be just a tourist searching the New York City skyline for wonders.

He turns from the ghost buildings and looks toward the bank of the river, at the benches where he used to unpack his peanut-butter-and-jelly sandwiches or his yogurt cup. "This place was my luxury suite for lunch in the summertime.... I used to come out here on the bench and just dream."

In the weeks after the attack, Moylan studied a *New York Times* article about the sequence of events and realized that, had he taken two or three minutes longer to get his coffee with Steidel at Starbucks, he still would have been in the elevator on the way to his office when the plane hit, and he wouldn't have survived.

Moylan turns back east, away from the water. Reflection can be healing, but he has work to do. He needs to get back to his office, five miles north in Midtown. "The funny sense that I get being here," he says, "is, life goes on. It's continuing."

"I Don't Remember That"

IT IS EARLY SPRING, dusk in Orange County, New York, and Moylan and Holly and their oldest daughter, Meredith, are driving the back roads of Warwick. Holly points out a place where George Washington slept. Meredith points out a dairy farm and creamery. We drive through the gaggle of geese and past the granite memorial to the people from Warwick who died on 9/11.

At dinner, we talk about past races, about what running meant to Moylan before 9/11. Meredith talks about watching her father finish one marathon on an ocean boardwalk, yelling, "That's my Daddy and he loves me," and years later joining him in center field of San Francisco's Candlestick Park for the end of a 5-K run. Holly and Meredith talk about how they enjoy staying up watching *The Gilmore Girls* and chatting when John goes to sleep. Holly wonders aloud why her husband—or any man—needs 100 T-shirts, and Moylan speaks mournfully of the "boxes and boxes" of his T-shirts she donated to charity.

I ask Holly and Meredith how long it took for them to get over the shock of seeing Moylan walk in the door, how they dealt with the hours of uncertainty.

"I wasn't uncertain," Holly says. "When we were watching the coverage on television, I told Meredith, 'Dad will be fine. He's a runner and he'll run right out of there. Besides, he called us from Hoboken before he got on the train.'"

Moylan blinks, shakes his head.

"No, I didn't call you. I didn't have my phone."

"You definitely called us," Holly says. "You borrowed a phone and called us to let us know you were coming home."

Moylan blinks again. "I don't remember that," he says.

"Yeah, Dad," Meredith says, "you called from Hoboken. To let us know you were all right."

STORYTELLERS

HAROLD KUDLER, M.D., is an associate clinical professor of psychiatry at Duke University and a nationally recognized expert on posttraumatic stress disorder. He hears part of John Moylan's post 9/11 story and says, "It's quite common for people in the middle of an acute stress response to have dissociative phenomena."

To Dr. Kudler, Moylan's elaborate memory of his family being traumatized as a result of not hearing from him makes psychological sense. "Sometimes," Dr. Kudler says, "the effort to create meaning and to create a meaningful narrative about what has happened to you actually becomes more important than the actual memory and might replace it. This story about coming home as a ghost and having everyone else scared might be a way to say, 'Boy, was I scared. I felt like a ghost in my own life. I wasn't even sure when I got home if I had survived that.'"

Moylan's responses during and after the attacks—his vivid recollection of details, his construction of false memories, his nightmares, his long avoidance of the World Trade Center site, his difficulty running afterward—are entirely consistent with symptoms exhibited by people facing extreme trauma, even the most resilient people, according to Dr. Kudler.

"There's a tendency to medicalize or pathologize responses," Dr. Kudler says. "It might be better to think that here's someone who is faced with a new challenge that's so radically different from the one he faced a few days earlier.

"Think of it like mourning. When you're bereaved, you wouldn't be able to invest in yourself, because you'd feel overwhelmed, and you'd sort of lose your center. For a while you wouldn't be able to do the things that reminded you of who you were, of the thing you did for yourself."

And Moylan's inability to go for his normal run?

"Running for him was something he did for himself, was important to him, and he made a point of always doing this regardless of anything else. Great exercise, recreational, self-affirming. But in the context of the disaster, when people are overwhelmed and filled with doubt, it's easy to see why someone wouldn't do those self-affirming things.

"And if he was angry, that anger may have drowned out his capacity to enjoy a simple pleasure like running, and take that simple time for himself. That anger could have drowned out a lot of those normal, good impulses."

When I tell Moylan what Dr. Kudler said, he is silent for a few seconds.

"He nailed me," he says.

PERSPECTIVE

HE WOULD WAKE in the middle of the night, certain that his house was under attack. He would dream that he was up in a tower and flames were licking at him. He would dream of having to make a terrible choice but not knowing what to do. He would dream of dying, "that I went through what those people went through." Noises startled him. "He was restless and jumpy and things would frighten him," Holly says. "If we were out somewhere and a child cried out, he'd jump, he'd be scared."

During the day, he thought of the people who had died. "I couldn't rationalize what had happened. People in the normal course of living, going to work, murdered. I thought about how they never got to say goodbye to anyone. I thought about my family, and about facing a decision to burn to death or to jump."

Every morning in the weeks after 9/11, he would get up and he would plan to run. But he never made it outside. He would make coffee, and sit on the couch, and sometimes watch television, and have his oatmeal, and when it was time to take his shower and catch his train, that's what he would do.

He couldn't stop thinking about chance, and fate, and wondering why he had survived.

At his company's insistence, he had two conversations with Red Cross officials, once in a group, once alone. He talked about how angry he was that there had been an attack. He talked about how angry he was that he had survived while others had died. He talked about how angry he was that he couldn't run. "And that about covers it," he says.

He reported for work on September 13, in Kemper's New Jersey office. The company assured Moylan and his coworkers that they would be reassigned to a building in midtown Manhattan, on a lower floor. The morning they reported for work there, on the 10th floor of Rockefeller Center, was the day authorities discovered an envelope filled with anthrax addressed to Tom Brokaw in the same building. Some of the Kemper employees left and never came back. Moylan stayed.

The nightmares continued. He kept jumping at the slightest noise. But Holly didn't say anything. "We had talked about counseling," she says, "and he just said, 'Let me see how things go.'" He knew that running would help him get over all his problems. So he got up every day, ready to run. But he couldn't do it.

Then one day, he could. Just like that. One of life's mysteries.

There were no grand pronouncements before he went to bed the night before, no stirring speeches at dinner. He was still angry. He was still scared. He still thought about the falling bodies. But on Columbus Day, almost exactly a month after the attack, he managed to get his shoes on, and to get out the door.

He made it four miles, and every step was difficult. His legs were heavy. He had trouble breathing. But he made it.

His first race was a half-marathon in Pennsylvania the next April. It was a clear day, warm, "almost like September 11," he says. "I remember that for the first time in a long time, I smelled grass, could smell flowers."

A few months later, in October, at a half-marathon not far from his home, he happened to overhear one of the runners mention that he was a firefighter. Moylan approached him. "He said he wasn't there, but he knew people who were. I told him I was in tower one. We both had similar feelings . . . about losing people. It was the first time I had verification that I wasn't the only person who felt like I did."

He ran the New York City Marathon in 2002 and 2003. He ran more marathons, more half-marathons. The nightmares faded away, as did his preoccupation with death and the randomness of fate. (He still jumps at the slightest noise, something he never did before 9/11.) One day, Todd Jennings, who lived near Moylan and who had just started running, spotted Moylan on the train "in his gray flannel suit and running shoes." Eventually, they started talking. About training regimens, and race strategy, and running in general. "No," Jennings says, "we never talked about 9/11."

Moylan and Jennings traveled to the Boilermaker 15-K in Utica, New York, in 2005, and the night before the race they went out for a pasta dinner. "He told me," Jennings says, "'I want to be remembered on my tombstone as a runner. Running is who I am.'"

There are things you can't control, no matter how much you worry and plan. Terrible things happen, and there's nothing you can do to stop them. Those are lessons that will change a man. For better or for worse.

After 18 years with the company, Moylan left Kemper Insurance in 2002 to go to work for Greater New York Insurance. He doesn't worry about what others think when he wears his blue suit and white running shoes combination in Midtown anymore. He ran a 3:22 marathon in 1982 and a 4:50 marathon in 2003. He still wants to get back to a four-hour time, "but I don't worry so much about time anymore." He still thinks about retirement and paying for his daughters' education, but it doesn't eat at him quite as much as it used to. He still calculates risk and calibrates the likelihood of disaster and does his best to protect himself and his family, but he knows there are some things beyond a man's control, and to worry about them is to waste precious energy.

When he finds himself irritated or impatient, he thinks of a terrible choice he never had to make, and he is grateful. Every morning, as he steps out his door, he is grateful.

"I told my wife, I should have a new birthday," Moylan says. "My new life started on 9/11. The fact that I survived is a gift. I know quite a few people who didn't. I made a promise to myself. I was going to live differently." He tries not to dwell on the past, or to look too very far into the future. But he has made one promise to himself. "Yeah, I'm going to go back to Iceland sometime. That's a plan now."

THE HILLS BEYOND

WEEKENDS, HE TREATS HIMSELF. Friday and Saturday nights, he soaks a pot of steel-cut oats in water so he can have homemade oatmeal after his runs. On Sunday, he sleeps till 5:30, has a cup of coffee ("my luxury"), and dawdles for a full hour before he heads out the door. He'll step out of his front door just as the sun rises above Warwick. He'll pass the Mobil station and the silent cows and the mooing cows, but that day he'll go at least 15 miles, so there will be other sights, too. He'll run by the VFW hall, where the old men always wave, and the fire station in town, where the guys always have a nice word to say. He might see a deer, or a porcupine, or even a bear. At mile seven, he'll run by a house where a snarling Rottweiler is tied to a tree, and he'll grip his pepper spray a little more tightly.

Just past that house, Moylan will ascend a gentle hill, heading east, and no matter how hard the run, no matter how he slept the night before or how he's feeling, as he crests the little hill, he'll slow down. It's his favorite spot on the weekend run—his favorite spot of any of his runs. It's just a little hummock, but when a man reaches it, he can turn to the right and look south, and he can see an entire valley stretching before him, and beyond that valley, forests and hills all the way to the horizon. He will still have another seven miles to go, and then his homemade oatmeal with the apples and bananas and raisins and cinnamon he allows himself on weekends. Then on Monday he'll think again about the day that changed his life, and on the day after that he'll catch the 6:42 train to Hoboken, and on the day after that he'll do it again. Or not. Who can really predict what will happen to a man, even a careful man, a man who takes precautions? That's another of life's mysteries.

Moylan will allow himself to walk a little bit on Sunday at the top of the gentle rise, to linger, to look at the valley and the forests and the looming hills beyond. He loves this spot.

"It's a nice place to get perspective," he says.

LEGENDS

A WICKED
GOOD LIFE

BY KENNY MOORE

[
*She's gone from small-town champion to Olympic
pioneer to single-named icon. But she
never sought fame or influence. Joan Benoit Samuelson
wanted something more precious—and has
spent the past two decades protecting it.*
]

JANUARY 2008

JOAN BENOIT was the first woman to run away from me. It was late in a
10-mile run through wet oak woods, two days before the 1983 World Cross-
Country Championships in Gateshead, England. I was 39, twice
an Olympic marathoner, in 2:20-marathon shape, and knew how to use it all.
Up a hill, she edged five yards ahead. I used it all. She had me by 15 yards at the
top. Down the other side she eased. I caught up. I did not share with her the full
significance of the moment. I remember a stab of dread at its implications. Only
one was positive. This 25-year-old woman with the dry wit and unshakable
rhythm was overdue.

One summer evening, as we talked over dinner at her seaside home in Maine,
she said, "I remember that run. It meant I'd be strong in Boston the next month."

Strong she was, and on April 18 she unleashed her full force over the Boston
Marathon course. It carried her through breakneck splits of 51:38 for 10 miles (a
5:09.8-per-mile pace) and 1:08:22 at the halfway point (a 2:16:44 marathon pace).
With those times she had to flag, and she did, suffering through the last six
miles at 5:47 pace. Even so, she finished in 2:22:43, two minutes and 46 seconds
faster than any woman had run a marathon before—faster than the world
record held by Grete Waitz of Norway. Suddenly my pride was a lot less
wounded.

The performance staggered both sport and runner. From that day forward, Benoit became a favorite to win the inaugural women's Olympic Marathon the next year in Los Angeles.

Benoit knew she was capable of winning gold, but worried that the public would try to possess her even more now, as it had after she first won Boston in 1979, at 21. "That was the first time there was all the attention, the commercial approaches, the foundations pursuing me. I really fell apart," she said. "I handled [the 1983 Boston victory] better because I'd been through all that before, and I'd learned."

As it turned out, she entered the tunnel leading into the Los Angeles Memorial Coliseum near the end of the Olympic Marathon with more than a gold medal on her mind. She was a minute and a half ahead of Waitz. She had it won. But alone in that dim, dusty passageway, sensing the 77,000 inside (and the nation) waiting to embrace her forever, it hit her: This is the first women's Olympic Marathon. This could really change my life.

Her first thought was, It's not too late. I can hide in here and not come out the other side. Of course, she could do no such thing. So she conducted a little bargaining session. "I thought, Okay, this isn't a world record, but it will be an Olympic gold medal. It seemed a trade-off. One couldn't be any worse than the other. I really didn't want to change my life, but I thought I could handle this one."

With that resolved, she strode out into the light and won in 2:24:52. She was filled with relief, vindication, and something more. Back in that tunnel she had essentially set a lifelong goal to not let the gold medal and attendant celebrity sweep away her identity. It was a vow to be herself.

It was a vow that would be tough to keep. Benoit burst out of that tunnel a Jungian archetype: she perfectly answered our demand for what a hero must be and do—suffering, and returning transformed. She was running not just for herself but to free women shoved aside when they tried to race this mythic distance. The marathon was always a riveting metaphor. Now here was a champion for real progress.

A few months after Benoit's Olympic victory, I traveled to Maine to visit with her for a *Sports Illustrated* article I was doing. The story was entitled "Her Life Is in Apple Pie Order," a play on a goofy photo of Joan and her new husband, Scott Samuelson, in their kitchen, displaying a pie with a happy face gouged into it. "It's not victory that she celebrates but being unharmed by victory," the article proclaimed. "She has been superbly grounded."

I wrote those words in the winter of 1985. When she then went on to set more records, when she became the beaming face of our sport, adored by so many that no one needed to ask, "Joanie who," I wondered, how could she not be swept up in all the symbolism, all the vicarious hunger? How could any old promise stand up against a world determined to drink in her heroism?

Returning to her home 22 years later, and just months after her 50th birthday, I thought it fair to ask Joan Benoit Samuelson if she really has been able to cling, through the injuries and the children and the drains of endurance sport, to her legendary balance. Has she kept the vow while evolving in the process?

"Tell you what," she said on this warm Maine night. "Hang with me this week and see how I've evolved."

THE SAMUELSON SANCTUARY is a white house on Flying Point, a glaciated granite arm extending into Maquoit Bay, a few calming miles from the bustle of downtown Freeport (think L.L. Bean HQ). The surrounding woods are pine, maple, and birch. House, barn, and grounds are arranged with an eye to the sea. The lawn sweeps down to a rickety dock on a cove. Kayaks are drawn up on marsh grass. A motorboat is moored far enough out to ride above the 10-foot tides.

The vegetable garden is protected by a picket fence overlaid with bare electric wires, charged by a solar panel. At night the current fades. In come hungry creatures. Scott, Joan's husband, catches a few alive in his Havahart trap. Earlier on this August day, he'd driven a furious, malodorous raccoon back into the woods. "He was huge and he was pissed the whole time," Scott recalls. "Abby wouldn't even get in the car with that one."

Daughter Abby, 20, is a sophomore at Bates College in nearby Lewiston, where she runs cross-country and Nordic skis. "She's also practicing her backward walking," Joan says, "guiding prospective students on campus visits."

Abby says she had hoped to declare a major by now. Her mother is entirely unconcerned. "That's why we have small liberal-arts colleges," she says, "for the time and the space."

On our first night together, Joan serves buttery beets, beans, and pungent salad greens, fresh from her garden. She is tanned and lean—leaner, it seems, than in her 20s, her great years when she won the two Boston marathons. Her fastest marathon, the American record until 2003, was the 2:21:21 she ran to defeat Norway's Ingrid Kristiansen in Chicago in 1985. Then she was a sprite, a waif in a Red Sox cap, and her strength the more astounding for it. Now her chin and nose are sharper. She's grown into the face of a great marathoner, and much more.

"I climbed Mt. Kilimanjaro in Tanzania in March," she says. "That was great. That's always been a goal." Asked her motives, she replies with the old dryness: "I climb mountains because they are there, and because there are a certain number of 4,000-foot-plus peaks in New England."

She pursues biking with a similar ease. "I was thinking about running 50

miles on my 50th birthday," she says, "but I aggravated a heel spur in the Oklahoma City Memorial Half-Marathon, so instead I biked 60 miles with a friend."

Her running has been up and down. Injuries, such as the one to her heel,
have nagged her lately, and almost with a sense of relief she cries, "The Olympic
women's Marathon Trials in Boston is my last goal in running!" The race, to
determine the three American women who will run the marathon at the Beijing
Olympics, is set for April 20, the day before the Boston Marathon. It will be Samuelson's fourth Trials, and while she holds no hope of making the team, she says,
"I want to break 2:50 at 50."

She begins to sketch her training plans for it when the phone rings for the
first of many times. She is in the throes of organizing the 10th running of her
creation, the TD Banknorth Beach to Beacon 10-K road race in her hometown,
Cape Elizabeth, Maine, a few miles south of Portland. This year, several current
and former elite runners are due, including Grete Waitz, Joan's old rival and
friend. Even as the race has gotten larger, Joan has remained its shepherdess,
involving herself in the most minute of details. She also takes part in the B2B, as
it's known, with Abby, son Anders, 17, and Scott. When thinking about the
upcoming race, Scott sighs, "What I hear from bystanders when I race is, 'Uh, the
rest of your family is in front of you . . . as usual!'"

Scott was way ahead on one crucial matter. The spring before, with Joan's 50th
birthday coming in May and her telling him "100 times" she didn't want a party, he
was forced into an act of genius. He sent everyone she knew two small envelopes and
a form letter. "I can think of little more important to Joanie," he wrote, "than friends,
family, and gardens (okay, maybe a little physical exercise) and I thought how much
she'd enjoy a gift that combines you and her gardens. I am creating the ultimate 50th
Birthday Seed Catalog of personalized seed envelopes from friends and family."

To keep it a secret, he rented a post-office box to receive responses. And
knowing her, he also asked everyone to include e-mail addresses. "Joanie will
want to write you all thank-you notes and I would prefer she send one group
e-mail to everyone, or I won't see her for a month or two."

Scott now staggers into the kitchen with an armful of albums that threaten
to topple across the table. "Everybody came through!" he says. "Al Oerter [the late
Olympic discus champion] painted a miniature abstract oil. Mark Parker [presi-
dent of Nike] must have worked hours on his ornate ink drawing."

The albums overflow with real seeds and metaphoric ones, photos, and
defining remembrances:

From Jane Seagrave and John Kennedy: Already roasted coffee beans. "If
anyone can grow these, you can."

From Valerie Tarantino: Victoria's Secret seeds. "Have you noticed Joanie has more 'bounce' in her step?"

From her friend Lynn: "When I'm on my second cup of coffee, wondering what my day will hold, I'll give Joanie a call. She's already baked four sheets of cookies, gone out for a 10-mile run, and put a pan of spanakopita together for a sick neighbor. I drink my coffee with more enthusiasm. There are always enough cookies for me!"

Joan's next words are a poignant confirmation of the multitasker's dilemma. "I have only looked at two of those albums," she says on her way to bed. "There are seven."

THE NEXT DAY, SHE DOES A TRAINING RUN with Beach to Beacon runners in Portland in the morning, then holds a press conference with the governor of Maine in the afternoon and TV interviews until 11 p.m. In between, she whips home for a run of her own and starts autographing 70 or so B2B posters. Race director Dave McGillivray has already signed them. "But," she moans, "he has a rubber stamp." She sets a pace to be done in two hours, but falls behind because she keeps adding personal notes.

The next afternoon, on the freeway heading to a Portland interview, her Black-Berry chimes. It is Alberto Salazar. "Oh, you're kidding!" she yells. This is Salazar's first contact with her since the miracle of his being resuscitated after collapsing with a heart attack at Nike's campus in Oregon in June. He guarantees that he was helped by a rosary blessed by Pope John Paul II and a crucifix blessed by Pope Benedict XVI. "Well, don't lose those," says Samuelson, the soul of practicality.

Salazar asks if she can fill in for him at a Nike event; Samuelson has been one of the shoe company's ambassadors at competitions and meetings for years. But on this occasion she has to decline, being booked solid. "But give my love to Molly and the kids . . . and take care of yourself!"

As we drive, I remind her of how she and Salazar escorted Lance Armstrong through the 2006 New York City Marathon. "I did the last 16 miles," she says. "Lance was focused beyond belief on every passing mile marker. I tried to take his mind off that, get him to not interrupt his rhythm. But at 25 and a half I knew it was going to be close. I said, 'If you want to break three hours, stay on my heels and you will.' And he summoned it. He made it. He went deep. What a cardiovascular system."

She parks her maroon Volvo station wagon and sprints in to the TV station. She's out in 25 minutes. "Darn, darn, darn!" she says. "I called Duncan Kibet Robert Kibet! He's only the race favorite. I hope he wasn't watching."

Now I must drive because she has to sign the remaining posters before the final meeting of her 70-member organizing committee. This is in a buzzing, fan-blasted room in the Cape Elizabeth Community Center. On time to the minute, Joan slips into a seat and nods to McGillivray, who is also the Boston Marathon director.

"It's not about event management now," he begins. "It's about crisis management." He brandishes a 149-page organization manual. "Communications?" he barks.

"We're a go."

"Medical teams?"

"All set."

"Race-day course helpers?"

"Seven hundred seventy-two."

Meanwhile, Joan passes out the posters to the right recipients. When finished, she asks to say a few unifying words. David Weatherbie, the B2B's board president and the son of Joan's former coach at Cape Elizabeth High, introduces her. "But before Joanie," he says, "I want to say this organization now has over 1,000 people putting on the race, and how wicked proud I am to be associated with each and every one!"

Samuelson stands. "Tonight we'll honor our volunteers . . . " she begins, but Weatherbie's gust of feeling has affected her. "I wasn't going to get emotional . . ." Her eyes stay dry, but she has to catch her breath. "You exemplify what any one group can do," Samuelson says, gaining control, "all across the world. You are a celebration of how running transcends and builds community!"

This seems about to be greeted with an ovation, so she wards it off with an order: "To the volunteers' party!"

ON THE WAY TO THE PARTY, we pass a bronze statue near Joan's high school. It depicts her carrying the flag after her Olympic victory. "This is why people ask if I'm dead," she says.

Joan turns onto a private lane, enters thick woods, passes stables and a mansion, and parks in a meadow next to ranks of other Volvos and Subarus. Below, an immense incandescent tent is filling with people. Barbecue smoke and music waft up the slope. The view is of great estates, sails on the glassine bay, Richmond Island, and the opening sea. This is the Maine that has been home to money and power down through the generations. Kennebunkport is but a bay and a headland to the south.

She explains the function's role: "We've always had the thank-you party the night after the race. But the volunteers were always exhausted by then. Only a few showed up, and it was this tired little party." That so chafed at Samuelson's conscience that she rescheduled the gala to provide the volunteers with a pre-race charge. "This is a test," she says. "I hope they have fun."

She thanks every parking guide, every little girl handing out raffle tickets. "I have to be kind of omnipresent for the sake of the volunteers," she says, almost apologetically, but it is clear that this is not a burden. This is her heaven. She wades into the tent to schmooze with the sponsors, of which there are dozens. There is a tent sponsor. There is a cheese sponsor.

I hang back and meet some of her friends. "I don't know how she talked me into it," says one, a doctor. "My young son had cancer. Joanie said, 'This is what you need to do.' She came and ran with me. She planned my training. She got me through it. She made me a marathoner."

"I always think I should send her a thank-you note for including me in something," says another, "and the next day there's a thank-you note from her!"

Three hundred volunteers attend, making it a raucous success. "On behalf of TD Banknorth Beach to Beacon," Samuelson tells them, "I thank you. This is a race for the people and by the people. I had a vision 11 years ago that led to this race, and I had another to have something fun for the volunteers, and that vision is realized tonight. Thank you for coming, thank you for understanding! Thank you for being!"

She concludes in a lower key. "Sometimes," she says in a tone almost of introspection, "sometimes the road we take makes such an impression that others are impelled to follow." This seems to describe not only the influence that came to her because of her great wins but how she welcomes the weight of it, the responsibility of it. All week, she will leave a paper trail of little crossed-out notes, trying to improve the thought.

At party's end, Larry Wold, who heads TD Banknorth's operations in Maine, walks away laughing at the preposterous view. "Not that this isn't part of Maine," he says. "It is. It is. It's just the wicked best part of it!"

That, of course, is the classic New England expression. "Wicked good" is all L.L. Bean feels it needs to say about its moccasins. It's a perfect contradiction, a thing so sublime as to be sinful. It suggests, too, the New England need to not want to enjoy something too much. Savor victory for an evening because when you wake in the morning, you will find it flown, and a new race beginning. That's certainly the Samuelson pattern.

Later that night, Joan is e-mailing before bed, her eyes closing. Scott comes in waving a flashlight. "The barn is filled with baby raccoons," he says. "One's even caught in an old lobster trap."

"No wonder that big guy you hauled away was mad," Joan says. "She's their mother." They investigate. The kits are downy but about half grown, too small to do without a mom, but too big to take in and nurse. Besides, they snarl and bite when neared.

"This is a disaster!" says Scott. The immediate options are to feed them or take them to where he dumped the mother. "But that's such a pain."

Joan is vexed. "This story is not about raccoons!" she yells. Tired, she just wants to simplify life's onrushing narrative.

Scott frees the one in the lobster trap. "Maybe they'll be gone in the morning."

As it happens, the raccoons are still there the next day, two asleep in an empty trash can. Scott carries the can gently across the road and into the woods, tipping it for ease of egress, and tiptoes away. Joan does a 30-mile bike ride.

ANDERS RETURNS FROM SURFING CAMP later in the day. He has his father's dark coloring and daredevil gene. In winter, he doesn't really change sports, just temperatures. He is a devoted shredder, a snowboarder. Fluent in Swedish, he spent six months as a foreign-exchange student in Stockholm to finish his junior year in high school. His e-mails home prove him a writer of promise. In a piece of fiction he wrote about a marathoner, one line jumps out: "He worked with pace and never grew too confident, always partially blind to his blatant gift." That, of course, is exactly his mother's relationship with her talent, but Anders says he was thinking more of a character in the novel *The Power of One*, by Bryce Courtenay. Even so, I repeat the sentence to Joan as we drive toward Cape Elizabeth. Her head snaps around. "Who wrote that?"

"Your son."

"My son?" Her face runs through about six expressions, and stops on sympathy. "Ahh, he's got it. The writer thing." She makes it sound like she'll have to shoot him a get-well card.

She visits the race expo and packet pickup, which is in full swing at her old high school gym. One greeter calls out, "Hiya, Joaniebaloney!" Boxes with the 6,500 entries line tables. Joan asks the guy manning the box with numbers 601 to 880 how he liked the party.

"My wife had diverticulitis and was in the hospital all week. I missed the party to be with her."

"Wow, thanks for being here today."

"You are welcome," he says, with the firmness of really meaning it.

That night she attends another, smaller soiree, this for families who host invited runners. Beach to Beacon is unusual in lodging runners in homes, rather than impersonal hotels. "Many of you will become fast friends—literally," Joan tells them. In the past several hosts have flown to Africa to visit their adopted runners.

On the way home, we get caught in a traffic jam on the freeway. Joan massages her tight right hamstring. "I should keep a tennis ball in the car for this."

I ask about her plans for breaking 2:50 at the Olympic Trials. "If I train seriously for it, train right, I should do it," she says. She did it easily in the 2006 Twin Cities Marathon, where she ran 2:46:27. And she covered the seven miles of the 2007 Falmouth Road Race in under-six-minute pace. A 2:50 marathon is exactly 6:30 pace. She's got the speed.

She's also had injuries. "One thing after another," she says. "In Oklahoma in a half-marathon in April, I felt an old injury in the calf and plantar fascia go at six and a half miles. I limped in, in 1:54:52."

I give her a look.

She gives me one back. "I know you say drop out. I have never dropped out of a road race, so I couldn't. To drop out of the Trials, that would kill me. But training right will need massage, will need taking more rest. The question is, can I do that? Can I back off, can I do stretching routines? Squatting in my garden is not what I should be doing. I know I'm going to have to try to take a three-month sabbatical, but, but..."

She almost shivers with horror at the prospect of reining herself in. "The problem is I cram in so much that... I cut things so close," she explains. "I'm naturally late for things because I cut things so tight. I'm not proud of that, but that's me. If I need to be there, if it's important for the kids, I'm always there, but it's always close."

The next morning, she attends the race's media conference and introduces two special guests, Grete Waitz and Canada's Jacqueline Gareau. "Jackie won the Boston Marathon in 1980," says Joan, "and I don't want to say much more than that, because it means mentioning Rosie Ruiz, who jumped in at the end and stole Jackie's laurels."

Afterward, we have lunch with Waitz at a seafood restaurant near the Portland docks. Having never been to Maine, Grete leapt at Samuelson's call to come to the race. They laugh about their various physical problems before the Los Angeles Olympic Marathon. Grete had a nagging muscle injury and didn't think she'd be able to run that morning. Joan was ready, but what she had survived to be there is properly legend.

In the spring of that year, her knee locked on a run. Rest and anti-inflammatories had no effect. Panicking and with nothing to lose, she went to Eugene, Oregon, and had Dr. Stan James operate on her—17 days before the Olympic Trials in May. "He and I had an agreement," Joan says. "If he got in there and found that it was bad, really in need of reconstruction, then he'd do it then. If not, I'd go right home.

"So I woke up in the hospital. Stan came in and said, 'I bet you're thinking it took massive repair. It didn't. I simply snipped a plica band that was caught in the joint."

"Then why am I here overnight?"

"Because your reputation has preceded you. I've been advised to force as much recovery on you as possible before you go out and test that knee."

He'd heard right. A few days later, she tested it to the obsessive tune of 17 miles. That caused such tissue damage to her out-of-shape leg muscles that therapist Jack Scott had to administer microcurrent stimulation for 14 hours a day. She arrived at the Trials in Olympia, Washington, not knowing if she could make the distance. She led all the way. "I had absolutely nothing left after 20 miles. If anyone had passed me, I think the whole field would have."

She won in 2:31:04. "The biggest win was the Olympics," she says, "but the race of my life was the Trials."

The story is a reminder of how placidly she could run her own race, ungnawed by doubt or what the competition was doing. She won in Los Angeles by roaring out to a big lead after only two miles. She didn't even recall some stretches later because she was "spacing out," in her words, supremely absorbed in maintaining the right flow for her, right rhythm, right breathing. "I felt smooth and strong," she says, "almost effortless. Never again."

Her true gift, therefore, in training and racing, was and remains being able to leave everything to the gods. She speaks of having a formal arrangement with them. "I promised myself if I was able to make it through the Trials and to the Olympics, I would give back," she says. So it's a done deal. Whatever her sport wants from her, she'll give.

As ever, when she takes a run, she hopes to get away from the obligations and planning and sheer thoughtfulness of her overcommitted life. If she finds that old spacey rhythm, she sometimes returns more refreshed than when she set out.

She still starts so fast, few companions are ready. Brad Hudson, one of the United States' top running coaches and a former 2:13 marathoner, ran with her in New York's Central Park last year. "I had to invent an appointment I'd forgotten so I could peel off and quit," Hudson says.

RACE DAY DAWNS MISTY and dank. The Beach to Beacon course record, set by Kenya's Gilbert Okari in 2003, is 27:28, an incredible time for this 10-K because the last mile climbs without pity. Sun graces the start at Crescent Beach, but at the finish at Portland Head Light the crowd waits in the fog that makes the lighthouse necessary.

The humidity, to employ an Anders Samuelson phrase, "is nearing solidification." A pair of Kenyans, Duncan Kibet and Evans Cheryiout, battle throughout the course, with Kibet barely winning, 27:51.7 to 27:52.1. Luminita Talpos of Romania is the women's winner in 32:20.

Anders is the first Samuelson, in 39:12, which would be faster but for the huge, sopping soccer shirt he wears. The crowd awaits his mom. McGillivray has broadcast a pledge to give a dollar to STRIVE, the race's youth charity, for every person who beats Joan, saying, "That's the only way to slow her down."

It doesn't slow her down. Only 363 of the 4,839 finishers beat her. She comes in together with (and hugging) Jacqueline Gareau in 41:57. Abby has no trouble handling Scott, yet again. At the award ceremony, McGillivray, saying he likes round numbers, rounds his gift up from $363 to $2,000.

Samuelson opens a long-prepared box. "And to Jacqueline Gareau," she says, "the laurel wreath she never got in 1980 in Boston!" Gareau joyfully mashes the leafy crown onto her curls, the picture of justice.

The crowd disperses reluctantly, struck by the sight of a schooner ghosting into the offshore fog bank. The lighthouse's foghorn is high-pitched, a mournful, muffled trumpet. "With great relief," says Joan, "we can now rest before the lobster bake."

At the race's final bash, Joan wears dressy black and sequins, which don't prevent her from wrenching lobster tail after lobster tail from their shells, and eating deeply. Hers is a Maine metabolism, pursuing its native diet.

Eventually Joan is called to speak. McGillivray says she will be in need of warmth this winter, training for the marathon Trials, so he gives her a symbolic sweatshirt. She takes the microphone, and after thanking each sponsor, says, "It's not always easy to live with a spouse you can't catch, but Scott I love you so."

As she steps down, the Olympic theme swells. There is no stopping this ovation.

WITH THE CRAZINESS OF THE PAST few days now over, it's time to relax. Two friends with whom Joan climbed Kilimanjaro, Wendy Hollister and Kari Rekoske, come for blueberry pancakes the next morning. They bring a beautiful picture of the three of them at Barafu Camp, Tanzania, with the mountain in the background.

"You have to go with a guide and porters," says Hollister, "one porter for your duffel, one for your water. They go up with these huge bags on their heads. They make a dollar a day."

Rekoske says, "It was five days up, and a day down. We had walking poles."

Joan was lucky she had Hollister. "Joanie got really, really cold," Hollister recalls. "I gave her my gloves. I gave her my jacket."

After Hollister and Rekoske depart, Joan types e-mail thank-you notes. Thus there is a moment to ask Anders and Abby whether being raised by Joan made for a great childhood.

"She incorporated us in all the trips and events she could," says Anders.

"And when she was planning them," says Abby, "she'd tell Nike she had to be back for this game or that meet. She made most of ours. Other kids' folks made half as many. Also, she'd sacrifice cool things to do in places because she'd hurry back. And that went double for the gardens. She can't be away from them long."

Samuelson is an accredited master gardener, though she doesn't compost using the orthodox series of piles, balancing green versus brown, kitchen scraps versus old leaves, nitrogen versus carbon. She gets her results by mulching everything she grows with seaweed that she and Scott have hauled from their shore and dried. This eelgrass (*Zostera marina*) grows in narrow ribbons. Her squash, artichokes, row crops, arugula, and peonies seem to push up though mounds of wadded cassette tape. Her celery has won a blue ribbon at the Common Ground Fair, Maine's biggest organic fair.

It would be uncharacteristic of her to garden for her needs alone. She contributes produce and time to the local Plant a Row for the Hungry organization, which donates more than a million pounds of food a year to local food banks and soup kitchens across the United States and Canada.

"I have a vision comparable in clarity to my B2B dreams a decade ago," she says. "It has to do with how the potato fields of Maine's Aroostook County have lain fallow for so long now that they have become organically certifiable soil. So I dream of Aroostook becoming a great center of organic cold crops. Broccoli, kale, everything."

The idea is warm and alive, waiting for a catalyst. Just how she will invest her time and energy has yet to be determined, but sustainable agriculture seems a natural for one so blithe to exhaust herself, as right for her as marathoning was in her youth. She is evolving wisely.

In other pursuits, such as raising her children and tending to her gardens, she's been fortunate to have a partner in Scott, whose love for the land equals that of his wife. "There have been years where I'm rototilling the snow to get those damn peas in," he says, chuckling. Theirs is a remarkable relationship. Each day Scott and Joan pursue their own callings, then meet back at the farm. "Joanie and I could never work together," he says. "Our friends crack up just trying to imagine that." Scott is a part owner and manager of an environmentally advanced water-treatment company, SeptiTech. Hers is far more the life that wears one down.

"The drain of her public appearances is seasonal and peaking this week,"

Scott says. But it's not always this pressured. "We're a skiing family," he says. "Almost every week in winter we head over to our cabin at Sugarloaf, and nothing gets done because we're out all day, and come in tired. That's our family time, together. That recharges Joan, and all of us.

"The question is what to do next, after Joan runs the Trials. How to balance her trips for Nike and the running-world obligations with sensible time at home."

That is precisely the question, and there's no precise answer. Joan has shaped her life to be doubly exemplary, to give back and to run her best, even though it's obvious that the two ends are so draining that compromise is inevitable. Accepting that is the single toughest thing for Samuelson.

At times, her headlong rush of activities is worrisome. It exhausts her, and she couldn't do it without her understanding support team. At first she's so rational, so expressive, she sneaks her mania past you. But after a while you begin to feel tired for her, and jump up to be useful. She should run for office or manage a political campaign. It's startling to think this soul once trembled because companies wanted to pay her to do commercials.

You wonder, as you do with the obsessive, whether she is happy. Happy when at rest. Is she trying to do good in so many ways that she'll lose herself? Is she literally wicked good? What is she trying to prove, after all she's done?

Truth is, it's not a case of wanting to prove anything. It never has been, not since her Olympic tunnel vow. She's living out her design, and her design climbs mountains because she sees them right there, unclimbed. If we understand that, we ought to stop wondering. We should just stand back in awe that this prodigy has come among us.

That afternoon we walk over to the beach. Scott, an osprey fluttering and wheeling over him, kayaks out to their white runabout, starts its 130-horse-power outboard, and brings it back to the dock. Soot, their big, old black Lab, knows where it's going and won't allow it to depart without him.

It takes 25 minutes over calm water, past islets that evoke the Baltic, past thousands of lobster-trap buoys to reach Cliff Island. As a child, Joan spent parts of her summers here. She grew up in its blend of everyone-knows-you safety and everyone-knows-you boredom. Abby and Anders have done the same.

The scene makes clear how Joan has kept her balance. She is inextricable from this island and this life, where vigorous families stay close, where neighbors feed each other, where hard work brings amazing possibilities, and where you can flow along at your own sweet, inimitable rhythm.

Everyone takes naps, Joan unconscious on a towel on the warm granite beach rocks, protected by Soot and family. No one has ever looked happier.

DUEL IN THE SUN

BY JOHN BRANT

> They had nothing in common. One was a
> humble farm boy from Minnesota. The other was the
> most electrifying distance runner of his time. In 1982,
> they battled stride for stride for more than two hours
> in the most thrilling Boston Marathon ever run.
> Then the drama really began.

APRIL 2004

IN FRONT OF SOME AUDIENCES, Dick Beardsley never even mentions the 1982 Boston Marathon. In fact, he barely touches on his running career at all. When he's delivering one of his regular talks to a 12-step group, for instance, he simply begins, "Hi, I'm Dick, and I'm a drug addict," then launches into the rending story of his disease and recovery.

When Beardsley finishes speaking, and the people are wiping away their tears and settling back into their seats after a standing ovation, then the host might explain how Dick Beardsley is the fourth-fastest American marathoner of all time, and that his race with Alberto Salazar at Boston nearly three decades ago remains one of the signature moments in the history of distance running; perhaps, in the history of any sport.

But other audiences, such as this one at the Royal Victoria Marathon in Victoria, British Columbia, know all about Beardsley's athletic career, and are eager—even hungry—to relive his legendary "duel in the sun" with Salazar.

There's a considerable amount of preamble. Beardsley is not good at leaving things out. He tells the crowd of 200 about getting creamed at his first high school football practice, quitting the team, and turning out for cross-country without knowing quite what it was. "Do they tackle you in cross-country?" he asked a friend. He explains how he ran his second marathon in a brand-new pair of running shoes that he didn't want to get dirty by breaking in, and that he prepared by fasting for four days because he'd read somewhere that fasting worked in ultramarathons, so he figured ...

Beardsley is blessed with the fundamental trait of the born entertainer: a complete lack of self-consciousness. He strides back and forth in front of the podium, laughing right along with the audience, as delighted as they are by his own buffoonery. His voice—honking, booming, unabashed—rolls around the conference hall in overpowering waves. Wearing jeans, a red pullover, and a blue fleece vest, whip-cord lean and with a lilt to his step, Beardsley might be mistaken for an athlete in his prime rather than a man of 48. You have to sit close to notice the hard miles showing around his eyes.

The crowd's laughter drowns out the canned rock music blaring from the expo next door. But when Beardsley shifts gears, traveling back to Hopkinton, Massachusetts, on the sunny noon of April 19, 1982, the room falls raptly silent.

Which seems only appropriate, because the 1982 Boston Marathon was great theater: two American runners, one a renowned champion and the other a gutty underdog, going at each other for just under two hours and nine minutes. Other famous marathons have featured narrow margins of victory, but their suspense developed late in the race, the product of a furiously closing challenger or rapidly fading leader. At the '82 Boston, by contrast, Beardsley and Salazar ran in each other's pocket the entire 26.2 miles, with no other competitor near them for the final nine miles. They were so close that, for most of the last half of the race, Beardsley, while in the lead, monitored Salazar's progress by watching his shadow on the asphalt.

Neither man broke, and neither, in any meaningful sense, lost. The race merely came to a thrilling, shattering end, leaving both runners, in separate and ultimately Pyrrhic ways, the winner. The drama unfolded in the sport's most storied venue, at the peak of the first running boom, when the United States produced world-class marathoners in the profusion that Kenya does today.

"An Epic Duel," "The Greatest Boston Marathon," "A Display of Single-Minded Determination and Indefatigable Spirit," read the next day's headlines. Since Beardsley was just 26 and Salazar 23, everyone assumed that this would be the start of a long and glorious rivalry, one that would galvanize the public and seal American dominance in the marathon through the 1984 Olympics and beyond.

But rather than a beginning, Boston '82 represented a climax. After that day, neither man ran a marathon as well again. And from that day since, incredibly, only two more of the world's major marathons have been won by a native-bred

American man. On that day, 156 runners, virtually every one an American, finished the race in a time of 2:30 or faster. By contrast, fewer than 60 runners have logged 2:30 or better at each of the past 10 Bostons.

So some of the younger members of the audience—including the elite runners who will lead tomorrow's Royal Victoria Marathon—listen to Beardsley's story with a mixture of curiosity, envy, and awe. Others in the crowd, those closer to Beardsley's age, listen on a different frequency. They know the enormous toll that Boston exacted on both Alberto Salazar and Dick Beardsley. If the glory of their marathon bore a heroic quality, so did their suffering afterward.

AT NIKE CORPORATE HEADQUARTERS in Beaverton, Oregon, Alberto Salazar descends to the ground-floor café of the Mia Hamm Building for a quick lunch. For the past several years, Nike has employed Salazar as a kind of coach-at-large, chartered to deliver that most endangered of species—the Great American Distance Runner—from the brink of extinction. On this drizzly October Tuesday, Salazar has spent the morning training the professional athletes in Nike's ambitious Oregon Project. This afternoon, he'll supervise the cross-country team at Portland's Central Catholic High School.

Both teams, he reports, are thriving. The Oregon Project's Dan Browne has met the qualifying standard for the 2004 Olympic marathon, and Central Catholic's Galen Rupp should repeat as the state cross-country champion. Meanwhile, other parts of Salazar's life are in similar bloom: his oldest son, Antonio, plays wide receiver for the University of Oregon football team, and his younger son, Alejandro, is a star striker for the University of Portland soccer team.

At 46, Salazar appears every bit the proud, happy family man and flourishing professional. His brown eyes are clear, calm, and bright, and his cheeks have lost a marathoner's hollowness. He no longer resembles "the young priest fresh from seminary whose face drives all the housewives to distraction," as one writer described him 20 years ago. Now Salazar looks more like a fit-but-comfortable middle-aged monsignor, a man still true to his religious vocation, but also at ease in the worldly realm of fund-raisers and cocktail parties.

A Japanese visitor approaches and politely asks for an autograph. Salazar graciously complies. "After Boston I was never quite the same," he says, after his fan has departed. "I had a few good races, but everything was difficult. Workouts that I used to fly through became an ordeal. And eventually, of course, I got so sick that I wondered if I'd ever get well."

Salazar's warm smile briefly turns wintry. For a moment, his poise falters and he seems like a traumatized man who, after exhaustive therapy, can finally talk about his past.

"It took me a long time to connect the dots," he says, "and see that the line stretched all the way back to Boston."

MONDAY, APRIL 19, Patriots' Day, broke warm and blue over Boston, perfect for just about anything except running 26.2 miles.

After driving out to the start in Hopkinton, Beardsley and his coach, Bill Squires, avoided the high school gym that served as the staging area for elite athletes. For the past four months, Beardsley had spent all of his waking moments, and some of his sleeping ones, thinking and dreaming about Alberto Salazar. Squires wanted to keep Beardsley as removed from the race excitement as possible.

So they camped out in the house of a town matron. Squires went into his usual patter. "How do, missus, beautiful day, lovely home, let me introduce Dickie Beardsley here from Minnesota. Dickie's a dairy farmer, got hay stuck in his teeth, but don't be fooled. In a few minutes he's gonna run the Boston Marathon, and just between you and me, he's got a shot to win it if he sets his mouth right and does the hubba-hubba on the hills . . ."

While Squires and the grandma yakked, Beardsley stretched, sipped water, made a half-dozen trips to the bathroom, and listened to a Dan Fogelberg tape. He punched ventilation holes in the white painters' cap that Squires had given him to ward off the sun and tried not to jump out of his skin.

At a quarter to 12 he heard the call for runners. He jogged out to the street, heading for the section at the front of the starting area roped off for elite athletes. But thousands of citizen-athletes stood between him and the starting line. He tried to fight through the crowd but couldn't make any progress.

Beardsley panicked. He felt as if he were caught in one of those sweat-drenched nightmares in which he was desperately trying to reach a critical destination, but couldn't move. (Decades later, after detox, Beardsley will be haunted by a similar nightmare: He's been in another accident. He's lying on a hospital bed and nurses are hooking him up to an IV-drip attached to a huge pouch of Demerol. He tries to scream at the nurse to stop, but not a sound comes out of his mouth.)

So Beardsley reverted to character. He started to make noise. "Hey, let me through! I'm Dick Beardsley, for crying out loud! I gotta get up to the front!"

The other runners, immersed in their last-minute preparations, eyed him coldly. Then someone recognized him, and word rippled through the crowd: "Look out, we got Dick Beardsley here! Make way, Dick's coming through!"

The crowds parted, and Beardsley, his nightmare dissolved into a dream, followed a clear path to the starting line.

Throughout the winter of 1981 and '82, as he had sat in front of the TV in the evenings, Beardsley pounded his thighs with his fists 1,500 times. He had read somewhere that pounding your muscles made them tougher. If he thought it might gain him a few seconds on the downhills, Beardsley would have tried curing his quads in a smokehouse. He knew that the marathon would be decided on the course's three long hills rising between miles 17 and 21. If he had any chance of beating Salazar, he would have to fly down the hills like a bobsled racer, capitalizing on the fact that Salazar outweighed him by 20 pounds. Conceivably, a series of rocketing descents might pummel Salazar's legs to the extent that Beardsley would be able to pull away from him before mile 25. If that plan failed and the race came down to a kick at the end, then Salazar, with his superior short-range speed, would do the pummeling.

Fifteen-hundred punches, each thigh.

BORN IN HAVANA but raised in the Boston suburb Wayland, Alberto Salazar, the world's greatest and most charismatic distance runner, was coming home from Oregon to run his first Boston Marathon. It was one of the most eagerly anticipated sports stories of 1982. He was fit and prepared, he announced to reporters upon arriving at the airport with his wife, Molly. If there were no injuries or unforeseen developments . . . well, the facts were plain: he was the fastest man in the race.

Six months earlier, Salazar had won his second consecutive New York City Marathon in a world-record time of 2:08:13, which had earned him, among other honors, a White House audience with President Ronald Reagan. In March, he had finished second at the World Cross-Country Championships. And just one week before Boston, he had run a blistering 27:30 in a 10,000-meter match race with the great Kenyan runner Henry Rono at the University of Oregon's Hayward Field.

The 10,000 had been Salazar's idea. He had lined up the appearance money for Rono, who had shown up in Eugene looking fat and blowsy, in the early stages of the alcoholism that would eventually destroy his career. But once the race started, he ran with his trademark ferocity. For 25 laps around the historic track, Rono and Salazar belted away at each other. Rono outleaned Salazar at the wire, by the width of his jiggling belly, the wags in the press box joked.

Rono's brilliant victory was essentially ignored. But Salazar's draining, word-class effort, just two seconds off Craig Virgin's American record, raised eyebrows. Occurring only nine days before the Boston Marathon, it violated every code in the sport's training canon.

Salazar didn't care. At the age of 16 he had determined that he would become the fastest marathoner in the world. Instead of the standard training—laying a foundation of endurance, then adding speedwork—Salazar did the opposite. He first honed his track speed to match that of a Henry Rono, then built his strength so he could maintain that pace over the length of a marathon. His goal was to demolish his competitors, run so far out in front of them that there could be no doubt of his greatness.

"I viewed every marathon as a test of my manhood," he says. "It wasn't enough for me to win the race; I wanted to bury the other guys."

AT MILE FIVE, THE LEAD PACK passed a pond where a couple was floating around in a canoe, enjoying the beautiful afternoon. Bill Rodgers poked Beardsley. "Hey, Dick, wouldn't you love to be out there right now?" As if they were two young executives commuting into the office, looking out the train window.

Then, a few miles later, Ron Tabb and Dean Matthews threw a rogue surge. It was way too early for a serious ante, but not so early that the contenders could afford to ignore it; they had to burn precious energy reeling in the pair. Beardsley laughed it off, but Salazar was genuinely steamed.

The crowds were huge. Most of the spectators cheered for Salazar, the native son. When Salazar waved at his fans, Beardsley did likewise. He waved and grinned as if this were the Fourth of July parade back home in Rush City, Minnesota, and the folks were cheering for him. Salazar was not amused.

Salazar wasn't finding much of anything amusing. He was booming along in the lead pack, looking strong, yet Beardsley sensed that he wasn't quite in sync. He also noticed that, despite the glaring sun and 70-degree temperatures, Salazar never drank.

There weren't any official, fully-stocked water stations. You had to accept cups of whatever a spectator might offer. As often as he could, Beardsley would grab a cup, pour whatever it contained over his painters cap, take a swallow, then offer the cup to Salazar. But he always refused it.

ON THE MORNING OF NOVEMBER 13, 1989, snow was forecast for the dairy-farm belt of central Minnesota. Before the storm arrived, Dick Beardsley, recently retired from his professional running career, needed to milk his cows, store the corn that he'd harvested the day before, and pick the corn remaining in his fields.

He rose at a quarter to four, blitzed through milking, skipped breakfast, and went to work loading the harvested corn in a grain elevator.

Like much of the machinery on a family farm, the elevator ran on a device called a power take-off, a revolving steel rod connected to the tractor engine. Normally, Beardsley sat in the driver's seat to engage the device; but today, trying to accomplish several jobs at once, he stood on the slippery tractor drawbar. The engine turned over unexpectedly, catching Beardsley's overalls leg in the power take-off. For a horrified moment, he watched his left leg disappear into the maw of the machine. Then he was caught in a whirlwind.

The shaft of the power take-off curled Beardsley's leg around it like a string around a spool, casting him into a devastating orbit. It crumpled his left leg, and flung his skull against the barn floor with each revolution. Beardsley screamed for help, but his wife, Mary, was in the house, too far away to hear. His head hammered into the floor as if it were a rag doll's. On each revolution he desperately reached for the shut-off lever, but it remained just a few inches beyond his grasp.

Beardsley started to slip away. It was an iron-gray morning, spitting snow, but he saw a brilliant light.

Somehow, the tractor engine died. Beardsley pulled his crushed leg out of the machine and crawled out to the yard, where Mary finally found him. Beardsley was relatively lucky; power take-off accidents kill more farmers than they maim. He came away with a punctured lung, a fractured right wrist, broken ribs, a severe concussion, broken vertebrae, a mangled leg, and a monkey on his back.

That first rush of Demerol in the hospital was unlike anything the straight-arrow, teetotaling Beardsley had ever experienced. He rocketed into another world—one without stress or strain or worry. It was so wonderful that if some higher power told him that he could go back, avoid the accident, but never take Demerol, Beardsley wouldn't hesitate—he would turn down the offer flat.

PAST THE 13-MILE MARK, and past Wellesley College and its gantlet of shrieking women, the lead pack melted down to Rodgers, Ed Mendoza, Beardsley, and Salazar.

At age 34, the great Rodgers, four-time winner of the Boston Marathon, had lost a step, and the frontrunning Mendoza would inevitably fade. The only concern was Beardsley, whom Salazar pegged as a talented journeyman. True, he'd run a few good marathons—a 2:09 at Grandma's in Duluth, the win at London the previous year—but he had no credentials on the track. Beardsley's best 10-K was a full minute and a half slower than his own.

And look at him there in his silly little painter's cap, slurping water from every kid he passed. Beardsley lacked gravitas. So let Beardsley and Squires think they could break him on the hills. Salazar knew they were dreaming. He was faster, tougher, and had prepared more thoroughly. The hills belonged to him.

A few feet away, Beardsley was thinking the same thing. He had spent the winter training in Atlanta, not to escape the northern cold, but because Georgia, unlike Minnesota, had hills approximating Boston's. In early April, he left Georgia to finish preparing in Boston, where he could familiarize himself with the marathon course. Shortly after his arrival, however, a northeaster blew into town, bringing heavy snow and a howling wind. Beardsley was scheduled for a key workout on Heartbreak Hill: up one side and down the other, eight times. Squires looked out the window and told him to forget it.

"Come on, Coach. Let's give it a try."

"I don't think I can even get us to Heartbreak, let alone have you run there." But Squires finally relented. He drove at a creeping pace through the deserted streets, delivering Beardsley to within three miles of Heartbreak.

"For chrissakes, Dickie, look at this snow. Let's go home. You're gonna slip and fall and kill yourself."

"Let me give it a shot, Coach."

Beardsley got out of the car and started running toward Heartbreak. He ran gingerly at first, but after a few steps picked up the pace. His footprints cut lonesome notches in the unblemished drifts; the icy wind scorched his eyes. Beardsley closed his eyes, moving on touch and sound and instinct, imagining—knowing—that at this desperate moment, Alberto Salazar was running someplace where it was warm.

He completed eight round trips over Heartbreak, just as planned. At the end of the workout, he quietly reported to Squires that he was ready. The hills belonged to him.

IN THE WEEKS AND MONTHS following the 1982 Boston Marathon, Alberto Salazar's decline was so gradual that it barely seemed like a decline at all. In the summer of 1982 he set two American records on the track, in the 5000 and 10,000 meters. In October, he won his third consecutive New York City Marathon. His time was a few minutes slower than at Boston, but he appeared to be his elegant, imperious self—the finest distance runner of his time.

But privately, Salazar worried. Before Boston he'd relished his workouts, ripping through them with the barest hint of fatigue. He was able to follow hard days and weeks of training with even harder ones; the ceiling for one training cycle became the floor for the next. But after Boston, the workouts yielded less and less pleasure. His legs felt heavy, his breathing shallow. It took him days instead of hours to recover from a maximum effort.

Salazar tried to convince himself that he hadn't blown it at Boston; that despite drinking so little, and running so furiously, he hadn't done himself lasting damage. He scoffed at the media for making such a fuss about his "duel in the sun" with Beardsley.

Throughout 1983, Salazar suffered one heavy cold after another. Deep, racking, bronchitis-style colds, one a month, lining up like winter storm fronts off the coast of Oregon. Consistent high-level training became impossible, and he entered the crucial Olympic year of '84 in dire shape. At the Marathon Trials, he struggled to a 2:12, second-place performance. It earned him a berth in the Games, but for Salazar, finishing second—especially in a race restricted to other Americans—was like finishing last.

He had a chance to redeem himself in Los Angeles, but the colds and malaise continued all summer. On the last night of the Games, it was Carlos Lopes of Portugal who ran into the Coliseum before the world's admiring eyes. Salazar finished an exhausted 15th.

Still, he was only 26, with many marathons and Olympics seemingly ahead. But the illness and weakness did not abate. Doctors failed to identify his malady, and Salazar, desperate to fight, remained impotent before an invisible enemy. He experienced insomnia, and went to the Stanford Sleep Clinic. He visited a cardiologist. He underwent surgery. He tried training in Kenya. Nothing worked.

But he stubbornly refused to stop running. Because running was how Salazar defined himself. Running was the means by which he proved his manhood. At the same time, on solitary long runs or during exacting workouts with close friends, the sport provided a shelter, a place to escape the pressure of constantly proving himself. Now, in his physical prime, his only outlet was denied him. He couldn't run, yet he couldn't stop running. Salazar reached the point where the best he could do was cover four or five miles in a crabbed shuffle.

"For much of the last 10 years, I hated running," he confessed to a reporter in 1994. "I hated it with a passion. I used to wish for a cataclysmic injury in which I would lose one of my legs. I know that sounds terrible, but if I had lost a leg, then I wouldn't have to torture myself anymore."

JUST PAST MILE 17, just before the firehouse at the base of the Braeburn Hill, Rodgers started to fade; just beyond it, Mendoza dropped away. Now it was down to Beardsley and Salazar. Beardsley stepped to the lead he would hold for the next nine miles.

As the hills unreeled, Beardsley launched one gambit after another. He would drive hard for 400 yards, then back off for 200. He'd repeat the cycle two or three times. But after a third fast 400, he'd slow down for only 100 yards. Then, hoping to catch Salazar flatfooted, he would surge. But Salazar covered every move. He stayed plastered on Beardsley's shoulder, throwing his own combinations. The sun was behind them, so Beardsley could watch Salazar's shadow on the pavement. When the shadow began to move forward, Beardsley speeded up just enough to stay ahead of it. Psychologically, he could not afford to let Salazar take the lead.

Heartbreak Hill came and went. The two runners remained joined.

BY THE SUMMER OF 1995, Dick Beardsley was taking 90 tablets of Demerol, Percocet, and Valium a day. He photocopied physicians' stationery, forged the prescriptions, and filled them at a dozen pharmacies in and around his home in Detroit Lakes, Minnesota. With meticulous care, Beardsley recorded his drug transactions in a small notebook, disguising the entries as bait purchases for the fishing-guide business he bought after recovering from his farming accident.

When Dick and Mary visited a friend's house for dinner, Beardsley excused himself from the table, went to the bathroom, and rifled his host's medicine cabinet for pain pills. He did the same at the house of his father, who was dying of pancreatic cancer.

Beardsley no longer drank water with the pills; he had trained himself to gulp them down dry, as if they were M&Ms or sunflower seeds. He spent all his waking moments thinking about pills—acquiring them, concealing them— much in the way that, years earlier, in the winter before the 1982 Boston Marathon, he spent all his time thinking about Alberto Salazar.

Amazingly, Beardsley was able to hide his disease, live a double life. Nobody in Detroit Lakes harbored suspicions. He appeared to be the same great guy as always: friendly, generous, outgoing, forthright, not in the least bit pompous despite his past as a world-class athlete. His fishing-guide business was thriving. He had become a popular motivational speaker for youth groups.

At the bait shop, or on a boat with a client, Beardsley never slurred his words or stumbled. He drove with obsessive care. He hid his pills in a secret place in his pickup truck and floated around in a private, secret cloud that insulated him from all trouble and anxiety. He was a week or two away from dying.

"After I got caught, during detox and treatment, the doctors just shook their heads when they found out how much I was taking," he recalls. "It was enough to kill an elephant. The doctors said that thanks to my running, I had a tremendously rapid metabolism, and an incredibly strong heart. Still, it was only a matter of time until one morning I just wouldn't wake up."

At home in the evenings, Beardsley would often nod off over his supper plate. One night, Mary said to him in frustration, "Do you think you could force yourself to stay awake and watch a video with me tonight?"

Worried that his cover might be fraying, Beardsley willed himself to watch the entire movie. The next day, while returning the video to the rental shop, he decided to surprise Mary with another movie. He spent a long time combing the aisles, studying various titles. Finally he found a film he was sure she would like.

At home, when he delivered the surprise, Mary stared at him. The video he had brought her was the same one they had watched the night before.

AFTER WATCHING THE EARLY PART of the race on TV, and discovering that an extraordinary contest was in progress—two runners, stripped down to bone and will, relentlessly moving down the streets of their city—the citizens of Boston turned out of their houses to witness the finish. Fathers lifted their children up on their shoulders and told them to pay attention, as an estimated crowd of two million turned out to watch some part of the 1982 Boston Marathon.

Beardsley had come off Heartbreak with Salazar breathing down his neck. The crowd pressed so close there was barely a path to run through. They were screaming so loud he couldn't hear himself think. He couldn't feel his legs. They seemed to belong to somebody else.

Twenty-one miles into the 86th Boston Marathon, and he was running a stride in front of the great Salazar, who must be hurting, too. Because if Salazar wasn't fried, he would have blown past him by now.

Five more miles was unthinkable. Beardsley decided he'd just go one more mile. That would be easy—or at least possible. Stay ahead of Salazar for one more mile. After that—well, he'd think of something.

He couldn't feel his legs. One more mile.

Meanwhile, Salazar was hurting. Shards of pain splintered up from Salazar's left hamstring. Sometime during the past few miles he had stopped sweating. His singlet had stiffened, as if covered in dried blood.

All that mattered now was not losing. That made things simple. He could forget about his time and focus on that single and sovereign goal. He might lose a 10,000-meter race to a Henry Rono, but he did not lose marathons, especially to a palooka in a painter's cap. Any moment now Beardsley might blow up and drop away like a disintegrating booster rocket. If he could maintain the pace, then it would simply be a matter of outkicking him.

Alberto Salazar feared no opponent, at least none that he could see.

JOSE SALAZAR, ALBERTO'S FATHER, was a passionate man. Journalists never tired of writing about Jose's romantic Cuban background: the fact that he'd been a close friend and fellow revolutionary of Fidel Castro, that he'd grown to hate the Communists, and, in exile, had dedicated his life to overthrowing his former comrade.

In 1988, Jose's church in Wayland hosted a guest from Europe bringing strange but exciting news: six teenagers in the Balkans of Yugoslavia had been visited by an apparition of the Virgin Mary. A devout Catholic well-disposed toward saints and miracles, Jose was fascinated. He undertook his own pilgrimage to the distant town, called Medjugorje. Upon his return home, Jose started sending Medjugorje literature to Alberto in Oregon. Alberto was the most devout of his four children, but also the one most in need of grace.

After a failed bid to make the 1988 Olympic team, Alberto Salazar had started a business career, owning and operating a popular, eponymous restaurant in Eugene. Despite the fact that he'd grown increasingly distant, surly, and abstracted since his running had declined, he regarded himself as a happy and prosperous man. He didn't need any of his father's Virgin Mary moonshine.

But one day in 1990, Salazar picked up a tract that his father had sent him. Within a few months, he was on a plane to Yugoslavia, embarking on his own pilgrimage. While in Medjugorje, Salazar was interviewed by a local priest. At long last, the former champion acknowledged his pain and emptiness.

He told the priest he was once presented with a wreath of genuine green laurels after winning a marathon. "My father took it with him and preserved it as a memento in a safe place," he said. "Several months later, this beautiful wreath, which marked a great victory, had lost its entire beauty.

"For sport is not simply a discipline," Salazar continued. "Sport can become a compulsion, another god. So long as one depends on it, he forgets everything else. If he loses this god, he has nothing else."

He flew home to the United States, sold his restaurant, moved his family to Portland, and went to work for Nike. A doctor finally determined that his chronic health problems were largely due to his overheating at the '82 Boston Marathon. The doctor prescribed Prozac, which resolved the worst symptoms of the pernicious strain of exercise-induced asthma and lifted Salazar's decade-long depression.

At age 34, he resumed training. In May of 1994, Salazar won the 54-mile Comrades Marathon in South Africa. Soon afterward, with nothing left to prove, he retired from competitive distance running, and began to coach.

DICK BEARDSLEY STILL COULDN'T feel his legs. Mile 24 had passed, so his one-more-mile scheme seemed to be working.

He kept watching Salazar's shadow. Suddenly, it loomed huge on the asphalt. Beardsley wondered if he was hallucinating. But it was the press bus roaring past to the finish line. The crowds were so thick that the bus had to travel the same line as the runners. As the bus went past, its mirror clipped Beardsley on the shoulder. Beardsley punched the bus in frustration. Then it was gone.

By the 25th mile, Beardsley didn't need to look for the shadow anymore. They had been running together their whole lives. He felt Salazar's presence more palpably than he did his own ruined legs. My God, he thought, one more mile, and I'm going to win this thing.

A half mile to go. Continuing to move in a disembodied, dreamlike cloud, Beardsley flashed on his father. For his high school graduation present, his father had given him an IOU plane ticket, good one day for a trip to the Boston Marathon. Tears started to well up. Beardsley told himself to cut it out, get into this, attend to business.

Beardsley tried one last surge, but as he bore down, a shout of pain arose from his right hamstring. The leg turned to rubber. You could see the knotted muscle bulging.

Salazar blew past him. This was wrong on every conceivable level.

Then the motorcycle cops roared past, following Salazar, forming a phalanx around the new leader. The motorcycles massed together and for the first time all day, Dick Beardsley lost sight of his opponent.

ON THE MORNING OF OCTOBER 1, 1996, Dick Beardsley attempted to fill a forged prescription at the Wal-Mart pharmacy in Detroit Lakes, just as he'd done scores of times over the last few years. The pharmacist was a fishing buddy. They always kidded around when Beardsley came in for his pills. But on this day, the pharmacist wouldn't make eye contact. Beardsley knew right away that he was in trouble. He did not flee, and he did not dissemble. He was booked on felony narcotics charges. His shocking arrest made headlines across the country.

Beardsley avoided a prison sentence, but he hardly escaped punishment. He underwent a long, harrowing detox and treatment that entailed methadone, lengthy stays in psychiatric wards, and rigid adherence to a 12-step program. Mary and Andy, Dick and Mary's son, stood by him, as did his friends in Detroit Lakes and the national running community. Through excruciating work—and the dispensation of grace—Beardsley regained his health, the trust of his family, his business, his public speaking career, and his sport.

In 2002, he ran five marathons, and six more the following year, with a postaccident personal record of 2:45:58 at the Toronto Marathon in October 2003. Each September, he puts on a popular half-marathon in Detroit Lakes. In 2003, the special guest at the race was Beardsley's good friend Alberto Salazar.

JUST WHEN BEARDSLEY THOUGHT nothing more could possibly go wrong, something did. A moment after losing sight of Salazar with less than a mile to go, he stepped in a pothole. That tore it, he thought; the best he could do now was crawl in. But somehow, instead of worsening the pain, stepping in the pothole stretched out the hamstring, straightening out the knot.

Beardsley started to sprint. He put his head down and pumped his arms. He found another gear. He felt like angels were lifting him up. A hard right turn onto Hereford Street. He caught a glimpse of Salazar, like a glimpse of the Pope in a motorcade, 20 yards ahead, then put his head down again.

At the top of the hill there was a hard left turn before the final straightaway. Salazar and the motorcycles made that turn and the crowd at the finish line went wild, screaming in their hometown boy.

Beardsley had to weave his way through the motorcycles. The cops thought he was finished, but here he was back from the dead. They looked pie-faced and astonished as he pushed past them.

Salazar glanced back over this shoulder, also thinking that Beardsley was gone. But instead he was right there, on his shoulder, bearing down on him. Salazar's eyes grew as big as headlights. He turned to the finish line, the last hundred yards, with Beardsley in hell-hound pursuit.

Up in the TV booth above the finish line, Squires kept screaming, "Dickie! Dickie! Dickie!"

It was all clear to Salazar. There was nothing else to consider but the finish line up ahead, somewhere in that insane jumble of people and police barriers and motorcycles. The fact that he did not lose was as ineluctable as a law of physics.

Hail Mary, full of grace. The pain and the jumble and a dry-ice cold all over. My God, Dick Beardsley was tough, but Alberto Salazar did not lose.

THE CAFÉ AT NIKE'S MIA HAMM BUILDING is just about deserted. Alberto Salazar's quick lunch break has turned into a two-hour retrospective of his life and career—just a few minutes less than it once took him to run a marathon.

Finally, Salazar rises from the table. In the lobby, before riding the elevator up to his office, he says, "At the time of the Boston Marathon, I didn't know Dick very well. And to be honest, for a long time after it, I sort of resented him. Well, that passed, like a lot of my stuff passed." He gives a terse shake of his head.

"Then in 2002, the Boston Marathon brought us back for the 20th anniversary of our race. We got to know each other. Now, among all the guys I ran with or against, Dick might be the one I feel closest to. I'll pick up the phone every few months and give him a call. I think he and I have a special bond. All that he's gone through . . . I'm not saying I can understand it, but maybe I can come close.

"We both give a lot of talks, to all kinds of groups, all over the country," Salazar continues. "Sooner or later, someone always asks about the '82 Boston. I don't mind—I like talking about it, and so does Dick. That's because we never discuss the race in terms of running a 2:08, or beating the other guy. It took us both a long, long time, but we finally realized that that's not what the marathon is really about. It's not what it's about at all."

"AFTER THE RACE, people came up to me and said, 'Gosh, Dick, if you hadn't had to fight through all those police motorcycles, you might have won,'" Beardsley recalls for his audience at the Victoria Marathon. "But I don't look at it that way. I ran the race of my life, 2:08:53. Alberto happened to run 2 seconds faster. All I know for certain is that I left everything I had out on that course. I didn't give an inch. Neither did Alberto. The way I look at it, there were two winners that day."

The crowd erupts in applause, as if they were at the finish line at Boston. Beardsley lets the cheers wash over him for a moment, then holds his hands up for quiet.

"Tomorrow, at your marathon, you're going to give it your all," he says. "When it's over, you can look back on a job well done. You'll be able to relax. You'll be finished.

"Well, the race that I'm running now, I can never relax, never be finished," Beardsley goes on. "The day I say that I've got my addiction beat, I'll be in greater danger than when my leg got caught in that power take-off. I can't let that day come. I just celebrated my seventh year of sobriety. These have been the seven hardest, and the seven most wonderful, years of my life. Every morning I feel like I'm getting up to run the Boston Marathon all over again."

AFTER THE FALL

BY STEVE FRIEDMAN

Think you know the story of Zola Budd?
Think again. Even if you remember how the barefoot
prodigy broke world records, became a symbol of
South Africa's oppression, and was blamed for
Mary Decker's Olympic nightmare, her story has more
heartbreak, more hard-fought redemption,
and considerably more weirdness than the legend.

OCTOBER 2009

LAST AUTUMN, at a pretty clearing nestled 3,333 feet above sea level in North Carolina's Blue Ridge Mountains, 194 female collegiate distance runners gathered to run a 5000-meter cross-country race.

Many were tall and slim, rangy and loose-limbed in the way of college-age distance runners. They came from North Carolina State and Clemson and Davidson and Miami and other colleges and universities, and it's a safe bet that no matter what burdens any of them quietly carried—anxiety about grades, boyfriend troubles, or any number of less specific but no less real woes—none had ever faced the combination of worldwide shame and personal loss that had battered the middle-aged woman in their midst.

She was neither tall nor slim nor rangy. She was 42, brown as a walnut, slightly thick in the middle. When the race started, she jumped in front. The young runners knew this was an open race, that oddballs could run if they wanted. But what was the runner in front thinking? Maybe she wanted to feel the sensation of leading a race. Maybe she would quit after a few hundred yards, then limp back to her grandkids and tell them about the day she led some real runners. Maybe she used to lead races, back in her day.

Some of the coaches looked at each other. She had a nice stride—there was power to it, and precision. She wasn't just a weekend jogger out for a laugh. The coaches could tell that, even if some of the young runners could not. She kept the lead even after a quarter mile. More coaches watched her, and for at least one of them, and maybe more, who beheld her curly hair, and her speed, and the way she had that little hitch in her style—elbows slightly too high, a little too wide—there was something familiar.

Her coach had told her to take it easy, that she didn't have to lead from the beginning. He had warned her against going out too fast. He had warned her that a gigantic hill sat in the middle of the course, and that if she went out too fast, the hill might swallow her. Now more coaches were looking at her, a middle-aged woman with legs like pistons and elbows flying. What they saw didn't make sense. She was decimating their college athletes. She ran the first mile of the race in 5:18.

No slightly thick, middle-aged jogger could maintain that kind of pace. She was slowing down. And now the giant hill in the middle of the course was looming. And the young athletes were tracking the sun-cured, curly haired rabbit down. They were clear-eyed, long-limbed, remorseless. They were on the big hill now, and they had caught up to her and they were going to pass her. Her coach couldn't help it. She had ignored his advice. Still, he couldn't help it. So Jeff Jacobs yelled. "Go, Zola!"

"Zola?" another coach asked, and stared at the runner. Other coaches stared, too. Zola? It was impossible.

Mention the name Zola Budd to the casual track fan and you'll likely get one (or all) of three associations: Barefoot. South African. Tripped Mary Decker. Those were the boldest brush strokes of her narrative, and they continue to be. But the legend of Zola Budd is, like all legends, simple and moving and incomplete. It is made of half truths, exaggerations, and outright lies. She did run barefoot—but so did everyone else where she grew up. She did refrain from speaking out against great and terrible injustice—but so did a lot of other people older and wiser. She did suffer stunning setbacks and tragic losses, but much of her misfortune was worse than people knew, the losses more complicated and painful than most imagined.

A lot of people thought she had disappeared and stopped running for good. But here she was.

"Go, Zola!" Jacobs yelled, and another coach took up the cry, then another. Was it nostalgia or a belated and overdue recognition of grit's enduring majesty? Here she was, doing what she had always done, even when no one was watching. Through all the fragile triumphs and shifting tribulations of Zola Budd's life—some well known, some known not at all—only one thing remained immutable:

running. Once she ran to connect with someone she loved. Then she ran to be alone. Running brought her international fame and then worldwide scorn, and then it brought her something few might suspect.

"Go, Zola, go!" The young runners closed again. Certainly they could hear the yells. What the hell was a Zola? It didn't matter. They had time, and nature and physics, on their side. They had young legs. They had grit themselves. They would show this middle-aged mom what racing was all about. They reeled her in, and she pumped harder, faster, and they reeled her in again. There was a long way to go.

Running had been fun for the curly haired athlete once, a long time ago, and then it had saved her when she needed saving most, and then it had almost destroyed her—all before she had even reached adulthood. Why was she running now? What was she running from? Or toward?

"Go, Zola!" the coaches yelled. "Go, Zola, go."

FRANK BUDD AND HENDRINA Wilhelmina de Swardt, whom everyone called Tossie, had five children before Zola. Their third-born child, Frank Jr., died of a viral infection when he was just 11 months old. When Zola was born six years later, Tossie was in labor for three days and received 13 pints of blood.

"The nurses told me the kid's a stayer," Frank, always good for a quote, would tell reporters years later, before things got ugly.

When Zola was young, her father was busy working at the printing plant his father, an English immigrant, had founded—and Tossie was sickly. The oldest of the Budd children, Jenny, became the toddler's caretaker. Jenny was 11 when her baby sister was born and she read to her often. Their favorite was *Jock of the Bushveld*. It's the true tale of a Staffordshire bull terrier, the runt of the litter who is saved from drowning by his owner and repays the favor by developing into a courageous and noble champion. When Zola started talking, according to family stories, Jenny was the first person she called "mom."

Zola was skinny and short and terrible at swimming and team sports, but Jenny liked running, so when Zola got to be old enough, she ran, too. They ran over the hills surrounding Bloemfontein, the South African city of 500,000 where they lived. The city sits at 4,500 feet, and when they ran in the morning, the air was chilly and clear. They ran barefoot, because all children in rural South Africa ran barefoot. They ran for fun. And they ran for something Zola would lose and not find again until decades later.

Then she got fast, and once the world discovered Zola and reporters started calling her things like "a prodigy among prodigies" and a "barefoot, waiflike child champion," running was no longer about fun. Once the skinny, undersized adolescent became a champion, and then a symbol, and then a target of the world's righteous wrath—at an age when other kids are entering college—running would be about everything but fun. Things were so much simpler when Zola was just a little girl, running barefoot through the hills with the big sister she idolized.

Later, there would be tales that Zola developed her speed racing ostriches, that her greedy father pushed her until she broke. Like many of the stories that swirled around her, they were half-truths. There were ostriches on the family property, more a large menagerie than farm, but she never raced them. And perhaps her father did push her—he saw how fast she was and got her a coach—but no one pushed her as much as she pushed herself.

It was a happy childhood. In addition to the ostriches, there were cows and ducks and geese. There were snow-white chickens her father bred and sold and a water-pumping windmill. There was a family Doberman named Dobie. There were mud fights in the summer, and in the winter, Zola and her brothers and sisters would build bonfires and stuff firecrackers into glass bottles, then light them, throw them, and watch them explode in the air. But Frank and Tossie didn't get along, and the shadow of little Frank's death seemed to always hover over the family. There were photographs of the missing baby all over the house, and every year during holidays, and on little Frank's birthday, Tossie grew quieter and sadder. For Zola, it was a childhood filled with mysterious woe and delirious joy. It was a normal childhood.

Zola's coach got her running more. Jenny became a nurse and wasn't around as much. She worked the night shift and she would come home just as the family was having breakfast. She would have a piece of cake or pie—Jenny always had a sweet tooth—and then she would go to sleep as Zola went off to school. When Zola needed to talk to someone, though, Jenny was always there.

Zola was fast, but not that fast. When she was 13, in a local 4-K, running as hard as she could, she came in a distant second. By the time she crossed the finish line, the winner was in her track suit, cooling down. Zola didn't like losing. But she had the rest of her life. Besides, it wasn't as if she was going to run for a living. There was school. There were her friends. And there was Jenny. All part of a normal childhood, which ended in 1980.

Jenny, then 25, had been in the hospital for a few weeks, being treated for melanoma. Zola was not allowed to visit. She was only 14, and Tossie knew how her youngest felt about Jenny. So Zola stayed home while doctors treated Jenny. Zola knew Jenny was sick, but she didn't know how sick.

Cara Budd, then 18, came into Zola's room at 4 a.m. on September 9. (Coincidently, it was Tossie's birthday.) Cara woke her little sister and told her the news. Jenny was gone.

Zola didn't cry or scream. She had always been quiet, had always kept her grief, and her joy, to herself. The only person she had really shared her feelings with was Jenny.

No one in the family talked about Jenny's death. A family that had never talked about its losses didn't talk about this loss. Zola? Zola ran harder than she had run before. She would get up at 4:45 and run for 30 to 45 minutes. She attended school till 1:30, then went home and did her homework, then she would run some more from 5 till 7. Frank and Tossie and their children just tried to carry on. There were four kids now: Estelle, who was 23, the twins, Cara and Quintus, and Zola. They had lost a baby and survived. And now they had lost Jenny. They would survive that, too. Zola? There was no one for Zola to talk to about Jenny's death, or her life, or how she was feeling. She ran harder.

That winter, she entered the same local 4-K she had lost the year before. This time she won.

She ran harder and still the pain of Jenny's loss stayed with her.

The next year, she won the South African junior championships at 800 meters, and the year after that, the South African national championships at 1500 and 3000 meters. She was still in high school and her normal childhood was just a blurry story, one that would be embellished and twisted and disfigured the more it receded into the past. A few years after Jenny's death, she ran 5000 meters in 15:01.83, faster than any woman had ever run it before, and life would never be normal for Zola again. She didn't know it, though. She didn't know the terrible places running would take her.

When she set the mark in the 5000 meters, she says, "that's when I realized, 'Hey, I'm not too bad.'"

She wasn't the only one.

JOHN BRYANT WAS A RUNNER, a writer, and the man in charge of the features department at London's *Daily Mail*. So in 1983, when he pored over some race results "lurking in the small print of *Runner's World*" and saw Zola's time, his response was akin to that of a geologist eyeballing a ribbon of diamonds in a fetid swamp. Impossible, ridiculous, too good to be true, an invitation to a Fleet Street sportswriter's doomed-to-be-dashed dreams. Absurd—but worth checking out.

"If the results were to be believed," Bryant would write 25 years later, "there was a teenage girl, running without shoes, at altitude, up against domestic opposition, who was threatening to break world records." (Budd's 5000-meter mark wasn't ratified because it had been set in a race in South Africa, then banned from international competition due to its apartheid policies.)

What Bryant didn't write: Budd was white. The racial angle, combined with the fact that Budd was South African, made the story irresistible. That the Olympics were coming up later that year and that South Africa was banned from participating set in motion a chain of events that changed Budd forever.

Bryant dispatched a reporter to Bloemfontein. Other reporters were there, too. They found the shy schoolgirl, watched her glide over the hills, elbows a little high and a little wide, saw pictures of British middle-distance superstars Sebastian Coe and Steve Ovett next to her pillow and above her bed, a huge poster of America's track sweetheart, Mary Decker (whose 5000-meter record Budd had bested by nearly seven seconds).

She was only 5'2" and 92 pounds, but already she was larger than life. The reporters wrote about Budd's parrot, who could swear in Sotho, a regional dialect. They wrote about Budd's speed, about the impalas and springbok in the city's game park who stared at the teen as she ran in the dawn's chill. Reporters didn't dig into Jenny's death or Frank and Tossie's rocky relationship. They didn't examine the crucible of grief in which Budd's speed had annealed.

At least one journalist, though, worried about the young runner. Kenny Moore, then with *Sports Illustrated*, described Budd's failed 1984 attempt to break the world record in the 3000 meters, at a race near Cape Town. After the setback, he wrote, "As photographers paced and growled outside, Zola sat hunched in a corner of the stadium offices, like a frightened fawn. If a true perfectionist is measured by how crushing even his or her perceived failure can be, Zola Budd is an esteemed member of the club. One wishes for her always to have loving, soothing people around."

Bryant's newspaper offered the Budd family £100,000 (then about $142,000) in exchange for exclusive rights to Budd's life story. The paper also promised to fast-track the teenager so that she would receive a British passport. That would allow her to run in the Olympics. (Budd could qualify because of her grandfather's British birth. It also helped that her father's business wasn't doing so well, and, as Bryant later wrote, that one of Frank Budd's two great life ambitions was to retire with £1 million in the bank. The other was to have tea with the queen of England.)

There were demonstrations when she arrived in England. People booed her. People shouted insults. She was a white South African, a privileged teenager from a racist nation, using a technicality to pursue nakedly personal ambition.

Few knew about Jenny, how running had once been Zola's way of spending time with her sister and then had become Zola's way of mourning her. Few knew of her father's failing business. She had never told anyone that. She had never been good at explaining herself. And she wasn't any good at it now.

"She was such a shy and introverted person," says Cornelia Burki, a South Africa–born distance runner. Burki, who had moved to Switzerland in 1973 and represented that country in the 1980, 1984, and 1988 Olympics, befriended Budd, 13 years her junior, at the race in South Africa where Budd set the world record at 5000 meters. She knew how Budd reacted to attention, how she shrank into herself. "All she wanted was to run," Burki says, "and to run fast."

But the world wanted something else. At her first race in England, the *Daily Mail* held a press conference beforehand and pumped in the sound track from *Chariots of Fire*. The BBC televised the 3000-meter event, which Budd won in 9:02.06. That single effort was fast enough to qualify her for the Olympic Games. A columnist for the *Mail* called Budd the "hottest property in world athletics." The *Daily Mail*'s chief competitor did not have access to the hot property. That newspaper ran a banner headline on its front page: ZOLA, GO HOME!

"To the world," a *New York Times* reporter wrote in 2008, "Budd was a remorseless symbol of South Africa's segregationist policies. To the *Daily Mail*, she was a circulation windfall."

And to the girl? "Until I got to London in 1984, I never knew Nelson Mandela existed," she told a reporter in 2002. "I was brought up ignorant of what was going on. All I knew was the white side expressed in South African newspapers—that if we had no apartheid, our whole economy would collapse. Only much later did I realize I'd been lied to by the state."

She wasn't a racist any more than any 18-year-old citizen of an apartheid nation is a racist. She wasn't an opportunist any more than any fiercely competitive champion is an opportunist. But was she a champion?

She captured the English national championships at 1500 meters. Later the same year, in London, she set a world record of 5:33.15 in the 2000 meters. It was an odd distance, rarely run. But it inspired a British journalist to articulate something a lot of other people were feeling.

"The message will now be flashed around the world," exclaimed a BBC reporter after the race. "Zola Budd is no myth."

NO MYTH, PERHAPS. But what a story! "The legs of an antelope," one reporter wrote later, with the enthusiasm and penchant for empurpled prose Budd seemed to inspire among the ink-stained, "the face of an angel and the luck of a leper."

She was a barefoot teenager, an international villain, the poor little swift girl. The best part? She would be competing in the 1984 Los Angeles Olympics against her idol, a former phenom herself, another runner who drove writers to breathless, pulpy heights.

Pig-tailed and weighing 89 pounds, Mary Teresa Decker, aka "Little Mary Decker," burst onto the international track scene in 1973, when, at just 14, she won a U.S.-Soviet race in Minsk. Over the next decade, she'd set world records at every distance between 800 meters and 10,000 meters. She was pretty. She was white. And she was American. But she had never run in the Olympics. An injury had kept her from the 1976 Games. The U.S. boycott prevented her from running in 1980.

A made-to-order archrivalry. Mop-topped schoolgirl versus America's sweetheart. The onetime wunderkind's last chance at Olympic gold; the only thing standing in her way, a skinny kid who had once slept beneath her poster. Another irresistible tale—and like all the fictions surrounding Zola Budd, it left out a lot.

For one thing, Budd was wary about Romania's Maricica Puica, the reigning world cross-country champion. For another, Budd had strained her hamstring training four days earlier, during a speed workout, and knew she wasn't at full strength. Finally, there was the ever-quotable, ever-ambitious Frank.

Zola was making lots of money now—from the newspaper deal, from fees for showing up at races, from pending endorsement deals. Frank was taking a huge chunk and wanted more. Zola told her father to knock it off, to let her be. Frank loved England, loved the high life. He was also harboring a secret that would later provide more tabloid headlines. Tossie, who had been incapable of comforting her youngest daughter when Jenny died, was doing her best now— she cared not a bit how fast Zola ran, nor whether she ran at all—but she longed for the quiet of Bloemfontein. Frank and Tossie's relationship, never placid, grew more turbulent. And two weeks before the Olympics, Zola told her dad he couldn't come to Los Angeles to watch her run. She was sick of his moneygrubbing, tired of his meddling, weary of the drama. So Frank stayed in England, stewing, while Zola and her mom flew to Los Angeles. And shortly after, Frank stopped talking to either his daughter or his wife.

The Olympic narrative was Decker versus Budd. The reality was a lonely, miserable teenager who knew too much. "Emotionally," Budd says, "I was upset, away from home, missed my family, by myself. It wasn't the greatest time of my life, to be honest. I thought, Just get in this Olympics and get it over with."

In the highly anticipated 3000-meter final, Decker set the pace, followed closely by Puica, Budd, and England's Wendy Sly. When the pace slowed slightly about 1600 meters into the race, Budd picked it up, running wide of Decker, then, as she passed her, cut back toward the inside to take the lead. Decker bumped Budd's left foot with her right thigh, knocking her off balance. Budd kept running, and Decker stayed close, clipping Budd's calf with her right shoe. There was contact a third time and Decker fell, ripping the number right off Budd's back. Budd kept running.

Boos rained down from the stands. Later, people would suggest Budd had pulled a dirty move, trying to cut off Decker and her other competitors. Others would say the maneuver showed the teenager's relative inexperience in world events.

It wasn't a dirty move. In fact, when a runner moves in front, it is incumbent on trailing racers to avoid contact. (Ironically, Budd says she made the move to get out of harm's way. "If you're running barefoot," she says, "it's best to be last or in front.")

The Coliseum echoed with more boos.

"I saw what happened," says Burki, who finished fifth in the race. "I saw Mary pushed Zola from the back. Zola overtook Mary and Mary didn't want to give that position in front. Mary ran into Zola from the back . . . As she fell down, she pushed Zola."

Budd pumped her elbows, kept running. She still didn't think she'd win—she says that she suspected Puica would soon pass her. But the full impact of the situation didn't hit her until she'd completed another lap and saw Decker stretched out on the ground, wailing. Puica and Sly passed Budd, but she passed them back. Then, she says, she started hearing the jeers and boos. The runners passed Budd again. Then another runner passed her. Then another. And another. Budd finished seventh, looking miserable. "The main concern was if I win a medal," Budd says, "I'd have to stand on the winner's podium, and I didn't want to do that."

In the tunnel, right after the event ended, Budd saw Decker sitting down and approached her. She was sorry about the way things had turned out. She apologized to her idol.

"Get out of here!" Decker spat. "I won't talk to you."

Burki saw that, too. "Mary was sitting there crying. Zola was walking in front of me, apologizing. Mary was screaming at her; I'll never forget that. Zola, being such a shy person, her shoulders dropped. It could have happened in any race, and it wasn't Zola's fault, but the blame was on her. For any young girl to cope with that, that was very difficult."

Later, at a press conference, Decker blamed Budd.

Officials disqualified her from the race (and an hour later, after reviewing the videotape, rescinded the disqualification). She skipped the press conference, boarded the bus carrying British Olympic athletes. In one seat was a young woman, weeping.

Budd had always been polite. "Why are you crying?" she asked the woman.

"Because of what they did to you," the young athlete told the runner.

A quarter century later, Budd still recalls the moment. "That was one of the nicest things anyone has ever done for me."

Budd's coach picked her up and took her to meet her mother. Budd had taken down America's Sweetheart. She had sidestepped sanctions against her native country—that amounted to cheating, said some. So many rich but false narratives about the young girl, and the only one who cared nothing about any of them was the person who cared most about her.

"It didn't matter to her that I didn't win a medal," Budd remembers. "She was just glad and happy that I was with her again, that we could be together." They stayed in her coach's suite at a local hotel. It was there that they received a telephone call from the manager of the British women's Olympic track team. She was calling to pass on the news that there had been threats that Budd was going to be shot. Two police cars were on their way. When they showed up, the officers had submachine guns.

"They picked me up at the hotel and drove me and Mom to the airport, right onto the tarmac, and watched as we got onto the plane. It was like a movie."

"I HAVE WANTED TO WRITE YOU for a long time . . ." Decker wrote to Budd in December 1984. "I simply want to apologize to you for hurting your feelings at the Olympics . . . It was a very hard moment for me emotionally and I reacted in an emotional manner. The next time we meet I would like to shake your hand and let everything that has happened be put behind us. Who knows? Sometimes even the fiercest competitors become friends."

Publicly, though, Decker was not quite so soft. "I don't feel that I have any reason to apologize," Decker told a reporter in January 1985. "I was wronged, like anyone else in that situation."

When she was a child and had endured her greatest loss, Budd ran harder. She did the same thing now, in the wake of Olympic infamy. Budd won world cross-county championships in 1985 and 1986, set world records in the 5000 and indoor 3000. But her parents divorced in 1986, and then she had absolutely no contact with her father. He had another life now. She ran harder. But what had once, a long time ago, provided Budd a refuge from grief now provided her detractors an opportunity to attack.

Well-meaning people asked her to speak out against apartheid. Movement leaders demanded she speak out. Why didn't she renounce her country's racist policies? She was naive, that was indisputable. She was also stubborn.

"My attitude is that, as a sportswoman, I should have the right to pursue my chosen discipline in peace," she wrote in her autobiography, published in 1989. "Seb Coe does not get asked to denounce Soviet expansionism; Carl Lewis is not required to express his view on the Contra arms scandal. But I was not afforded that courtesy and it became a matter of principle for me not to give those who were intent on discrediting me the satisfaction of hearing me say what they most wanted to hear."

But now, on her terms, she would speak her piece. She wrote in the same book: "The Bible says men are born equal before God. I can't reconcile segregation along racial lines with the words of the Bible. As a Christian, I find apartheid intolerable."

That was a nice sentiment, but for many, too little, too late. In April 1988, the International Amateur Athletic Federation (IAAF) told the British Amateur Athletic Board (BAAB) that it should ban Budd from competition because she had appeared at—but not competed in—a road race in South Africa.

She had suffered insults and accusations for years. Why does a runner, plagued for miles and years by a creaky knee, or a pebble in her shoe, or an aching tendon, finally quit? Is it a new pain, or just too much of the same?

A doctor examined her in London and declared her "a pitiful sight, prone to bouts of crying and deep depressions . . . [with] all the clinical signs of anxiety." She decided to fly back to South Africa, to Bloemfontein. She told the press back home, "I have been made to feel like a criminal. I have been continuously hounded, and I can't take it anymore."

Back in Bloemfontein, away from the angry eyes of the world, she met a man, Michael Pieterse, the son of a wealthy businessman and co-owner of a local liquor store. They married on April 15, 1989. Zola invited her estranged father to the wedding (she had reached out to him once before, but he had maintained his silence). She asked her brother, Quintus, to give her away at the ceremony. When Frank heard that, he told his son that if he accompanied Zola, Quintus would be written out of his father's will. Zola promptly disinvited her father to her wedding, which prompted him to tell a reporter, "I no longer have a daughter called Zola." (Pieterse's father walked Zola down the aisle.)

In his will, Frank Budd stated that neither Tossie nor Zola and her sisters should be allowed to attend his funeral, if he died before them.

Five months later, in September, Quintus discovered Frank Budd's bloody body at his house. He had been shot twice, by his own shotgun, and his pick-up truck and checkbook had been stolen. The next day, a 24-year-old man was arrested. He claimed that Budd had made a sexual advance, and that it had triggered the killing. (The killer was later convicted of theft and murder, but given only 12 years due to "extenuating circumstances.")

A murdered father who apparently had been leading a secret life. Worldwide enmity. She ran. In 1991, in her native country, she ran the second-fastest time in the world over 3000 meters. With repeal of apartheid and South Africa's return to the Olympics, Budd raced in the 3000 meters at the 1992 Games in Barcelona. She didn't qualify for the final. In 1993, she finished fourth at the World Cross-Country Championships.

And then, as far as the world was concerned, she disappeared. As far as the world was concerned, she stopped running.

ALL THE TEENAGERS were chasing her. She had grown up too fast, and now she was being chased by runners half her age.

The course wound over hills, at altitude. It must have seemed high to the girls who had been training at sea level. To a runner who remembered the chilly dawn of the African veld, it must have felt like home.

"Go Zola, go!"

Once reviled, once booed, the antiheroine of all sorts of compelling but not-quite-complete stories kept going. No one was booing now. People were cheering, yelling her name. She kept going and the young runners fell behind and she won the race in 17:58. Afterward, the coaches from the teams surrounded her. They wanted to meet the legend.

"They had heard about her," Jeff Jacobs said. "But who had ever met the real Zola Budd?"

THE LEGEND COMES TO THE DOOR of her Myrtle Beach, South Carolina, house barefoot, of course, in shorts and a T-shirt that says DOES NOT PLAY WELL WITH OTHERS and has a picture of Stewie, the cartoon baby from *Family Guy*. She walks a little bit bowlegged. She has agreed to meet because she has always been agreeable, even when she didn't understand what she was agreeing to. She says she's working on that.

She is finishing her dissertation to obtain her master's degree in counseling. She's also working as an assistant coach for Coastal Carolina University's women's track team, which allows her to travel with the team and compete in open events. The men's head track coach, Jeff Jacobs, coaches her. She says that people who have gone through pain can help others understand and endure pain. She says that long-distance runners are privy to a special relationship with pain and solitude and grace, and adds, "I doubt that sprinters have that."

She ran her first marathon in London in 2003, but dropped at 23 miles, depleted. She ran a marathon in Bloemfontein in 2008 and logged 3:10. Last year, she entered the New York City Marathon and ran 2:59:51. She's planning on racing a half-marathon by year's end and a marathon next year. In the meantime, she wants to compete on the masters circuit, "in as many local cross-country races and local 10-K and 5-K races as possible." But that's not the focus of her life. She had a baby girl in 1995 and twins, a boy and girl, in 1998, and she's just a mother, she says now, just a wife. Yes, she knows it's 25 years since she was blamed for destroying the dreams of America's Sweetheart. No, it wasn't her fault. Yes, she knows people are still curious about it. She is pleasant without being effusive, charming without being gushy.

She says that her accomplishments mean little, her disappointments even less. She smiles. It's a shy smile, almost an apologetic one. She doesn't want to push her kids. She knows what it's like to be pushed. She treasures the moments of her childhood when no one was pushing her, before she had discovered her gifts, before the world had discovered them and adored them and twisted them to its own purposes.

No, she says, she never quit running, just competing. She can't imagine not running. The time she loved it best was before anyone—even she—knew how fast she was.

"I never strived to be the best in the world," she says softly, still smiling, remembering those happy days. "I just ran every day. I just ran."

Her mother died four years ago, and that was hard, and sad, but it was good, too, because all of Tossie's children and grandchildren got to see her, got to say goodbye, to show her that she was beloved. Zola got to tell her mom how much she had always loved her, how much her support had meant, how when the world cared so much about how fast she ran and what country's colors she wore and whom she was competing against—about all the stories—it meant so much to have a mother who didn't care at all, who ignored the stories, who just cared about who Zola was.

It was so unlike Frank's death in 1989. Tossie and Zola had to comply with his will, so they couldn't attend the funeral. Plus, there were the ugly stories in the papers. That was hard, too, and sad, and there was nothing good about it.

Fatherless, motherless, Budd has run through it all, elbows a little too high, a little too wide, and most of the world didn't know, or care, and that made the running something better, something closer to what she had when she was young. Running helped her deal with her father's death, as it had helped her deal with all the people calling her names and telling her she was things she was not. It helped when she discovered that her husband was having an affair four years ago. The story of Zola Budd was resurrected. New banner headlines, at least in South Africa. New sordid details—the other woman had been a socialite and beauty pageant contestant nicknamed Pinkie. Michael had bought a house for her. She had called and threatened Zola. Zola says that Pinkie poisoned and killed one of her dogs.

She filed for divorce, and she told a reporter, when Michael denied that he had done anything wrong, "Why do all husbands deny it? I have no idea. But I have more than enough evidence that he is having an affair. More than enough."

But she had been through worse, and when Michael got rid of Pinkie, Zola and her husband reconciled.

Not that she has forgotten. "Marriage is like cycling," she says. (She has recently taken up mountain biking.) "There are only two types of cyclists, those who have fallen or those who are going to fall. Same with marriage, those who have had problems and those who are going to have problems."

For someone whose mere name serves as shorthand for international drama, she could not seem more placid, more accepting. "Running and other stuff passes away," she says. "It's old news. The legacy you leave for your kids, that lasts."

She still holds British and South African records, at junior and senior levels. Her name is in the lyrics of a song once popular in her homeland. The reliable, long-distance jitneys in her hometown are called Zola Budds or just Zolas.

She doesn't display any of her old medals. "They're in a box somewhere in South Africa, I think."

She says the happiest times of her life were when her children were born. Where do her running victories rank in her spectrum of life's happy moments? She barks a heavy laugh, as if that's the most ridiculous question she has ever entertained, in a lifetime of entertaining ridiculous questions. "They don't."

She wants her children to grow up doing whatever they want to do. Anything at all, as long as it makes them happy. "Well, artists are never happy, are they? But fulfilled, I want them to be fulfilled."

How does she think she'll be remembered? She laughs again, but this time it's an easy, light sound. "I have no idea. I never thought about that."

She doesn't mention her victory in the cross-country race. She doesn't talk a lot about running. Yes, she thinks she was treated unfairly, but it was a strange time and her country was doing terrible things. No, she's not a racist, and no one who knows her would ever think she was. No, she never became friends with Mary Decker, but they did make peace.

"Both of us have moved on and running isn't so important in our lives," she says. "We're both a bit more wise."

Which isn't to say that running isn't important at all to the champion. She might be placid, she might be serene, but she did hire a college coach to train her. She does compete against women half her age. The family received a two-year visa to live in the United States last year. Zola wanted to expose the kids to another country's educational system. But she also wanted to try the masters running circuit here. They chose Myrtle Beach because they wanted to be on the East Coast, which makes it easier to fly to their homeland, and because Michael loves golf, and there are more public golf courses in the Myrtle Beach area than almost anywhere else in the world. Zola does not play golf. "It's dangerous if I play golf," she says. "It's better for everyone if I don't play."

She doesn't watch sports on television. She does not watch the Olympics. She has watched her Olympic duel with Mary Decker only once, the day after it happened.

She wants to give her children what she once had as a child, before the world discovered her, before there was a story. She says she understands adolescents who cut themselves, "because physical pain can be better than emotional pain." She remembers a time before she was aware of any emotional pain, when she was just "that young kid who plays barefoot on the farm."

She talks about that kid a lot, about life on the farm, about the time when no one knew about her speed, when no one cared.

When she is asked about Jenny, she grows quiet for a moment. She remembers that her sister's favorite color was green. She remembers that Jenny had her own dog, a pinscher named Tossie (after her mother) who followed her everywhere, and she remembers Jenny's sweet tooth, and the way she would eat her pastry while the rest of the family sat down to breakfast, before she went upstairs to sleep.

She remembers Jenny reading to her, and running beside her. She remembers the story of the little runt, *Jock of the Bushveld*, and how he grew up to be a brave, beloved champion. She remembers how when Jenny died, Zola attacked the hills and trails with a vengeance she never knew she possessed.

"Her death made everything in my life, even eating and drinking, seem of secondary importance." Budd wrote in her autobiography. "Running was the easiest way to escape from the harsh reality of losing my sister because when I ran I didn't have to think about life or death ... There is no doubt that the loss of Jenny had a major effect on my running career. By escaping from her death I ran into world class ..."

"[The family] did not talk about her death a lot afterward," she wrote in a recent e-mail. "I started training a lot and that was it."

Jenny has been gone for 30 years, but at the moment it's as if she's in the next room, in front of one of her morning pastries, or in her bedroom, pulling her curtains closed, getting ready to sleep. Budd talks about her sister quietly, and matter-of-factly, and then she quietly and matter-of-factly weeps.

"If Jenny hadn't died," she says, "I probably would have become a nurse."

She talks about her father, too, and recounts the visit she made to his gravesite, where she made peace with him. She knows he suffered, too. She doesn't believe her father made any advances against his killer.

Asked about her father in 2002, she had told a reporter, "Back then South African society didn't accept homosexuals. It took a terrible toll on him." Today she says, "If he had been around now, he could have been more open about who he was."

The intimate details that the world knows about Frank Budd are largely due to Zola's fame. She knows that. She knows that his actions are part of the Zola Budd story. What she also knows—what the world doesn't know—is he was a good dad, before all the money and fame and fighting. So much of what the world knows about Zola Budd is the simple story, the one with cartoon villains and epic struggles and bright, bold lines dividing right and wrong. But things were always more complicated than that. Frank Budd was greedy and pushy, and that fit into a simple story, but he was other things, too. The world doesn't know that Frank Budd watched a cow chase his little 10-year-old girl and the family dog, Dobie, and that he remarked on how fast she was, before anyone else had, and that the two of them laughed and laughed at how afraid of the cow she had been. The world doesn't know that he constructed a little duck pond for his youngest child and that she would tell him stories about how she took care of the ducks, that she fed them just like he told her to, that she and her father loved each other and were happy once upon a time before the world discovered her gifts, before the gifts became so heavy. She sheds a tear for her dad, too.

Running was so much fun when she was just a child, then it became a release, and finally, a means to attain things she never wanted—money and political symbolism and international fame. It became so important. It became part of a larger narrative. And it wasn't her narrative.

And now, even though she still is intensely competitive, even though she sometimes runs too hard for her own good, she is preparing for a return to competition that may bring with it a lot of scrutiny that she never welcomed nor enjoyed, and it's okay, because she's got her balance about her now. She knows what's important. She knows what's hers.

She'll do her best in the upcoming marathons. She'll do well in the masters circuit, too. That's the plan. Truth be told, she plans to kick some serious American ass, not that she would ever say that. She might be shy and sensitive and misunderstood and have the face of an angel and all that. But she is still a champion.

But that's not why she's running. Not to win. That was never the main reason she ran. That was never the real story.

Most people don't think too much about why they run. They never have to, because running simply feels good and helps them. Zola Budd, though, has had to think about why she runs.

She runs not for medals or glory or to set anyone straight, either. Not to make anyone understand her. That never worked.

She runs for the thing that running once bestowed upon her, a long time ago, and that running almost snatched away. She is running to get it back.

"I run to be at peace," she says.

THE POWER
AND THE GLORY

BY MICHAEL PERRY

When Ryan Hall was in eighth grade,
God told him to run. A decade later, he was a
2:06 marathoner and an Olympic favorite.
His story is almost beyond belief.

SEPTEMBER 2008

RYAN HALL will be happy with second place.

In his prayers, he thinks of entering Heaven, and imagines running through the gates as if into a great stadium filled with people raising a joyful noise. He hopes to be just off the shoulder of the leader, but he won't attempt a late kick. "The goal of my life," he says, "is just to follow in the footsteps of Jesus as closely as I can."

At the risk of committing light blasphemy, let it be said the Son of God may want a new pair of shoes. Not only did Hall win the U.S. Olympic Marathon Trials, he was the fastest qualifier in American history, taming a tough New York City course in a Trials-record 2:09:02. It was only his second race at the distance; his first was the 2007 Flora London Marathon, where his 2:08:24 was the fastest debut by an American. Returning to London in 2008, he ran 2:06:17, breaking his own record for the fastest marathon ever run by an American-born citizen. Three marathons, three benchmarks. When Ryan Hall toes the starting line in Beijing, he will be operating at a level of possibility not seen since the days of Alberto Salazar.

Even so, it's hard to imagine a race that can supplant the memory of Hall's win at the Trials. It wasn't so much breaking the record as the galvanizing manner in which he broke it, dusting an all-star pack and covering the final miles less like a marathoner than an amped-up slugger circling the bases after a walk-off homer.

But then, in this glorious hour, the darkest news: 20 miles back, his friend and fellow competitor Ryan Shay had fallen dead. Just four months earlier, Hall's wife, Sara, had served as bridesmaid when their mutual friend Alicia Craig married Shay. All four were record-breaking distance runners with Olympic dreams.

A year later, of the four, only Ryan Hall is set to run beneath the rings. How will he approach the moment? The story will be variously framed: the athlete running for the memory of a fellow racer, the fallen friend, the grieving family; the underperformer who switched genres and scorched his way into history; the man caught in a dialectic in which his most transcendent moment is forever tethered to grim mortality.

Hall prefers another story—the only story, he says, the one that helps us understand why he might remain modest in triumph and strong in tragedy. He calls it the greatest story ever told.

IT'S SUNDAY MORNING, and Ryan Hall is late for church. This is not to imply that Hall is slothful. Quite the opposite. He rose at dawn. For a 15-mile run. Under normal circumstances he knocks that distance down with time to spare before services commence. But this morning he was running in the company of an NBC television crew, and they needed B-roll and interview footage. By the time it was in the can, the Summit Christian Fellowship church choir had taken hymnals in hand. They are currently in full throat, accompanied by an electric bass and a drummer on a trap set. The words to the hymns, superimposed over scenes of ocean waves and sunsets, are projected on two pull-down screens flanking the riser. As the verses flip by, the congregation—60 or so people seated in a room decorated with plastic ivy, artificial Christmas trees, and strings of white lights—sings along. As the last hymn prior to worship builds to a crescendo, two men stationed on opposite sides of the room fire handheld confetti cannons. The final notes of praise rise through a powdered rainbow tumbling down.

The church is located across from the Big Bear Disposal Site & Recycling Center. Big Bear Lake, California, is an enclave of the sort and size that operates at the tipping point between the American small town as defined by central casting (old-timers staking out well-worn counter seats at the Teddy Bear Restaurant) and a resort town developed to snag outsiders (Starbucks, faux Alpine lodges, a go-cart course). Set far away from the rest of the world in the San Bernardino Mountains (at roughly the same elevation as that crucible of marathoning, Kenya's Great Rift Valley), it can be fairly characterized as sleepy on an off-season Sunday morning, and anything but when the ski-booted masses descend at peak time. Today is one of the quiet Sundays. The spring sun has baked a pitchy scent from the needles fallen beneath the tall pines surrounding the church, and the pickups and minivans of the families within sit on the asphalt lot outside. The church building itself is a humble one-story structure painted pale green—you might miss what it is, should you fail to spot a Calvary's trio of small crosses planted near the entrance. There is another even smaller cross visible just below the peak of the roof. Before you see either of these, you will probably see the white banner tacked to the siding. In blue letters it reads, RUN, RYAN, RUN!

BIG BEAR LAKE IS OUT THERE, twinkling in the sun, penned in by a dam on one end, and by mountains to either side. If you drive up from San Bernardino, you'll want to dose on Dramamine for the switchbacks on Highway 18. The climb terminates in a fork at the dam where Highway 18 splits to run the south shore, Highway 38 the north. Toward the far end of the lake, a bridge called the Stansfield Cutoff reunites the roads, enclosing the water in a 15-mile loop. In a sense that loop is Ryan Hall's road to Damascus, where the Bible tells us the Christian-killer Saul of Tarsus pulled a spiritual U-turn and became the loyal apostle Paul. For purposes of conversion, the Lord knocked Saul flat and struck him blind. Happily in Hall's case, he settled for just tuckering the boy out some.

"In eighth grade I was kind of at a crossroads in my life," says Hall. You're about to roll your eyes, looking at this pure-faced blue-eyed 25-year-old with the blond hair, and then he smiles and adds, "I didn't realize it at the time, you know." Hall speaks in a southern California patois that, accurately or not, will remind a Midwesterner of surfboards. His sentences are heavily leavened with "like" and he will deploy "gnarly" as an adjective without irony. His gaze is considerate and thoughtful, and apparently incapable of guile. But do not think pushover—he emanates the steadfast resolve of the true believer. If by way of introduction you reveal that you do not believe as he believes, his countenance remains warm and open, but you will catch just a shade of the patient indulgence believers reserve for those yet a-wandering.

"My parents were strong Christians," he continues. "I definitely believed, but I wasn't really strongly pursuing my faith. I was playing baseball, basketball, football—I was into, like, the cool crowd at school. And then one day traveling down the mountain to a basketball game, I got this random—I describe it as a vision, but you could call it an idea, whatever—this thing pops into my mind where I am looking out at Big Bear Lake, and I think, well, it would be a great thing for me to try and run around that."

It's tough to put this in context now, what with the mind-bending marathon times in the books and Beijing right around the corner. But Hall wants you to understand that the power of the vision lay partially in the fact that he was not being asked to do something to which he seemed naturally inclined. "I never really had any interest in running. Like, in middle school, whenever they made us run the mile, I'd complain just like everyone else. But at that moment it became something that was very captivating . . . it really grabbed me."

By now, of course, the story about the kid who circumnavigated Big Bear Lake in basketball shoes has become central to the Ryan Hall legend. He ran the route with his father, Mickey. Mickey says they made one stop in 15 miles, and he knew already the boy had something special. The kid was worn out at the end, but back home while unlacing his shoes, Ryan says he too knew this was more than a one-off stunt. "At that point, the trajectory of my life completely changed. All of a sudden I stopped doing baseball, basketball, and football, and started running full time." And somewhere out on that loop, something else alchemized: "It was at that point that Jesus really became my best friend. That's when our relationship took off . . . and it was a direct result of him bringing running into my life."

At Summit Christian Fellowship, the people are praying. The highest profile congregant has yet to present—he is re-creating that famous day for the cameras—but the flock understands what might be keeping him. After all, they are the ones who hung the banner. They know: God told Ryan to run.

SURELY OUR FEELINGS regarding athletes who choose to bring their faith to the field reflect the state of our own souls. Fellow believers will likely rejoice at God's word made manifest in the form of peak performance; nonbelievers will at best dismiss the testimony, deride it at worst. Ryan Hall believes he was chosen by God to run for God. One of Hall's favorite Bible verses—the one he scribbled on the autographed poster just inside the door of the Teddy Bear Restaurant in Big Bear Lake—is from the book of Isaiah. Those who wait on the Lord, will run and not get tired. The Lord has taught Hall not to overlook that key word: wait. The divine plan doesn't always run parallel to mortal hopes and dreams.

Consider Ryan Hall's earthly father. Mickey Hall is trim but solid. He is sitting midway up the aisle at Summit Christian Fellowship, and the hand he drapes across his Bible could swing a big hammer easily. In fact, he grew up framing houses for his father. Mickey's father drove the crew hard. "Head down, butt up!" he would say. "If you're not in that position, you're not making money." By age 42, Mickey's dad had enough scratch to retire, and "Head down, butt up!" had become the family motto.

If ever a man had the makings of a stage father of the first degree, it would be Mickey Hall. Ultracompetitive ("Maybe what you would call overcompetitive . . .

I wouldn't let my grandmother beat me in a game of cards!"), drafted as a pitcher by the Baltimore Orioles in his first year of college, and given to obsessive use of a stopwatch (long before he was calling splits for Ryan on the track, Mickey would time the boy and his four siblings as they cut and split firewood), you might anticipate his reaction when he took his son for a run one day and discovered that his progeny was a prodigy.

You'd be wrong. "I tried to convince him to play baseball," Mickey says, laughing. "He could really throw!" But Ryan wanted to run. So Mickey stopped coaching baseball and started a track program (Big Bear had no track or cross-country team)—and began to deploy that stopwatch the way God intended.

Fraught waters, the whole father-as-coach thing. But Mickey has never forgotten the backstop his father built in the backyard when he was 11. "I would go out and throw half an hour every day at that thing," says Mickey, and he wound up getting his shot at the bigs. Butt up, head down, yes, but the marvelous thing, Mickey says, is that his dad always assigned work and play equal par. He put down the hammer and took the kids to the beach for volleyball. He taught them to surf and kicked Mickey loose of the construction crew so he could make baseball practice. When Ryan Hall tells the story of the firewood and the stopwatch, the smile on his face tells you the memory is less Dickens and more "can-do" Bobbsey Twins. And it drives him still.

GOD MAY CALL YOU to run, but that doesn't mean you're on the fast track. You're the man, God told Moses, then sent him off on a four-decade detour. So even in Hall's immediate and revelatory promise as a runner, his father saw the potential for trouble.

"As a tiny ninth-grader competing against juniors and seniors he ran 4:35 in the mile," says Mickey. "I never had to push him. If anything, when Susie and I had to discipline him, we'd threaten to take away his training time." Mickey spent more time riding the brakes than cracking the whip. "I was with him for every workout in high school, and my tendency is to go too hard. So when he would go too hard, I would say, 'Whoa, we're done,' and he'd say, 'No, Dad, I can do more,' and I'd say, 'I know you can—you're not.'"

Mickey Hall's fastball was clocking 90 miles per hour when his college coach asked him to pitch three innings of a preseason game. At the end of three, the score was tied zero–zero. The coach asked him to pitch one more. Still zero–zero. One more, said the coach. And back in he went, head down, butt up, inning after inning in a meaningless game, until the ninth, when his shoulder went *pop!* and the Orioles flew away forever.

Under his father's guidance, Ryan won four individual state titles in high school and ran a state-record time (4:02) for 1600 meters. The recruiters were circling, and after much prayer, Ryan felt God directing him to Stanford. God also decided it was time to give Ryan a little taste of Job. Before preseason camp even began, he suffered an iliotibial-band injury. "From the moment I started at Stanford, I was off my game," he says now. "I was struggling with school, I was struggling with my running . . . I'd wake up in the morning with this heavy burden feeling, like uhhhh, things are not what I had pictured." He slept poorly, ate poorly, and gained 10 pounds. In the absence of his father's governing hand and despite the advice of his college coach, he treated recovery runs as one more chance to hammer. Midway through his sophomore year, he was a bona fide flop. He abandoned Stanford for a quarter and returned home. He figured running the familiar roads would help him get things sorted. Help him recover the groove.

It turned out quite the opposite. "I got more depressed. I remember waking up in the morning, trying to go for a run this one day, it was snowing outside, and I just could not get myself out of bed. Went out, and was trying to, like, just do a short, easy run. And I jog, like, half a mile and I start walking. And I just walked home, 'cause my spirit was just crushed. Because I wasn't running well, I didn't see myself as having much worth."

This time there was no road-to-Damascus moment. No blinding revelation. Hall gave himself over to prayer and pondering. "I realized the only things that were going well in college were my relationship with my girlfriend and my relationship with the Lord," says Hall, who had begun dating champion miler Sara Bei and befriended a circle of like-minded believers through his involvement in the Stanford chapter of Athletes in Action. "I decided that God had called me to go to Stanford." He returned to the university. "I was no longer a runner who happens to be a Christian," he says. "I was a Christian who happens to run."

Things didn't instantly change. "I still had a subpar track season that year," says Hall, who cites the end of his 2004 Olympic dreams as a low point. "But I was happy. I knew I was where I was supposed to be, and finally got to a point were I really enjoyed my time up at Stanford." Before he graduated, in 2006, he'd won an NCAA championship at 5000 meters, led Stanford to a team cross-country title, and married Bei. Things were looking up.

TODAY AT Summit Christian Fellowship, the pastor isn't in the pulpit. He has given the microphone over to his wife and left for the parsonage, where he's washing lettuce and chopping chicken salad. It is Mother's Day, and at the end of service, the pastor and several male parishioners will serve a luncheon to honor the mothers in their midst—Ryan Hall's mother included. The Hall family work ethic and competitive genetics may be patrilineal, but it was Susie who led Mickey Hall—and thus the rest of the Hall family—to Jesus. Mickey was an atheist in flip-flops when he followed Susie to church one day. Took a while, but in the process of writing a college paper about why the Bible was hoo-hah, he wound up a believer. And when Susie began volunteering on behalf of disabled children, Mickey noticed. In fact, when you sort out the chronology, you discover that Mickey turned down cash from the Orioles before his injury. He had seen the joy in Susie's service, he says, and he was already doubting the little white ball could match that. Now he has been working 21 years as a special-education teacher, and if you want to see his face light up, cut the track talk and ask about those students of his.

Mickey Hall has watched friends thrive in the big leagues. But when he recounts his baseball stories, there is no trace of "I coulda been a contender." He revels in the telling. You look at him now worshipping beside the wife who showed him another way, and you see there is no room for regret in the joy. He is fond of quoting 1 Corinthians: "run the race in such a way that you might win." Compete with all your heart, he tells his children, Ryan included. "But don't make it bigger than it is—it's just a sport."

A woman makes her way to the front of the church. She has asked that the congregation pray over her. There is trouble on her face, tears coming down. From her modest podium, the pastor's wife calls on the Lord, and several parishioners close around the woman, some praying with a palm raised to heaven, others laying their hands on the petitioner. Somewhere amid the supplication, Ryan Hall quietly seats himself in the back row.

HALL DOESN'T TAKE missing church lightly, but with his training and travel, absenteeism has become an occupational hazard. This has led him to examine the life of Brother Lawrence, a 17th century Carmelite monk who taught that godly people should weave worship into work. "Brother Lawrence was one of the guys who pioneered that thought about doing every single little thing for the Lord and staying connected with him throughout the day in prayer," says Hall, who often listens to an audio version of the Bible while driving, or on his iPod while running. "Rather than study the Bible at some appointed hour, I try to make worship much more just a natural flow and part of my day," he says. "A big challenge for me is to pray without ceasing, as the Bible tells us. So I pray when I am out running. Or doing dishes. When my mind is wandering, I try and hone it back into praying. I'm not very good at it yet."

Brother Lawrence also preached Christlike humility and warned of the consequences of pride. How does Hall reconcile these lessons when his job requires crushing the competition? "There's obviously a gray area," he says. "You gotta have confidence. The question is, what are you putting your confidence in: your own ability? And what do you believe about your ability? Do you believe you've done something to deserve it? Or is it a gift? I believe I have a gift from God. But then I also have to train really, really hard. So I see it as being a good steward of the gift God's given me . . . it's my obligation to God to develop this talent the best I can. So, I try and make that my focus rather than wanting to beat people. Not that it's not fun to win, because it is . . .

"I think part of it, too, is just being content with whatever the Lord has for my life."

But whither motivation? If all outcomes—win, place, or no-show—are God's will, does Hall have permission to lose? "I don't know," says Hall, after some thought. "I don't have all my theology figured out. I don't know if God has someone in mind to win the Olympic Marathon either. Only one guy can win that race, and everyone in that race wants to win and it's their dream to win, so what does that mean for the rest of us who don't win? The 99.9 percent of us who will never get a gold medal in the Olympics? Does that mean that we're all failures, and that all the training we did our whole life building up to it was a waste? Definitely not."

In the course of her homily, the pastor's wife reveals that she will be traveling to Beijing to see Ryan run. She does not want to go to China, she says. She has been telling the Lord so. But the Lord does everything for a purpose, she says, and somewhere in China that purpose will be revealed. Hall listens impassively but attentively. Wearing khaki cargo shorts and an Asics T-shirt, he looks preternaturally fine-tuned, the way all athletes do when at rest among the schlubby rest of us. Every move is economical. His hand rests on his Bible, and his Bible rests across his right thigh. There is no dust on Ryan Hall's Bible. It is hardly tattered, but the gilding on the pages is scored and worn. When he opens it to follow the sermon, it falls open easily to reveal well-thumbed page corners and verses underlined in pen. This Bible is not a prop. You can see him turning to it again and again. When racing for Heaven, one must train to the finish.

"I don't think I have an exact point in my life when I accepted Christ," says Hall. "I can remember doing it—you know, as a kid—over and over again 'cause I was kind of afraid the first time didn't count or whatever. I wanted to make sure I was covered. What I have learned as I have gotten older is that it's such a daily thing. It's not a one-time decision and that seals the deal. It says in the Bible to work out your salvation daily with fear and trembling... it's a long journey and it's not like you instantly get to this holy status. I am very much still in process, as I think all Christians are. All people are, really... we're all still growing."

WHEN THE SERVICE CONCLUDES, everyone makes their way across the church parking lot to the parsonage, where tables have been set beneath the shade of the pine trees. Ryan sits next to his father, and the resemblance is strongest when the two men smile in unison. Their upper lips peel back to reveal a generous set of incisors, and you think of Gary Busey minus all the crazy.

Big Bear Lake has always turned out for ball games, not for track meets. In fact, when Hall won his state cross-country titles, he wasn't eligible for a letter because there was no team. Nowadays the posters all around town say RUN, RYAN, RUN! but when he began, the sight of a teen pounding out miles was unusual enough that some lowered their car windows to holler, "Run, Forrest, run!" When Hall and his parents relate these stories, amusement trumps animus. "There just weren't funds for a track team," says Mickey. "Besides, he was getting to do everything we wanted him to do without being on a team." Now, thanks to Ryan's high profile and the efforts of a local reporter who raced for Mickey in high school, Big Bear Lake has both track and cross-country teams, and Ryan has lent his support to the Lighthouse Project—a local organization dedicated to creating "child-honoring communities." Farther afield, Ryan and Sara are members of Team World Vision, a charity designed to promote self-sustaining communities in Africa. The couple speaks eagerly of the time when they will be able to serve as missionaries in Africa.

As Hall eats chicken salad with a plastic fork, fellow church members stop by to say hello. They call him "Ry" and happily tell visitors stories about the little boy they knew. The fellow across the table couldn't give two hoots about Beijing and keeps steering the conversation back to trout fishing and his half-wolf dog.

The utter lack of obsequiousness is a reminder that the Lord need not rain down disappointing splits and shinsplints to keep his servants humble. His touch can be ineffably deft. A man who has been studying Hall from a distance leans to his wife's ear and asks a question. "Yes!" she says, brightly. "He's going to the Olympics!" He leans to her ear again. "No, no," she says, still beaming. "In cross-country!"

YOU CAN ASK A MAN QUESTIONS. You can observe him about his daily business. You can even sit beside him in church. But in your heart you know it's presumptive to think your brief window can illuminate his soul. It is likewise tempting to posit a natural connection between spirituality and long-distance running. Even at the basest amateur level, running is predicated on periods of extended isolation, meditative rhythm, and regular access to the deoxygenated edge of failure (where the best revelations reside). Hall has been quoted saying that he saw the scarred body of Christ during the last two miles of the 2007 London Marathon. And yet, one shouldn't get carried away. When he speaks of his faith in his laid-back California accent, it's unlikely he'll knock you off your seat. Hall is neither fiery nor overly eloquent in defense of his faith. Remember his words to describe the moment God spoke to him at Big Bear Lake? "I describe it as a vision, but you could call it an idea, whatever . . ." Disarming but not disarmed, he acknowledges skepticism even as he remains resolute in faith.

"It's not my goal to convert anyone, you know," he says in a conversation at the Olympic Training Center in Chula Vista. "I think Jesus invited people to hear what he had to say. I think he told people what was in his heart. I want to be authentic with people . . . for me not to share why I run or what gets me through hard moments in races would be cheating them. But I'm not going to force someone to hear something they're not interested in hearing."

"Do the work, Ryan. Leave the rest to God." Over and over his father has told him this, but he would dearly love to win in Beijing. He is not impervious. After losing to Alan Webb in the mile at the 2001 Arcadia Invitational, he flung his shoes and went for a long run barefoot. After the Pac-10 Cross-Country Championships in Arizona, Mickey and Susie found him weeping in the bushes. Last year, prior to the Trials, he told his mother he had promised God he would have a better attitude whenever he didn't do well. "I told him, 'Expect to be tested on that,'" says Susie Hall, eyes twinkling. "And then he had three bad races leading up to the Trials. He needed to be humbled. People relate far more to the disappointment than the celebration." (True enough, but oh, that finish at the Trials.)

The day before we attended church in Big Bear Lake, I accompanied Hall on a pair of recovery runs at the Olympic Training Center. To keep things fair, I rode a bicycle lent to me by 5000-meter specialist Ian Dobson. Terrified I would veer in too close and be forever known as the man who ruptured the Achilles of the most promising U.S. marathoner in two decades, I followed at a safe distance, which is to say I watched Hall run from a perspective shared by 99 percent of his recent competitors. I was struck by the immaculate nature of his footfalls. Each heel came to earth perfectly square, with no hint of pronation. "His stride was gorgeous from the beginning," says Mickey Hall. "His legs would just flow." His torso, on the other hand, is held parsimoniously erect as if to provide the heart and lungs a stable work environment. The stiffness continues in the specific alignment of his thumbs, pointed forward from atop his fists. His elbows are held at right angles and sweep back and forth just above the iliac crest, crossing at the same plane every time. His left elbow wings out a tad—a teensy imperfection held over from an early habit of crossing his body with his arms. Mickey spotted this early and mostly cured it by tying Ryan's elbow to his side.

But Mickey is right: everything is extraneous to those legs. You can see them in footage from the homestretch of the Trials, turning over in a pinwheeling lope, each foot meeting the earth right on axis, then looping up and away to fly forward again. The legs are all business right to the finish, even as the arms begin to loosen, even as Hall's head begins to swivel to acknowledge the noise of the crowd. The closer he draws to the line, the more evident it is that this is a finish for the ages. Hall begins to gesticulate, pointing to the sky, raising his arms high, even slapping hands with the people crowding the course. At first it seems uncharacteristic based on what you know of Hall and his mellow Christian demeanor. Then you notice the blazing intensity of his eyes and the inclusiveness of his open arms, and you realize he is not exulting, but exhorting. He is not celebrating triumph over man but rather triumph in the Lord—in short, this is a man in rapture. Hall often refers to running in terms of sanctuary, and here he is now, Brother Lawrence in a singlet, twining work to worship, running 4:55 splits, praising God full tilt right until he breaks across the line and the only thing left to do is bow quietly down, the work all done, the victory won.

IT HAS BEEN A LONG DAY for the Hall family. After the church luncheon, the television crew and I return to their house for a final round of interviews. Susie spreads photo albums on the kitchen table (should you ever qualify for the Olympics, know that the picture of you wearing an Olympics sweatshirt, a diaper, and your sister's tap shoes will wind up on TV) and serves fresh-baked apple muffins as she runs around the house gathering mementos from Ryan's career. She has to dig around some. "We don't keep a shrine to Ryan," says Susie. "We have five children. We could fill the walls with his things, but we try to celebrate the gifts each of them have." Ryan and Mickey sit down together and talk for the cameras some, then do a father-son run for yet more B-roll. Finally Ryan—who has learned the lesson of rest and follows a strict regimen of icing, recovery, and massage—leaves for an appointment with his masseuse.

So now the final piece of gear is packed as sunlight slides through the pine trees at a flattening slant. In the living room, Mickey Hall cues up footage of Ryan's triumphant finish in the Trials. Susie and Ryan's grandmother Madeline join them, and for a while everyone just watches, eyes raised to the screen. Eventually, Susie speaks. "You know, for three days before every one of Ryan's races, Mickey fasts and prays. He prays that it will be a good race and a safe race." Up on the screen Ryan is surging for the finish, strong as a bolting deer, glorifying the Lord with each step. You think of Mickey, on his knees and hungry (so weak one time he fell and wound up in the ER), beseeching that same Lord that he might deliver every runner safe to the finish line. And yet we know full well watching the footage now, that even as Ryan Hall was pointing to the sky and the crowd was making a crazy joyful noise, his friend Ryan Shay was dead. The following night Mickey dined with Shay's father-in-law. "What do you say to someone who's lost their son?" he says, shaking his head. "What do you say?" The questions are not new, and hang in the air. God's mystery will be revealed, answer the believers; grim coincidence, say the nonbelievers.

Hall has at times gone out of his way to play down attempts by outsiders to over-personalize the tragedy by casting him and Shay as best friends, but in the month following the Trials, he and Sara quietly moved in with Alicia in Flagstaff, and Hall will tell you that he trains for the Olympics with Shay's memory a constant companion. It would be easy to nudge the narrative toward that end. To set the possibility of Ryan Hall ascending the center dais as Ryan Shay's spirit made visible. It could happen, and Hall will be thrilled if he runs to victory. But he knows first and foremost he must run to honor the Lord.

Ryan Hall's grandmother is suddenly at my elbow. Her face is troubled. All day she has been a sparkling presence. A petite woman with glittering eyes, her family loves to tease her for her vociferous cheering at Ryan's races. In private company she is quick to laugh and often punctuates her asides with a knowing grin. But now the house is quiet—Mickey has his son paused up there on the screen—and the glitter in her eyes has gone wet.

"I want you to know . . ." says Madeline, faltering. "I want you to know that this family prays, and prays for many things. That it will be a good race, that it will be a safe race, but they never . . . they never . . ." She stops now, holding her hand to her mouth as her eyes fill with tears. It takes her a moment to gather before she can speak again.

"They never pray to win."

DETERMINED

BY CYNTHIA GORNEY

[
*Deena Kastor is a great cook, a wine lover,
and a budding author. But after some intense training
in the California Sierras, all she wants to be is faster.*
]

OCTOBER 2005

WEDNESDAY was designated an easy day in Deena Kastor's summer training schedule: coffee at dawn; walk the dog; run 12 miles at 8,200 feet in an average 5:50-per-mile pace alongside Meb Keflezighi, the only other American to have won an Olympic Marathon medal in recent decades; drive home; nap; run a late-afternoon five-miler at a really languid pace, like 7:00. So this makes Thursday a hard day. The Thursday workout begins in a park in the middle of Mammoth Lakes, California, where Kastor and Keflezighi both live. The town is at 7,800 feet, which causes the unacclimated to suck wind after climbing a single flight of stairs, and at 8:30 in the morning the sun is brilliant down the length of the playing fields and baseball diamond. A half dozen men are standing in the grass with fly-fishing rods, practicing casts. A woman wrestles a twin stroller from the back of a mini-van. Three 12-year-old boys in soccer cleats pummel each other against a chicken-wire fence, waiting for the rest of the team.

Out in the parking lot, hopping distractedly from one foot to the other, Deena Kastor looks like one of the soccer boys, except, at 5'4" and 104 pounds, skinnier. She also has expensive yellow-lens wraparound sunglasses, which they don't. Her hair is tucked up into a black cap. She's studying her husband, Andrew, who is walking the length of the pavement with plastic cones and a rolling distance-measure chalk marker. "You're marking every 200 meters, right?" she says.

Andrew Kastor looks over at her and lifts his eyebrows. "I don't know," he says dryly. "I'll put the cones somewhere—177, how's that? Your 177-meter split."

Deena makes a face at him. She does some knee lifts, swings her arms around, lunges a few times. She starts telling a story about the time she got a rock in her shoe during mile 11 of the 2004 Olympic Marathon Trials, but Andrew tells her to quit stalling and run. "This is why I need a training group," Deena says. "When I'm by myself I just kind of mosey."

"Come on," Andrew says.

What happens next resembles nothing so much as a motionless deer suddenly startled into flight. Deena's body springs up and forward, there's an explosive rotation of lean, extended legs, and each footfall is light and quick as she accelerates past the first cone. The soccer boys scramble onto the fence to watch. The fly-fishermen stop midcast to stare. The woman with the stroller drops it to the concrete and shades her eyes as Deena sails by, Andrew pedaling hard beside her on his mountain bike. "Holy moly," the woman says, and smiles. "She is booking."

At the 400-meter cone Deena slows, trots, turns around, and picks up the rock-in-shoe story exactly where she left off. She doesn't appear to have broken a sweat. "Finally I had to sit down on the curb to get it out," she says. Then she takes off again. She looks floaty. She's the fastest American female marathoner in history, but she's training for Chicago, in October, where she wants to run a sub-2:20, which would beat her own U.S.-record-setting PR by more than a minute and kick off her third decade of championship distance running—at 32, Deena Kastor has been a national-class competitor for two-thirds of her life—by making her one of the six fastest female marathoners in the world. She's run Chicago only once before, in 2002. It wasn't pretty, and she's out for vindication. "Good form," Andrew says. One more 400. "Relax," Andrew says. One more 400. "Make sure you don't have any rocks in your shoes," Andrew says. Back and forth, 1:20 rests between repeats, Andrew bicycling with the stopwatch. "Shoulders down. Chin back. Everything forward."

To the west, although it's summer, the eastern Sierra peaks are still snowy, and a great slope of snow and granite looms above the grass and pine trees of the park. Every day, Deena swears, she's dazzled by the landscape all over again. Andrew and her running partners like to tease her for being the gushy one on the trails: they're all cranking out 5:30s in thin alpine air and Deena's saying, Look at the flowers, look at the mountain, look how beautiful. "Nice and smooth," Andrew calls out, and checks his watch; six miles into her workout, Deena's running her 400s in 69 seconds each. That's a 4:36-per-mile pace, well under the 5:19s she'll want for Chicago, but what she's trying to do now is teach her body some of the speedup lessons it will need for that fast, flat, mid-autumn race. In Chicago there will be none of the terrain variation that would put different muscles to use midcourse and favor a mountains-trained runner like Deena;

in Chicago, absent some freak weather pattern, there will be no shattering heat to make a 2:27 time the moral equivalent of sub-2:20. That 2:27:20 won Deena the Olympic bronze in Athens, and although everybody who watched that race agreed that Deena ran it brilliantly, picking off heat-flagged competitors on a course whose pavement at one point registered 130 degrees, the bagged Olympic medal is now kept in a basket on the Kastors' kitchen counter, half-buried under the detailed splits tables Deena parses to figure out how much faster she might have run in Athens if not for the hills and the heat.

She nails another 400 now, and she and Andrew both look at their watches. "Sixty-seven," Andrew says, and hands her the bottle of Cytomax. "Definitely the fastest one so far."

"I need to sharpen my legs up," Deena says. "I feel good. I just don't feel, like—springy."

She prances in place, shakes loose her arms, and heads out easily toward one of the park's wooded trails. Twenty minutes of cooldown, 15 minutes of ice-water bath, an afternoon weight-training session at the gym, another run at the end of the day. Andrew's not her formal coach, more the combination therapist-masseur-cheerleader-worrier, but he knows the training routine by heart; usually he's the one reminding her not to overdo it. "She doesn't have a lot of gifted raw speed," he says quietly, watching Deena disappear into the pines. "Sixty-nine-second 400s, for her, is moving." Then he grins and slings his bike onto the rack on the back of their car. "But she can do them all day."

WHEN SHE WAS 18 or so and already a veteran in the sport—she'd been running, and winning state and national titles, since middle school—Deena used to entertain younger runners at training camps with a mental game at the end of the day. Deena called this the "fantasy run." She would tell them to lie down and close their eyes. "I would just guide them with my words," Deena says. "I'd say, 'We're at a trailhead. The sun is beating down, and you can feel it on your back. We're hopping over creeks, and charging up hills.' My favorite part was where we turned around and made our way back to the trailhead. We would stop at a creek and lean down. Some would say they were running with somebody, some said they were by themselves, but we would all balance on a rock, in the middle of the stream, and grab some cold water and splash it on our faces and make our way back to the trailhead where we started."

An interesting thing about this, Deena remembers: some of the kids, trail-running only in their own imaginations, would react the same way she had discovered she did—still does, in fact. Their heart rates would increase, and they'd break into a sweat. "The ones that had focus," she says. "You could tell."

The passion in Deena's voice as she spun out those verbal runs stayed with Bill Duley, one of her early running coaches, who owns a running store in Agoura Hills, the Southern California town to which Deena Drossin, her name before she married, had moved with her family when she was 8. "You really felt her love for running during those things," recalls Duley. "And the kids just loved it. 'Deena! Do another fantasy run!'"

Duley first began working with Deena when her parents, neither particularly athletic but both big believers in the benefits of organized youth sports, delivered her to the kids' cross-country team he was putting together. Deena was 11 then. She'd played soccer, joined a softball team, taken ice-skating lessons; she liked the skating, but showed no evidence of being any sort of athlete. "I wasn't good at anything," Deena says. "In soccer I was the clumsy one that would go for the ball and my feet would get in my way, or I'd score for the other team. In softball I was making daisy chains in the outfield and I'd hear people yelling my name."

She had never impressed anybody as being speedy, either. Her father, Paul, a businessman, had been a volunteer coach during Deena's various athletic ventures, and he had a succinct reaction to his wife's suggestion that a running team might help Deena make new friends. "I said, ugh, she's going to get killed," Drossin recalls. But he assented, and eventually Bill Duley sized up his new charge. "Skinny little prepuberty girl with no muscle tone," Duley says. "Lanky. She hadn't grown into her frame yet. Her movements weren't real coordinated. But she just kept going. While running a 400 she hadn't prepared for, she wasn't real fast—but she never slowed down. Then she did the same thing in the 800. I said to myself, There's something here."

Clueless and cheerful, Deena entered her first meet three weeks after joining the team. She ran the 800, tucked in at the shoulder of the much-vaunted local age-group champ, came in right behind her, and watched the girl collapse to the ground. "And I'm already eating my Snickers bar," Deena says. That was pretty much how it went from there; more than 20 years later, Deena still pulls out an 11-year-old's vocab when she describes the way her body took to distance running. "Awesome," she says. "Right from the beginning. The first long run was four miles into the mountains. I had never known those trails existed, and I was so excited. We ran past Ronald Reagan's old ranch, and I thought that was the coolest thing."

Her physical stamina was exceptional, as it turned out—as an adult, Deena still impresses physiologists with the unusually high cardiovascular efficiency her system displays—and before her 12th birthday, Deena had won her first

National Cross-Country Championship. By the time she was ready for college, she had won five state titles and made the Foot Locker Cross-Country Championships every year in high school. She was recruited around the country and finally settled on the University of Arkansas, where the camaraderie among the team runners seemed strongest—that mattered to her more than anything, she says. She racked up a very good collegiate record, but not a great one. She won repeatedly at the Southeastern Conference, but not nationally. She was an eight-time All-American, but never won an NCAA final. She wobbled as a runner; she refocused much of her time and energy on the short stories and poetry she was composing for the school's creative writing program, and for a while, still a student, she dropped running completely and started up a part-time baking enterprise for restaurants around the college town of Fayetteville.

It was a lively business, and Deena took it seriously. She was waking at four o'clock in the morning, baking scones and pies and cakes in a smokehouse kitchen she had gotten permission to use for free, and then delivering her products around town while they were still warm. She made bagels the traditional way, boiling them before they were baked. She made heart-shaped shortbreads dipped in espresso-flavored chocolate and pistachios. She came up with a catchy name, Sweet Expectation, and by the time she had decided to scale back the baking and finish out her last season as a university runner, it was clear to Deena that she had a plausible business waiting after college if she decided to pursue it.

But she didn't. She chose the giant gamble instead. Milan Donley, an assistant Arkansas coach at the time, had been watching Deena carefully throughout her collegiate career, and in 1996, as she was finishing her senior year, he offered to call Joe Vigil to see whether he would take her on as a postcollegiate trainee. On the surface, this looked like a bit of a reach. Vigil was a national legend, recently retired from nearly 30 years of coaching at Colorado's Adams State. The small group of runners he now coached was all-male, fast, and willing to submit to his hardcore, high-mileage program in the distinctly unglamorous town of Alamosa, Colorado. But Donley, who earlier had worked with Vigil as an assistant, had seen how well Deena could perform when she was on. He felt the right coach might make something remarkable of her abilities—provided she held nothing back. "I suppose I did everything I could to discourage her," Vigil recalls. "I said, 'Alamosa's a small place, at altitude, windy, the winters get to 30 below.'" She was from Southern California, he reasoned; that ought to put her off. "Finally I said, 'Look, if you're serious, come visit for a day or two, see if you like the place. We'll talk.' Well, my wife and I got home from the Atlanta Olympics, and lo and behold she'd moved in, two days before I got here. She wasn't going to look back. She was going to make it go."

She would give it four years, Deena had decided; she still didn't think she knew quite how good a distance runner she could actually be, and listening to Donley finally persuaded her to spend the necessary time finding out. "He said, 'How will you know unless you try?'" Deena says. "His point was, 'You already know you can do the bakery. But you can't open a bakery and then 10 years down the line decide you want to try running again.' He said, 'Don't give yourself a month. Go somewhere. Commit yourself.'"

A fax from Deena had arrived in Alamosa some weeks before she did; its contents were not reassuring to the dubious Vigil. Still trying to make up his mind whether to take Deena seriously, he had asked her to send him a list of her training goals. "She wanted to win a national championship in cross-country," Vigil says. "She wanted to be a senior world-level cross-country runner. And like any runner, she wanted, one day, to be an Olympian." He chuckles. "These were sort of lofty goals."

THAT STORY ABOUT DEENA swallowing a bee midrace, during the 2000 8-K World Cross-Country Championships in Portugal, and going on to finish the race anyway. True?

"No," Deena says. "I chewed it up and spat it out."

She's padding around her dining room in blue jeans and socks, the cordless phone jammed under one ear. Aspen, her beloved 9-year-old Labrador, was roughed up this morning by a cranky neighborhood dog; Deena's trying to reach the vet to see whether Aspen's bleeding ear needs stitches. "It was the World Championships," Deena says. "I had given the team a pep talk when we were in the starting area—you know, 'There's six of us on this team, and when it starts to hurt out there, think of the other girls that are relying on you, and push a little harder.' So, 500 meters from the start, this bee flies into my mouth. It stings my uvula, the thing that hangs in the back of your throat. I got it to the front of my mouth, spit it out, and kept running. Luckily I'm not allergic, but I could feel my throat closing up, and by the back side of the third loop I blacked out, still running. I ended up stumbling over some roots and kind of coming to when I hit the ground. When I got up, I saw the women in front of me, so I tried charging after them to make up my distance—the whole time, I'm thinking, My team is relying on me, I gave them that pep talk."

This is actually a very good Deena story, as it turns out, not just because it's about tenacity at a level unfathomable to most people—she did finish, 12th in a field of more than a hundred, and helped the American women place third—but also because of the way she tells it: lightly, matter-of-factly, and as though the main point to be remembered, the main really annoying thing, is that she was extremely well prepared for that race. "I was fitter than I had ever been," she says. Deena spent eight years under Joe Vigil's guidance, making the Olympic team twice (she ran the 10,000 at the 2000 Games) and compiling one of the all-time great résumés in American distance running. The formal relationship ended when Vigil stepped back from coaching full-time after Athens. But he still watches out for her (recently Vigil mailed Deena a handwritten list of train-ing goals to consider as she prepared for Chicago), and Deena sometimes makes her career recap sound like a long series of blunt performance assessments with a plainspoken, affectionate, intensely demanding coach.

On the 2002 Chicago Marathon, for example, only the second marathon of Deena's life (at the first, the year before in New York, she ran 2:26:58, the fastest marathon debut ever by an American woman): "I ran Chicago five seconds faster than New York. But I didn't count it as a personal best, because I was much more fit than that and should have run faster. It was cold and windy that day, and I let it get to me. All I remember is freezing, like my legs were frozen sticks pounding against the pavement. I suffered the entire way."

On the 2003 London Marathon, which she ran in 2:21:16, shaving five sec-onds off Joan Benoit Samuelson's 17-year-old American marathon record: "I had some of the key points in the race written on my hand. I fell off pace a little bit, and thought, My gosh, if I just fell off pace, I can get back on pace."

On the USA Outdoor Track and Field Championships in June 2005, in which she entered the 10,000 despite a freak misstep in her front yard six weeks earlier that nearly broke a bone in her left foot and forced her to take a month off from running: "I just wasn't fit enough." She came in fourth, missing the chance to compete for the United States at the World Track and Field Championships in Helsinki. "I didn't make the team. I'm fine with that. What I'm shooting for is to run fast in Chicago. I'm happy to focus on my goal, rather than dwelling on what I'm not doing."

On the afternoon in early 2001 when she realized she might finally try marathons, after years of insisting she had no interest in any race that demanded a whole month of physical recovery afterward: "I was visiting my parents' house. It's nine miles from the beach, and I'd never run the whole way there and back before. I started out slow, maybe eight-minute miles for the first few, and on the way back I started getting this euphoric feeling. I'm starting to climb, I'm start-ing to feel so good, and I get to where I know I'm at like mile 15 or 16, and I'm just hammering, and I'm having the time of my life. I called Coach Vigil. I said, 'I just finished an 18-mile run, and I feel great. I think I could do a marathon.' And he said"—here Deena flashes an enormous smile, mimicking the sublimely happy man on the other end of the phone—"'Oh, how I've waited to hear those words come out of your mouth.'"

Deena squints at the entrance to her bedroom, scratching Aspen on the head. "How do you get a bloodstain out of a carpet?" she asks. The carpet is off-white, except for the patch that at this moment is not, and covers the whole main floor of the two-story wood house where the Kastors live and where Andrew, a massage therapist and runner Deena met in Alamosa, keeps his office. There's a blue-and-white tiled kitchen, a deck looking out into the woods, and an artist's easel that holds a big unfinished acrylic painting of a woman's feet clad in flip-flops. The painting is Deena's. She's never studied art or painted before, but there's a good art store in town, and she thought it would be fun to try. ("I'm a little obsessed by feet," she says. "I think toes and feet are so cute, and I happen to not have cute feet. I'm hoping that when I stop running, I will.") She's also composing a cookbook. She's decorating the beach house she and Andrew just bought in Southern California. She knows a lot about wine, which the Kastors store in a special 200-bottle closet they had built downstairs. (It's not temperature-controlled; "We drink them too quickly.") She plans to open a wine and cheese shop someday—small, she thinks, with her baked goods for sale, and little bistro tables. She and Andrew keep a framed blackboard in the dining room, on which Deena rewrites a new message every few days; yesterday it was a quote attributed to Mahatma Gandhi, "You must be the change you wish to see in the world," and today it's the menu for dinner, to which two guests have been invited, and which Deena intends to whip out after the day's third workout:

Pork Tenderloin with Apple Sauté
Tri-Pepper Risotto
Brocollini & Asparagus
Vanilla Ice Cream with Raspberries & Fudge
Wine!

JOE VIGIL LIKES TO SAY Deena's single greatest athletic gifts are in her head—"that nine inches above her shoulders," as he puts it. This is more complicated than it sounds. All elite athletes are disciplined and somewhat obsessive about dedication to their sport, but both Vigil and Deena's new coach, a 34-year-old Philadelphia-based marathoner and former Vigil trainee named Terrence Mahon, say part of the reason for Deena's extraordinary longevity as a competitor is her odd genius both for focusing and for letting go. She runs 140-mile weeks and structures her waking hours around meticulously programmed daily training and recovery plans, but she can't remember most of her own PRs. She knows her track goals for a given year precisely—"14:45 in the 5-K, and in the 10-K I'd like to run 30 flat"—but she doesn't know what the world records are at those distances (14:25, as it happens, and 29:32), and doesn't seem to care. "It is true, she forgets her best times," Mahon will say in an e-mail, a few days later, answering a query about Deena's curious disinterest in the sorts of statistics one would think might keep a world-class racer awake at night. "She is an in-the-moment runner, and once the race is over, it is forgotten. She takes a mental break and then goes on to the next goal. It is not that she places no value on her personal bests—it's just that they no longer serve as motivators for where she wants to go in the future. She needs bigger incentives than that."

In the gym, now that her dog is attended to and settled back home with disinfectant on the bloodied ear, Deena's doing V-sits. At one point in the pet hospital the veterinarian had loosened his grip and Aspen tried to lunge from the operating table, nearly knocking Deena over; for a moment, as she grappled with her frightened dog, Deena's slenderness made her seem fragile and tippy and small. But here she looks like an angled carpenter's ruler, all long limb and muscle. Her V-sits are perfect. She snaps off dozens of them, moves to the exercise ball for a while, begins lifting the 45-pound bar for a series of body squats. She's adding bar weight gradually, still tentative about stressing her foot; she trained through the injury by running full workouts on a submerged treadmill that took most of the weight off her foot. "We brought music in," Deena says. "I have such a great support system. Andrew played lifeguard and DJ while Terrence was coaching from the side of the pool."

When no one else was around, Deena says, she entertained herself during the long underwater runs by singing, which she also likes to do while taking the daily ice baths at home. She likes belting out Madonna songs. "But not if anybody's listening," she says, and hoists herself onto a hanging sling to do some dangling leg lifts. She does some overhead lat pulldowns. She lifts some free weights. She says hey to Meb Keflezighi, who has wandered into the gym for his own workout, and they pull out the rope-and-PVC-pipe ladder Deena designed for the special quick-stepping exercises she likes, and with the ladder stretched out over a length of gym floor, two of the fastest marathoners in the current American competitive ranks take turns playing a kind of manic hopscotch against each other, demanding military-style pushups as punishment for any imprecision that nudges a rung with a foot. The rules are insanely complicated and fast: one hop between ladder rungs, double-time grapevine steps between ladder rungs. "Drop and give me 10!" Deena cries, spotting Meb on a misstep. He grimaces, but obliges at once. As he counts out his pushups, Meb fixes his gaze on Deena's feet; she's high-stepping and boingy and twinkletoed and laughing, but her concentration is absolute, and Meb, soundly beaten, shakes his head in admiration. "She's a work of art, isn't she?" he says.

PURE HEART

BY AMBY BURFOOT

> Running was his love, and Ryan Shay
> used it to chase an Olympic dream as passionately
> as any athlete has. That pursuit ended tragically—
> but an even deeper love lives on.

FEBRUARY 2008

IN A WAY, THEY were like so many other couples visiting New York City as newlyweds. With no kids to keep an eye on, they could stroll the city streets hand in hand, go for a run in Central Park, drop into glitzy stores, and shop without worrying about the family budget. But Ryan and Alicia Shay traveled to New York last fall with more than sight-seeing and idle fun in mind. Ryan had a race to run.

It was the U.S. men's Olympic Marathon Trials, the quadrennial event that would produce America's team for this summer's Olympics in Beijing. And at 4:30 a.m. on Saturday, November 3, 2007, the morning of the Trials, Ryan and Alicia slid out of their Manhattan hotel bed for a race that wouldn't begin until 7:35. Ryan had to grab a quick breakfast, though, and then catch the 5:20 bus to the start at Rockefeller Center. This was no time to be late.

Ryan had prepared most of his 28 years for this day. He was not yet 10 when he began racing blustery cross-country meets in northern Michigan. In high school, college, and beyond, few could match him. The longer the distances, the greater his success. The marathon seemed his perfect event, demanding, as it did, precise attention to detail and endless 140-mile training weeks. Tougher than the rest? That was Shay. More dedicated. More single-minded. More solitary.

For many runners, the sport provides a social outlet. At Shay's level, though, there is little company, not when you're aiming for a 2:11 marathon and a spot on an Olympic team. For the most part you have to go it alone. But that was okay. Ryan embraced everything about his sport, his event, and the quest for a life-

160

changing Trials performance. He knew what it demanded: one day, one race, one man against the distance.

Alicia Shay didn't go to Rockefeller Center with her husband of not quite four months. Ryan said it wasn't important; he'd rather see her in Central Park, where the marathoners would run five loops. They said their goodbyes at the 5:20 bus.

A few days later Alicia recalled the moment. "I thought of all the things I could tell him for encouragement," she says, "but in the end, I decided to just say, 'I love you.'"

"I know," he replied with a kiss. "And I love you, too."

WITH ITS POPULATION OF 990, Central Lake, Michigan, located about 225 miles northwest of Detroit, is the kind of hamlet where the WELCOME TO sign says HOME OF THE 1980 CLASS D GIRLS SOFTBALL STATE CHAMPIONS. Downtown measures two blocks by two blocks and is anchored by Rocket Rob's Village Pizza and Crossings Bait Shop. "I tell people it's the Mayberry of the North," says Quinn Barry, a Central Lake high school teacher and coach. "It's a town full of hardworking people who feel a strong connection to each other."

The Shay family moved to Central Lake from Nashville, Michigan, when Ryan was nine. Ryan was a scrappy kid from birth. He didn't have any choice. Not when he was the fifth child in a family that would grow to eight. Not when his only older brother, Case, five years his senior, was fast, tough, and unbridled. "I was just a punk kid back then, and no great brother," says Case, now a teacher in South Korea. "Ryan and I had a sibling rivalry. He wanted to do everything I did, and I beat the crap out of him plenty. He couldn't keep up with me at first, but he liked challenges and had a high tolerance for pain."

While Ryan couldn't match Case for many years, he never stopped trying. He mimicked everything Case did—high-jumping, guitar-playing, schoolwork—always aiming to surpass his older brother. "He finally started beating me in running when he was about 20, a sophomore in college," Case admits.

Ryan seemed to have only one gear, full-speed, which he applied to everything. Barry was one of the first to witness Ryan's raw competitiveness, recalling it with a mix of smiles and horror. In eighth grade, Ryan played on the Central Lake basketball team. In one game, he scored nearly half the Trojans' points, but the team lost. In the postgame handshake lineup, Ryan blasted each opponent with a curse word. Barry, the school's athletic director, yanked him aside and explained the error of his behavior. "But I really wanted to win tonight," the young athlete protested. Then he made his apologies.

It was as a runner, though, that Ryan left his mark at Central Lake High, whose cross-country and track teams have been coached by his parents, Joe and Susan Shay, for two decades. Joe, 58, is a former quarter-miler grown portly. He moves and speaks slowly, suffers from diabetes, and doesn't look the part of a driven track coach. He has more the philosopher's approach to the sport, with a library exceeding 100 track and running books. He has examined each carefully, looking for new wisdom to inform his coaching. Susan, 56, is the Central Lake school librarian, more angular, quiet, and private than her husband. All eight of their children ran for Central Lake, most with distinction. But Ryan far outshone the rest. He won 11 state titles, including four straight Michigan state championships in cross-country, a mark that's never been matched. His final one was perhaps the most memorable. He not only won the small-school title, but his winning time was faster than every Michigan high schooler's, including the kids from the well-heeled suburban towns down south.

The titles aside, Ryan's self-confidence proved he had big-time ambitions beyond his small-town roots. Once, when a classmate expressed admiration for a medal Ryan brought home from a regional meet, he told her, "Someday this is going to be a gold medal from the Olympics."

Yet, for all his victories, Ryan felt few understood his passion for excellence or his attraction to distance running. The locals couldn't fathom why a teenager would bull his way through 10-mile training runs in blizzards and sub-zero temperatures. Ryan was 15 when his father gave him a copy of *Pre*, the biography of American distance legend Steve Prefontaine. Before he died in a car crash, at 24, Pre was known for seizing control of races like no American before him. He'd run boldly from the front and might have won an Olympic medal if he had been willing to settle for silver or bronze. He wasn't. He went for the gold, and came close, fading to fourth in the final meters of the 1972 Olympic 5000. It took Ryan just a few days to read *Pre* cover to cover.

"What did you think?" Joe asked his son later.

"At last, someone who understands me."

Soon the walls of Ryan's bedroom were covered with Pre stories and posters, and he began training even harder. He stuck to an unwavering schedule: run in the morning, go to school, run at practice, and come home and complete all his homework before eating. He'd never allow himself to touch dinner until his studies were completed. It wasn't a family rule; it was his own self-imposed discipline. In 1997, he graduated from Central Lake with a 4.0 GPA. He was also class president and covaledictorian. "He had such a sense of purpose and so much discipline," says Joe, a touch of wonder in his voice. "He simply wouldn't allow himself to be distracted by outside influences."

MIDTOWN MANHATTAN WAS STILL DARK when the buses arrived at Rockefeller Center. The 131 men running the Trials filed out and trudged down to the concourse level, beside the famed skating rink. Meb Keflezighi. Alan Culpepper. Ryan Hall. Dathan Ritzenhein. Abdi Abdirahman. Brian Sell. They were all here and they represented the greatest assemblage of American distance talent ever gathered for one marathon. Some folded themselves into chairs, some sat against a wall, some sprawled full-length on the floor, looking bedraggled and groggy, conserving every kilojoule of their energy supply. In fact, they had never been more focused or adrenaline-charged. Four years had passed since the last Trials. It would be another four years until the next. Carpe diem. Seize the day. Carpe viam. Seize the road. It was time.

Stretching guru Phil Wharton assisted several runners through easy leg exercises. Ryan Shay was one of the last he worked on, just enough to get the blood flowing. They were friends, both living in Flagstaff, Arizona, and Ryan had received regular treatments as he increased his Olympic Trials training. Before sending Ryan off, Wharton said, "Run patient today."

"That's the plan," Ryan offered back.

Ryan's coach, Joe Vigil, was more emphatic. He had coached Deena Kastor to an Olympic medal in 2004. He is a master in the art of starting-line advice. While he expected Ryan to know what he needed to do by now, Vigil left nothing to chance. He had trained Ryan to run a 2:11 marathon and thought he was ready to do just that. "Stay away from the front, but stay in the hunt," he told his runner. "It's a breezy morning, a good day for following."

Vigil's final words: "Run with confidence. Run with emotional control."

FOR A KID FROM A SMALL, REMOTE TOWN, Ryan Shay drew plenty of attention from big-time colleges. He made recruiting visits to three—Tulane, Arizona, and Notre Dame. Ryan's weight—as much as 170 pounds in high school—and muscular upper-body build drew attention from the runners he met. On his trip to Arizona in 1997, he met Abdi Abdirahman for the first time. Abdi initially assumed that Ryan was a football linebacker. Ultimately, Ryan chose Notre Dame. "He liked that it was a top-25 academic school and a top-10 running school," says Nate Shay, who later followed his older brother to South Bend. "Those two things were both really important to Ryan."

Still, not everything came easily when he got to college. In high school Ryan often ran alone and won races by huge margins. Notre Dame was different. Before Ryan's first race in a Fighting Irish singlet, his coach, Joe Piane, instructed his runners to stick together for three miles. After that, they were free to run as hard as they wanted. "He must have misunderstood me," recalls Piane with a knowing twinkle in his eye. "He stayed with everyone else for about three strides before taking off. Afterward, I asked him about it. He said, 'Coach, I came to Notre Dame to run fast.'"

He showed a similar bluntness in the classroom. Early in his freshman year he submitted a 10-page paper for an English class. In it he explored his running dreams and the ways to achieve them. He titled the paper, "American Distance Running: Getting Lapped in the Fast Lane." The paper began, "My goal in life is to become an elite distance runner. I want to indulge in victory and be able to tell myself that I am the best at what I do." It went on to excoriate high school runners for not training hard enough—"The youth of today are basically lazy, and distance running is a lot of hard work"—and postcollegiate runners for not believing they could beat the East Africans. He concluded the paper by invoking Steve Prefontaine, who ran "to see who has the most guts," and by saying that he and others must follow Pre's example. "This is what will make Americans great runners," he wrote. "This is what will make them heroes for eternity."

Ryan was 18 when he handed in the paper, and he lived by its precepts. At Notre Dame he gained All-American honors nine times across three seasons: cross-country, indoor track, and outdoor track. There was no time of the year when Ryan wasn't training and racing hard. Among his Notre Dame teammates, the stories of his effort are legion. Ryan never ran a mile slower than six-minute pace. No one could stay with Ryan on his cooldowns—or wanted to. He once helped lift Notre Dame to a conference title with a bum leg that had tormented him for two months. "He was the most tenacious runner I ever had," says Piane, Notre Dame's coach for the past 33 years.

The favorite tale is one that still stirs disbelief. During one of his infamous blizzard runs—he never let weather of any kind interfere with a workout—Ryan had completed just three miles of his scheduled 16-miler when a car knocked him down at an intersection and ran over his shinbones. Bouncing up, he checked himself out and felt fine. He still had 13 miles to go, and damned if his training log wasn't going to report that he had finished every one of those 16 miles.

When he later returned to his apartment, he told his teammate, Sean Zanderson, what had happened. Zanderson searched Ryan's face for a telltale grin.

None. He looked at Ryan's shins. Bruised and bleeding. He told Ryan he'd better get himself over to the hospital for X-rays. "Yeah, I guess you're right," Ryan said. But first he insisted on doing his extensive postrun stretching routine.

Appropriately, Ryan's best college track race came at the University of Oregon's Hayward Field, the track made famous by Prefontaine's many beat-me-if-you-dare efforts. Ryan was the fourth seed in the 10,000 meters of the 2001 NCAA Track & Field Championships. The first lap unfolded at a pace so pedestrian that he found it sacrilegious. Would Pre ever run this cautiously? No way. So he surged to the front and stayed there for the next 24 laps, winning by a wide margin. "If I was ever going to win a big race," Ryan said afterward, "that was the place I wanted to do it."

A LITTLE BEFORE 7 A.M., the runners began shuffling up the Rockefeller Center stairs to the street level to begin their warmups. Like all marathoners, they checked the weather first. It wasn't nearly as bad as most had feared 24 hours earlier, when forecasters were predicting that remnants of Hurricane Noel would strike Manhattan with heavy rains and wind gusts to 40 or 50 miles per hour. Vigil was right: It was breezy. But just breezy. No rain.

Ryan warmed up in part with Abdirahman, a race favorite and an occasional training partner in Flagstaff. They did strides on 50th Street, between Fifth and Sixth avenues, then wished each other well before removing their sweats and taking their places at the start. "He was in good spirits. There was nothing wrong with him," says Abdirahman. "He told me, 'Abdi, you're the class of the field. Just believe in yourself, and run your race.' I actually thought he had a good chance to make the team. He had a great strategy: he was going to stick with Brian Sell."

Moments before the start, Ryan Hall, another favorite, appeared out of nowhere. Hall had been delayed in his final preparations. Now he was looking for a spot on the front line. He saw Shay, whom he knew, and figured his friend would open up a space for him. Shay did. "Good luck," Shay told him. "Go get 'em." Hall was wearing mostly blue, with a number 2 attached to the side of his shorts. He was the second seed in the field, based on his qualifying time. Shay wore a white singlet and black shorts, with the number 13 pinned on them.

Behind the small but elite field, the Gothic-style towers of St. Patrick's Cathedral reached upward.

RYAN SHAY HAD HEADED OFF TO COLLEGE with one primary goal—to become the best runner possible. And he would let few things distract his focus. As in high school, he had little time for girlfriends while at Notre Dame. He dated and had relationships, but none that endured. Dating wasn't his big concern. Training harder, getting faster, making it to the Olympics—now those were worthy aspirations. "Ryan was always so disciplined about everything he did, especially his running," says his sister Sarah. "He was too serious to be the playboy type."

After graduating from Notre Dame in 2002, Ryan needed a new way to nurture his running. At the time, veteran U.S. coaches Bob Larsen and Joe Vigil had just launched a small group called Team Running USA. They wanted to help talented postcollegiate runners stay with the sport and climb the rungs of international success. Among the first to sign on were Deena Kastor and Meb Keflezighi, both of whom would go on to medal at the 2004 Olympics. Larsen and Vigil subjected prospective team members to a battery of physiological tests at the U.S. Olympic Training Center in Chula Vista, California, but also conducted in-depth interviews. They considered character just as important as VO2 max. They wanted team members to have the drive, purpose, and vision of a Deena or a Meb.

Ryan met several times with Vigil to discuss joining the group. Vigil has a Ph.D. in exercise physiology and doesn't jump to hasty conclusions. He interrogated Ryan to judge if he had the right stuff, wondering, in particular, about a proposal that Ryan made: he said he wanted to go straight from the 10,000 meters to the marathon. No top-tier American distance runner had done this in 20 years—not since Alberto Salazar in the early 1980s. "Okay, but first sleep on it," Vigil told the ambitious 22-year-old. "When you have, get back to me, and we'll talk some more."

Ryan didn't need more time to think about his marathon dream, but he let several weeks pass before he called Vigil back. He didn't want to appear rash, a quality Vigil disdained. When the timing seemed right, Ryan picked up the phone and dialed the man who would coach him for the next five years, becoming a second father of sorts. "I want to focus on the marathon," he said.

Vigil didn't actually care about Ryan's choice of events. He only cared about commitment. "I was a little surprised by Ryan's decision," Vigil admits. "But he was so determined. I'm a very hard-driving coach, but he always did the work. He had a tremendous appetite for hard work."

Ryan moved from South Bend to Mammoth Lakes, California, the high-altitude community where Team Running USA members do much of their training. One day Vigil assigned a 15-miler and sent his new runner out on some unfamiliar trails. Ninety minutes later, Shay hadn't returned. Vigil got into his four-wheel-drive pickup truck and began scouring every dirt road in the area. He drove for hours and never located Shay, who eventually staggered into town in the late afternoon. Vigil figured that Ryan had run 15 miles and walked 31.

The next day was a "hard day" of interval training, 10 x 1000 meters. Vigil suggested that Ryan skip the interval repeats, given the calamity of his previous day. "Ryan wouldn't even consider it," says Vigil. "He figured if it was an interval day, you did your intervals. You didn't make excuses."

The work paid off. Ryan ran his first marathon in October 2002, finishing 15th at Chicago in an impressive 2:14:30. Four months later, he made headlines when he won the 2003 USA Marathon Championships in Birmingham, Alabama, in 2:14:29. He was the youngest national marathon winner in 30 years. "Ryan was one of the first to get the ball rolling for American marathoners," says fellow Michigan native Greg Meyer, who won the Boston Marathon in 1983, the last American to do so. "He showed the way for the young guys who have followed him, like Ryan Hall and Dathan Ritzenhein."

More importantly, Birmingham would be hosting the Olympic Marathon Trials a year later. Shay's course tour and victory gave him a leg up on the competition. Suddenly, he was being mentioned as a possible Olympian. The dream unraveled when he sustained a hamstring injury in the final weeks of his training for the Trials. Then he aggravated the hamstring midway through the race and limped to the finish in 22nd place (2:19:20).

Shay was just 24. At the time of the next Trials, he'd be 28, a marathoner's peak age. He'd have four more years of Vigil's inspiration and another 20,000 miles of high-altitude training. He'd tinker with other aspects of his program. Perhaps he would drop the upper-body weight work; it only seemed to bulk him up. He could improve his diet to get leaner and meaner. He'd return to the track to lower his 10,000-meter PR. He'd keep looking for the best place to train—in California, Colorado, Arizona, wherever. He was a ramblin' guy, single and unattached. No commitments. Except for the one he had made to himself a decade earlier: to work harder than anyone else.

The four years would pass quickly. When the 2008 Marathon Trials rolled around, he'd be ready for the race of his life. He was sure of that.

FROM ROCKEFELLER CENTER, the marathon course turned south for a quick spin around Times Square, as glittery as the rest of New York was dark on this gray morning. The race favorites ran cautiously, worried about the dim light, the 90-degree turns, and the pockmarked streets. They had but one goal: to stay on their feet until they reached the smoother roads of Central Park. That's where the race would begin.

No one paid much attention when a couple of little-known runners spurted to the lead in midtown. The big guns ran in a large, slow-moving cluster. They covered the first two miles at a 5:30 pace—practically a walk. That changed abruptly when the group reached the park at its extreme southern end and turned left for the first of five clockwise laps. Brian Sell dropped the pace to an honest five minutes per mile. Everyone had expected this of Sell, a bulldog runner like Ryan Shay, unwilling to accept a piddling marathon pace. Now it was official—the race was on.

Alicia Shay had positioned herself near the five-mile mark on the east side of the park, just south of the Jacqueline Kennedy Onassis Reservoir. It was a great vantage point. Here, the east roadway and west roadway are separated by just 500 yards. This meant that Alicia could sprint across the gap in less than two minutes. She is herself a champion distance runner who had recently won the USA 20-K title, and she was wearing her racing flats. She figured she'd see Ryan at five miles, seven miles, and every two to three miles after that.

At 8 a.m. Alicia stood on the inside of the park roadway and craned her neck leftward, to the north. The runners would be appearing any moment now. Hundreds of other marathon fans had stationed themselves in the same vicinity. She didn't recognize the first two runners to flash past—Michael Wardian and Michael Cox—but suspected they would soon drop back. She lifted herself up on tippy toes, and held her breath, waiting for the big group of prime contenders. That's where she hoped to see her husband. In the lead pack, near its rear. Running as relaxed and economically as he could. His strength was his strength, and the longer he could conserve it, the better his chances.

Here they came. Sell and Abdi and Hall and Meb and a couple of dozen more. Yes, and her Ryan. He was running exactly where he was supposed to be, at exactly the right speed, five minutes per mile. That was the pace he had trained for, the pace he and Vigil had agreed upon. "Ryan looked great at five miles, smooth and controlled," Alicia remembers. "He was at the back of the pack, right where he wanted to be." She dashed across the park to the seven-mile mark, with high hopes and expectations.

RYAN SHAY BOUNCED BACK nicely from his disappointment at the 2004 Trials. In March 2005, he won the Gate River Run 15-K in Jacksonville, Florida. It earned him his fifth USA national road championship in 26 months. Eight months later, he had a rare bad race in the ING New York City Marathon, when he strained several ligaments in his foot and finished 18th. But he knew what had happened; he could fix it.

The evening following that race he joined friends at Rosie O'Grady's, an Irish bar in midtown Manhattan. Among those gathered was a recent Stanford grad and, like him, an NCAA 10,000-meter champion—someone, though, whom he had never before met. Her name was Alicia Craig.

A willowy, freckle-faced beauty and self-described "Wyoming girl," Craig had grown up among cowboys and rodeo riders in Gillette, Wyoming, and at her family's 14,000-acre Wyoming cattle ranch. Result: she's not one to be easily impressed by macho posturing. She had heard about Ryan's tough-guy veneer. That night, in a long conversation, she detected no trace of it. "He was so gentle and transparent and easy to talk to," she says. "We had so much in common, it was almost crazy. I found that he was one of those people who, after you spend time with them, you feel better about yourself."

Still, she left the restaurant and returned to her California training base with no thoughts that a relationship might blossom. She figured that she and Ryan would simply see each other on the national distance-running circuit. He had a bolder vision. A few months later, he moved to the Woodside, California, house where Craig was living with a handful of Team Running USA members. Ryan had heard that these guys were logging some long, gnarly workouts, and wanted in on the action.

Ryan Hall, a recent Stanford grad, lived nearby with his wife, Sara, and was one of the team members. Hall had never met Shay before but vividly recalls their first runs together. "We did a fast, hard 10-mile tempo run on a Saturday," he says. "The next day was a long run, and Ian Dobson and I were taking it easier. But Ryan was out there hammering again. Ian and I looked at each other like, 'Is that guy crazy or what?' I soon learned that he was simply the hardest-working runner I've ever met."

The team house didn't afford much privacy, not with a half-dozen other runners in residence, but there were fleeting moments. One night, after everyone else had gone to bed, Ryan got out his guitar and began singing for Alicia. "He was obviously trying to impress me, because he was nervous and jittery and sweating so much," she says. "I wanted to tell him it was okay to stop, for his own sake. But he stuck it out in typical Ryan fashion. He played and sang for two hours, and many of the songs—George Strait and other country-western tunes—were among my favorites, even though he couldn't have known that. It was just the sweetest thing."

The two hadn't even had a date yet, but their friends could see the growing attraction. Alicia's teammates began teasing her, warning her to be wary of that Shay fellow. His brothers, receiving e-mail photos of Ryan and Alicia, noted that the smirk was gone from his face, replaced by a look they had never seen before.

"You could only call it a glow," says Nate. "It was obvious that he had met the right woman, and he knew it. His life until then had been one long suffer-fest, what with all the moving around and the hard training every day. I think he was so relieved to finally meet someone he could open up to."

Soon there was an official first date, but only after Ryan polished his burgundy Ford F-150 pickup truck for hours. And a second date. And the night when Ryan held Alicia's hands, looked in her hazel eyes, and told her why she was the most amazing person he had ever met. "A lot of people thought Ryan was quiet and guarded," she says. "But he was the exact opposite with me. He was so open and soft. He prided himself on always giving 100 percent, and that's the way he loved me, 100 percent. I've never felt anything like it."

Alicia's family noticed the difference. Her sister Lisa Renee Tumminello, 38, was worried about Alicia's health at the time. In her last year at Stanford, Alicia had fallen hard in a freak dorm accident, and suffered two years of head and neck pain and frequent waves of nausea. Her running had plummeted to an all-time low. Suddenly, that didn't seem to matter so much. "As she grew closer to Ryan, Alicia developed a giggle I had never heard before," says Tumminello. "She was filled with a childlike joy. She and Ryan were so playful with each other."

At Thanksgiving 2006, Alicia took Ryan home to Wyoming for "the Ranch Test"—the scrutiny of her parents, siblings, uncles, and aunts, together almost 20 in number. She didn't realize that Ryan planned to ask their permission to marry her. At an opportune time, Alicia was dispatched on an errand with her young nieces and nephews. Ryan faced the adults of the Craig family in the kitchen, his hands folded stiffly in front. "He didn't have anything planned or scripted," says Tumminello. "But you could see that his face was so full of love, and he didn't hold back anything. He said he wanted to care and provide for Alicia for the rest of his life. About halfway through, he realized he still had his baseball cap on his head, so he pulled it off and apologized. That was funny because no one in my family would care about that kind of thing. He was just so adorable."

That night Ryan scoured the Internet and ordered a diamond engagement ring. He planned to propose at Christmas. But having passed the Ranch Test, he couldn't contain his excitement. Two nights later, in a Colorado cabin, he dropped to one knee, popped the question, and slipped his honking Notre Dame ring onto Alicia's slender ring finger. "It was the cutest thing," she says. "Of course I said yes." Then Ryan reached for his guitar, and this time, as he sang their favorite songs, there was no tension in the room, just tenderness.

They were married on July 7 in Jackson Hole, Wyoming, with Mount Moran towering over them in the brilliant, sunset sky. When Alicia picked the date, she had been merely trying to arrange her wedding around a cousin's wedding the previous week. She didn't realize that 7-7-07 had become a popular date for many young couples. Ryan detected another pattern in the numerals. The Beijing Olympic Games would begin on 8-8-08. He thought this a good omen.

Over the next three months, as he intensified his training for the Olympic Marathon Trials, she detected nothing unusual. Sure, he had some aches and pains, as you would expect from running 140 miles a week, but nothing more. His last blood test before the Trials was his best ever. Competitive to the end, he couldn't resist lining up his results against Alicia's and pointing out all the areas where he "beat" her.

On November 2, the day before the Trials, Ryan and Alicia joined Ryan and Sara Hall for an easy jog in Central Park. Sara and Alicia had been Stanford teammates, and Sara was one of Alicia's bridesmaids. The men chitchatted about nothing of great import and stopped after four miles. "Sadly, I don't remember much about that run," Hall says. "He seemed the same old Ryan."

The women logged an additional four miles, entertaining each other with stories of their husband's prerace idiosyncrasies. Sara said her Ryan refused to eat in a restaurant before big races; she had to travel with a hotplate to cook spaghetti in their hotel room. Alicia said her Ryan could turn downright goofy before his races, the last thing you'd expect from such a straight-laced, routine-driven guy.

That evening proved a case in point. After a dinner out with Alicia's parents and a brief stop so Ryan could buy Alicia her favorite chocolates, the couple retired to their hotel room. Ryan couldn't resist a playful game with Alicia. He grabbed her hand and wouldn't let go. She had to visit the bathroom? Too bad, he wouldn't release her—not at first anyway. When she returned, he locked onto her again. "One of his missions in life was to make me laugh," she says. "We had such a wonderful, light-hearted evening. I thought it meant he'd run well the next day."

ALICIA DIDN'T SPOT RYAN at the seven-mile point, but was untroubled. The pack remained large and tightly bunched. No question, Ryan had burrowed himself into the midpack, content to let the others drag him along. When you did that, the running became effortless, and you preserved something for mile 20 and beyond. Ryan was in the perfect place. Alicia hurried back across the park, to about the nine-mile mark, to give him a big cheer there.

Her cell phone rang. It was Phil Wharton. He had ominous news. A friend had just phoned to say that Ryan had fallen. It appeared that he hit his head.

Wharton was racing to the location just north of the Central Park Boathouse. "I'll call you right back," he said.

Wharton arrived just as EMTs and paramedics were pushing Ryan's stretcher into an ambulance and closing the doors behind him. He spotted a woman visibly upset. "She said she was a physician but not associated with the race," Wharton recalls. "She had tears in her eyes. She said she had been giving him CPR for eight minutes, but couldn't revive him."

As the ambulance pulled away, Wharton called Alicia. "They're taking Ryan to Lenox Hill Hospital," he said. "I'll meet you there."

Alicia asked a policeman for directions, and now she was truly glad to be wearing those racing flats. She tore across a small greensward, exited the park just north of the Metropolitan Museum of Art, and flew across Fifth Avenue after a quick traffic check. She turned south on Park Avenue and converged with Wharton on opposite sides of 77th Street, just a block from the hospital. It probably took her just six or seven minutes to get there from Central Park. At the main desk, she asked where Ryan was, and just kept moving.

She got to the room, but something seemed amiss. There was too much commotion. "It was chaos," she recalls. Doctors flitted about frantically. She couldn't see Ryan, and figured she must be in the wrong place. To be sure, she pushed through to sneak a look. It was Ryan. Someone was working over his chest.

A doctor led her from the room and explained that Ryan's heart had stopped beating. They couldn't get it restarted. The words didn't sink in. They made no sense. No heart beat? How could that be? Ryan had a head injury. Even if it were true, she had heard so many stories and seen so many TV shows. Those defibrillator paddles, they always got the job done. "I didn't believe the doctor," she says. "I figured he was one of those people who always assumes the worst. I knew Ryan was going to be okay."

She waited for the good news. It never came. A few minutes later, one of the doctors said, "I'm sorry, there's nothing more we can do."

The room slowly emptied. Alicia had Ryan to herself. For an hour, maybe more, she held his hand the way he had held hers the night before. She expected him to open his eyes any minute. She hugged him and waited for him to start breathing again. "I was convinced he would," she says. "I knew he would. He felt so alive. He was so warm. It was as if we were lying in bed holding on to each other."

AT THE END OF NOVEMBER, ALICIA SHAY returned to the home in Flagstaff she had shared with Ryan. Friends and family members had warned her not to. She admitted to being "so scared" the first time back. Then she realized that she felt more comfortable in Flagstaff than anywhere else, with all their mutual friends and the places they frequented and the reminders of Ryan throughout the house.

Lauren Fleshman, her former teammate at Stanford, was coming for the month of December. Ryan Hall, who ended up winning the Olympic Trials, and Sara planned to visit in January. And there would be others after them. "It's going to be a very full house," she says with a hint of laughter. "I don't have enough beds for everyone."

There's a brief pause. It has been nearly one month since the morning that her husband died. Then she continues. "I'm doing okay," she says. "Nothing can take away the pain I feel over Ryan's loss, and I know someone else might be filled with anger, but I'm 100 percent amazed every day by the Lord's grace, power, and love. And I'm so thankful for my amazing family and all my friends."

Alicia then talks about her own running and her future. She says she gives Ryan credit for her comeback and strong performances in 2007. "He knew how much I loved running, and he wouldn't let me quit, even when I was very down," she says. "He was my best friend and my number-one fan."

She wants to keep running, and to pursue her dream, the same as Ryan's: to make the U.S. Olympic team that will compete in Beijing this August. "That's what he would have expected. I can't expect anything less of myself. I won't expect anything less."

Alicia will race the 10,000 meters at the U.S. Olympic Track Trials in Eugene, Oregon, on Friday evening, June 27. She'll be running on Pre's track, the one where Ryan scored his biggest track victory in 2001. The symmetry is too perfect. But it's a brutal system, the Trials: one day, one race, one woman against the distance. Nothing is guaranteed. Nothing. In last summer's national championships, Alicia finished fourth. She'll have to move up at least one position. And because of what happened to Ryan at the Marathon Trials, the whole world will be watching. That's a lot of pressure.

"After what I've just been through, pressure is nothing," she says. "Other peoples' expectations mean nothing to me. I have my resolve—that's the important thing. And I have Ryan's passion. He believed racing should be joyful, and so do I. The only hard thing will be running my race without having Ryan there."

She sounds resolute, if a bit shaken, much like the last time many people saw her. That was at Ryan's funeral, two weeks earlier in Central Lake. In the

evenings leading up to the funeral, Quinn Barry and several others had organized a series of memorial runs around the Central Lake High track, which was
ringed with flickering luminarias. You didn't have to run. You could walk. You
could just show up and bow your head. "I knew that people would want a place
where they could come to remember Ryan," said Barry.

For four nights, they came. Friends. Family. Old classmates. Current Central Lake students. Coaches who knew and admired Joe and Susan Shay and
their years of devotion to youth track. Townsfolk who didn't know Ryan or any
of the Shays, but had heard the stories and understood the loss, not just to the
immediate family, but to every small town where big dreams are too easily
punctured.

On Thursday night, the night of the final run, a thick rain and mid-30s temperatures couldn't keep nearly 200 people from paying their respects. Roger
Send and his daughter Amanda, 17, drove from Traverse City, 40 miles to the
south. They had met Ryan at a cross-country race the previous year. "He told me
how to use energy gels to improve my endurance," said Amanda. "And he said I
should never let anyone discourage me about my running. I should always stay
positive and focused." The Sends knew that Ryan had fallen at the 5.5-mile mark
in Central Park, and they had decided to finish his marathon for him by logging
20.7 miles on the Central Lake track. It took them nearly four hours, but they
reached their goal.

On Sunday, eight days after the Olympic Trials, Ryan Shay was laid to rest
after a packed memorial service at the Harvest Barn Church. Ryan and Alicia had
been there several times and enjoyed its rousing, 10-person instrumental-and-
vocal praise band. The service lasted almost three hours and included eulogies
from three important Joes in Ryan's life: Joe Piane, his Notre Dame coach; Joe
Vigil, his professional coach; and Joe Shay. Speaking in a soft, tremulous voice,
Joe Shay told the congregation that his son was a tough, determined man, "but I
prefer to think of him in words such as tender, loving, sincere, caring, and
loyal."

As the service was about to end, the church band prepared to play a final
song, "Blessed Be Your Name." The minister looked down at Alicia to ask if she
wanted the original, upbeat version, or, given the somber circumstances, would
she prefer a "calmer" version?

Alicia didn't hesitate. She made the only choice possible. Up tempo.

LEADING MEN

BY KENNY MOORE

[
Steve Prefontaine was a stubborn front-runner.
Bill Bowerman was the stubborn, successful coach who thought
he could change him. Both won—and both lost.
]

APRIL 2006

THE TALENT AND THE TEMPER

AFTER THE 1968 MEXICO CITY OLYMPICS,** Bill Bowerman hung his serape and sombrero on a nail and thought about how to make the best use of the next four years. One of his top priorities was to get more help for his University of Oregon track program. Bowerman had had dozens of graduate assistants in the 19 years he had been coaching at Oregon, but it was never a fully paid position. Perhaps the time was right to remedy that condition.

Bowerman decided to hire Bill Dellinger away from Lane Community College. Dellinger was an Oregon grad, a former Bowerman runner, and, in 1964, a medalist in the Olympic 5000 meters. As a coach, "Dellinger was good in the running events. He'd tell his boys that when you get really fit, running's easy, running's like brushing your teeth," Bowerman said. "Of course, that wasn't training. Training is like having your teeth cleaned an hour a day." Dellinger would be the first of Bill's assistants to work directly with runners of distance. In the fall of 1968 that was significant, because entering his senior year at Marshfield High in Coos Bay was one Steven Roland Prefontaine.

In the spring of 1968, as a high school junior in Coos Bay, Oregon, Prefontaine had set the state two-mile record of 9:01.3. Bowerman had arranged for two of his Oregon runners, the two-miler Arne Kvalheim and the miler Roscoe Divine, to take a 10-mile training run with Pre. "I had just beaten [Gerry] Lindgren with my 8:33 national record," recalled Kvalheim, "and Roscoe was in 3:57

shape, and this kid took us out on the beach and kept saying, 'Am I going too fast for you? Can you keep up?'"

They not only could, they felt like leaving him standing, but reined themselves in for the sake of their mission. Later they would learn that Pre was bursting out in a cockiness that had been long suppressed. His father, Ray, a carpenter and welder, had met and married his mother, Elfriede, in Germany while he was with the occupation forces after the war. Elfriede spoke German around the home, so Ray did, too. When Steve started school, he knew more German than English, and suffered for it. "Kids made fun of me," he would say, "because I was a slow learner, because I was hyperactive, because of a lot of things."

In the eighth grade, he found he could run well. All it took was being able to stand the discomfort of effort. His need to measure up, in the elemental ways demanded by his Oregon logging town and port, turned into a need to surpass. As a sophomore, he finished sixth in the state cross-country race, but not before wildly trying to steal the race from the favorites with a quarter mile to go. Earlier, he'd announced to his folks he was going to the Olympics someday. He knew it. He could feel it.

His mother, who'd grown up in a Nazi Germany where the last thing you wanted to do was stand out, blanched and ordered him to never talk that way again. She insisted he was an ordinary little boy. His father gently, gradually explained to Elfriede that the great thing about this country was that it was okay to dream big, but some part of Elfriede never absorbed that. Later, when her son enumerated the errors of the Amateur Athletic Union (AAU) for eager reporters, it would gall and mystify her. Plenty of other people had the same problems. Why couldn't they be the ones who stood up and exposed themselves to authority's eye?

In fact, Pre's bluntness was pardoned by anyone who grasped how good he was. In his senior year at Marshfield High, all boasts were quickly followed by proof. He broke the national high school two-mile record by nearly seven seconds with an 8:41.5. But even though Dellinger came to watch many of his races and Marshfield coach Walt McClure was nudging him toward Oregon (and was training him with workouts that Bowerman had suggested), Prefontaine wasn't getting anything from Bowerman himself like the recruiting pressure that he was receiving from a hundred other schools. Finally, though, Bowerman wrote him a letter.

It was a handwritten note. "I could barely read it," Pre would recall. "It said if I chose to run at the University of Oregon, he had every confidence I could become the greatest runner in the world." Pre signed on. Then he hopped on a plane with McClure to Miami for the 1969 national AAU meet. That's where I met him, the night before his three-mile.

The race was run in 90 degrees and 80 percent humidity. Gerry Lindgren and Tracy Smith ran away early and dueled to the line. Smith barely took it, though both were timed in 13:18.4. Pre began strongly but fell back to seventh with a mile to go. He looked doughy and white; his was not the kind of body to endure these conditions. But then he started passing people on sheer will and drove himself into fourth place, in 13:43.0. Since Juan Martinez, who finished third, was Mexican, Pre had made the national team.

Later that summer, in Stuttgart, Germany, in the Western Hemisphere versus Europe 5000 meters, he hung with Lindgren and East Germany's Jürgen May until the last two laps and clocked his best time to date, 13:52.8. We went on to Augsburg for the West German dual. Pre led all the way to the last turn, whereupon the cadaverous Harald Norpoth of West Germany exploded around him and won effortlessly.

Pre was mad from the instant he crossed the finish line. On the victory stand, while receiving their medals, Pre got into Norpoth's face. "I think it's chickenshit," he hissed, "for an old guy like you to let a little kid do all the work and humiliate him in the end." The crowd saw how hot he was, and started to jeer. Norpoth replied eloquently without a word, lifting his gold medal to the crowd and then holding it right under Pre's nose. This was a dual meet, and the win was the thing, not politesse.

Six weeks later, Pre drove his light blue, jacked-up '56 Chevy the 108 miles up the Umpqua River from Coos Bay to Eugene and registered at Oregon. He soon met a freshman classmate, Mac Wilkins, then a javelin thrower. Together they strolled into Bill Dellinger's office, to say hello and find out the time of the annual welcoming picnic at the Bowerman home.

As Dellinger welcomed them and gave them material on academic requirements and class schedules, Wilkins spotted a glass-framed photo on the wall and realized what it was. "Wow," he said softly.

Dellinger saw where he was looking. "My finest hour," he said. "Tokyo, on the victory stand."

Pre went over, peered at Bob Schul wearing Olympic gold and Dellinger wearing bronze, and started stabbing his finger at the picture. Wilkins thought he was going to break the glass. "That's the guy!" Pre yelled. "That's the chickenshit guy who sat on me in Germany!"

Wearing silver, of course, was Norpoth, whom Pre had sworn to hunt down and defeat. "He's a smart runner," said Dellinger. "In fact, I like to think that picture is of the three smartest guys in the race. We didn't chase after [Ron] Clarke when he tried to surge away, and we didn't try kicking from 400 out like crazy [Michel] Jazy."

"I would have run like Clarke," Pre announced loud enough to be heard down the hall. "I would have made it hard all the way!"

Clarke, an Australian who broke 17 world records during his career, was a front-runner out of principle. "No matter who I was racing, I tried to force myself to the limit over the whole distance," he once told me. "It makes me sick to see a superior runner wait behind the field until 200 meters to go, and then sprint away. That is immoral. It is both an insult to the other runners and a denigration of his own ability." Pre believed in this front-runner's creed.

"Notice," said Dellinger, "Clarke isn't in that picture. Clarke got ninth."

Later, Bowerman asked Dellinger what the excitement had been about. Dellinger sketched the scene. "Ah, with the talent," Bowerman sighed, "comes the temperament." He sighed that occasionally over the years, but more often in the Prefontaine era. This had been Pre's first salvo in a debate over front-running.

A Rube Awakening

THAT WEEK, AFTER AN ORIENTATION run with some upperclassmen, Pre went with them to the sauna, where they discovered Bowerman. Still coming down off his trip to Europe, Pre told how the AAU's Dan Ferris had put the U.S. team in an unsanitary hole of a hotel in Augsburg, while Ferris himself lived high on the hog across town. As Pre was getting worked up, Bowerman stood as if he was leaving, but then sat down right next to him, covering his key ring with his towel. Many eyes noted the keys. Many glances were exchanged.

"Apropos of the AAU," Bowerman said, "I'm sorry to tell you that the USOC has again refused to recognize the NCAA-backed Track and Field Federation. The AAU is still our governing body. I don't know how those old men figure to keep from stagnating if they don't let in new blood." He stood again. "It's understandable. They're crotchety old men, those kings of Olympic House. They don't want to change. It hurts to change."

Bill slapped his keys on the inside of Pre's thigh. "Doesn't it hurt to change?" he asked in his merry way, pressing down as the heated brass did its work.

"Sometimes it hurts more," Pre finally shouted, "just to sit and take it!"

Bowerman didn't expect this. As he went out the door, the others could see he was impressed. Pre, inspecting the welt, came to a realization. He turned on everyone there. "You didn't warn me!" he yelled. "What kind of teammates are you? You set me up!"

"Welcome to Oregon," someone said when the hysterics had died down enough. It apparently was a few days before Pre could feel it was an honor.

As Pre and Bill assessed one another, Bill, for one, noted similarities. Both were from small towns. Both were blunt. Bowerman sometimes called Pre Rube for his hopeless candor, but did so with a wink because it applied to him, too. "Or at least it did before I grew old and crafty," he said later.

How do you handle a hardheaded man? At their first goal-setting session, Prefontaine announced to Bowerman that it was great that Bill was the finest coach of milers, because that was the race he wanted to ultimately rule. Bowerman asked how fast he hoped to run. Pre said, "3:48."

Knowing the record was 3:51.1, Bowerman kept his counsel, only noting that 3:48 was 57 pace. But over the winter and spring of 1970, he observed that whereas Pre was hugely gifted over longer distances, and capable of fully recovering from most workouts with a single night's sleep (no extra easy days for him), he didn't have anything like the foot speed of a Roscoe Divine or a Jim Ryun. Speed, unlike stamina, can be improved only so much by training. Pre would never quite crack 50 seconds for a quarter mile.

"But that winter," Bill recalled years later, "all he wanted to do was train for the mile, run the mile. It got to where on our spring trip to Fresno, when I put him in the two-mile, he didn't want to run it. 'I'm not a two-miler,' he said, 'I'm a miler.' I suggested to him that he might want to give some thought to which university he'd be running for if he didn't try this particular two-mile, because it wouldn't be ours."

At that, Pre had turned and run out of the room. In 15 minutes he was back. He said, "Okay. Fine. Got it," and won the two-mile in 8:40.0. After that one quick test of the waters, Pre was never seriously defiant of Bowerman again.

In April 1970, running all alone in the three-mile in a dual meet against Washington State University, Prefontaine clocked a blistering 13:12.8. He was a natural three-miler and so good that any immediate concern about what kind of kick he had was rendered ludicrous by the pace he could sustain. "The man was designed," Bowerman grinned years later, "to run away with things." In the success of that breaking away, Pre had brought something unprecedented to the Bowerman stable at the University of Oregon. Bowerman himself would have to come to terms with it.

SIMPLY UNSTOPPABLE

IN JULY 1972, EUGENE HOSTED its first Olympic Track and Field Trials, which would produce the team for that summer's Games in Munich. The nerve center for runners was neither the track nor the athlete-thronged dorms. It was downtown, where flocks of ectomorphic, prominently veined competitors flitted through the Athletic Department store and were persuaded to stop, sit down, unlace, try on, and perhaps reconsider. The fledgling Blue Ribbon Sports, which would become better known as Nike, was taking exuberant advantage of its Bowerman-provided opportunity to introduce its running shoes to the nation's finest. The little store was jammed even without customers. Jeff Johnson, Bob Woodell, Geoff Hollister, and the rest of the company had converged here to get shoes on their feet.

Phil and Penny Knight were hot-pressing customized names on T-shirts to give athletes with their shoes. "How do you spell your first name?" Phil asked one marathoner. "D-U-M-P," he said.

"Okay," Knight said, arranging the letters. "What's your last?"

"Nixon." Thus did Tom Derderian run off in an emblem of the Trials' zeitgeist.

The crowd on the last day numbered 23,000. They were there mostly for Pre, and they rose to him in the last mile of the 5000-meter final, when he broke three-time Olympian George Young with ruthless laps of 63.4, 61.5, and 58.7, and cut seven seconds from his American record with 13:22.8. His great sense of theater led him to grab a "Stop Pre" shirt (that Lindgren had been booed for warming up in) and run victory laps in it. The sight of their champion parading the arena wearing the metaphoric pelt of the vanquished foe (Lindgren didn't make the team) made for atavistic hysteria.

Through all this drama, high and low, Bowerman abandoned his usual practice of watching from high in the stands. Instead, he was a presence on the infield, a genial general, welcoming new members to the team of Olympians he was taking onward. There, he pulled every string for them. Just as the 200-meter finalists were bending into their blocks, ABC wanted a delay for a commercial. Bowerman overheard the TV cameraman's walkie-talkie ordering him to run onto the track and take a slow shot of every tense face, thereby blocking the start until ABC was ready. The cameraman trotted to obey, but before he reached the track his camera refused to go any farther. He turned to see Bowerman standing on his cord. Bowerman nodded to starter Ray Hendrickson and the sprinters were started on time—meet time, not media time.

The Bowerman-Dellinger race plan for Munich, conceived with Dellinger's experience in Tokyo in mind, was for Prefontaine not to simply surge and slow, as Clarke had done, but to free himself with inexorably faster laps late in the race. His battle against Young in the Trials, when he'd run the final mile in 4:10, was a dress rehearsal, but everyone involved knew he could run faster.

Dellinger, both to enhance that ability and to learn exactly what Pre could stand, put him through training to simulate that long last mile. There were three key workouts. One was a set of four three-quarters in 3:12, 3:09, 3:06, and 3:00, with one lap recoveries, followed by a bunch of repeat miles. One was warming up, going to the line, and running, all alone, a four-minute mile. Pre did it in 3:59.0, changed shoes, and continued with his day.

The last workout gave him real concern. It was two essentially back-to-back runs of a mile and a half in 6:30, with an 880 jog in between. These were brutal because the pace dropped every half-mile, from 70 to 65 to 60. No one could stay with him on both of these six-lap efforts, so Dellinger asked young Oregon miler Mark Feig and me to alternate halves (I had qualified for the Olympic Marathon and would also be going to Munich). I drew the two-flat final 880 of the first run. Pre kept the pace but you could see he was going all out to hold it. He finished and looked so chartreuse Dellinger was about to say, "Knock it off for today." Pre didn't let him.

"The next one will be easier," he said, and threw up a sticky yellow mass all over Dellinger's new Adidases. "Didn't give those last three Danish time to digest." The second one was easier.

MUNICH GONE WRONG

ON AUGUST 19, we flew to Munich, were bussed to the banner-bedecked Olympic Village, and checked out our rooms in the United States' 14-story building. Groups of four or five would share apartments. We found everything comfortable and clean. But our coach was looking beyond our creature comforts.

"Since the war I'd been conscious of security," Bill would say later. "So I walked around the Olympic Village and there was none. As guards they had boys and girls dressed in pastels or Bavarian uniforms, not one with a weapon. The back fence was nothing, six feet, chain-link, no barbed wire. The Germans were trying to erase the memory of Hitler and Berlin in 1936. I went to Clifford Buck, our USOC president, to whom the Oregon Track Club had sent our fat check, and said we needed some real security on our building. If we let visitors just walk in uninvited, the place would be picked apart."

Buck told Bowerman to write him a letter, which Bill did. "We should be able to keep out thieves, harlots, and newspapermen," he wrote. Buck sent the letter on to the Olympic Village mayor, Walther Troger, who, Bill would say, "took rather strong umbrage." Troger informed Bowerman and others with similar concerns that the Munich Organizing Committee, under International Olympic Committee member Willy Daume, was determined to minimize police or military presence. These were intended to be the "Happy Games," the ultimate statement of how peaceful and free life was in postwar West Germany. "Let's pray it stays that way," said Bowerman to all and sundry.

"The Germans were outraged that one of these whippersnappers from America would say their security wasn't good enough," Bill's wife, Barbara, would recall. "So they went to the IOC and complained about Bill. From then on Bill was caught between the IOC and the Germans. But what happened then was something that happened to Bill strangely often his whole life. Something that started out simple became a great prophecy."

The early track events were eye-opening, especially if you were a 5000-meter runner studying your competition while they ran the 10,000. Finland's Lasse Viren was tripped and fell hard midway through the 10,000 final, almost taking American Frank Shorter down with him. Viren arose 40 yards behind, gradually caught the pack, and went on to beat Belgium's Emiel Puttemans in a world record 27:38.4. Pre sat with Dellinger and watched in silence. Viren was not ghostly and corpselike like Norpoth, but tall and ran with an eerie smoothness, the exact opposite of Pre's chesty power. You would never have guessed Viren had covered his last 800 in 1:56.6. "Better hope that guy has shot his wad," Arne Kvalheim told Pre.

That night, Bowerman left the Olympic Village and went out on the town. Barbara's hotel put on a Bavarian dinner, so Bill didn't go back to the Village ("feeling guilty about it," Barbara would say) until quite late. He slipped into his ground-floor room and lay down. It seemed to him his head had just touched the pillow when there was a pounding.

Shorter was the only one in our apartment five floors above who had heard anything. "I was out on our little balcony," he recalled later. "I'd dragged my mattress out there and had been sleeping there for a week or more. I heard a sound like a door slam." It brought him from fitful sleep to apprehensive alertness: "That's a gunshot." It was about 4:45 a.m.

A few minutes later came the pounding on the coaches' door. Bowerman groggily opened it. Before him stood an Israeli racewalker, Shaul Ladany. "Can I come in? Can I stay here?" asked Ladany distractedly, puffing, pushing close.

"What for?"

"The Arabs are in our building."

"Well, tell them to get out."

"They've shot some of our people," Ladany told him. "I got out through a window."

"That," Bowerman said later, "changed the whole complexion."

Bowerman was the first of the U.S. delegation to know we had become caught up in the Olympics' great loss of innocence. He called the U.S. Consul. "We've got a problem in the Village," he said. "I want some security."

Thirty minutes later there were two U.S. Marines at the U.S. entrance and two in the halls. "We secured the building," said Bowerman. "But I got a call about 6 a.m. from the IOC. They said, 'You've done it again, Bowerman, bringing Marines in here. We want to see you first thing in the morning.' I said I'd be glad to be there."

By 7:30 a.m., German security forces had begun to flood the Village streets. We would eventually learn that eight members of the Black September faction of the Palestine Liberation Organization, dressed in track suits and carrying rifles in sports bags, had scaled the back fence of the Village and forced their way into the Israeli men's quarters. They shot and killed Moshe Weinberg, a wrestling coach, and mortally wounded weight lifter Yossef Romano. They took nine other athletes and coaches hostage in the two-story duplex. The terrorists tied and gagged their captives, took up defensive positions, and shortly after 5 a.m. tossed a list of demands from the balcony to a policeman. To show their seriousness, they threw Weinberg's body out the window onto the sidewalk.

Thus began a day and long night of terror. The German authorities finally helicoptered the Palestinians and captive Israelis to a nearby airfield, where they falsely promised a plane would take them to Cairo and the prisoners to Tel Aviv. But at the airport, the Germans horribly botched an ambush. All nine hostages were killed.

The Games were postponed for 24 hours, but few felt like competing. "If they loaded us all into a plane right now to take us home," said a devastated Prefontaine, "I'd go." Instead, Dellinger persuaded Pre to come away into the countryside. He drove Prefontaine a full hour, well into Austria, where they stopped and inhaled truly Alpine air. To keep Pre from running himself to death as therapy, Dellinger had them take a jog together. This was September 6. Assuming the Games went on with only a day's postponement, the 5000 semifinals would now be on September 8 and the final on the 10th.

"I knew I didn't have to worry about Pre's bouncing back emotionally," Dellinger would say, "because he was so pissed that all this was giving Viren an extra day to recover after the 10,000." Dellinger goaded him a little more, pointing out that since he was, at 21, the youngest in the race by two years, every veteran in there—say, defending champ Mohamed Gammoudi of Tunisia or Harald Norpoth—was going down the list of entrants, coming to his name, and writing him off as a cocky kid who was going to be thrown back into babyhood by the attacks. Personalizing it like that was working, Dellinger saw.

Pre qualified for the 5000-meter finals, and on the last day of the Olympics, he and 12 others were leaning over the starting line. Pre's plan was unchanged. With four laps to go he would begin a mile-long drive to run all pursuers off their feet. The field was the strongest ever assembled, the best being Gammoudi, Puttemans, Norpoth, Viren and his countryman Juha Vaatainen, as well as Britain's Ian Stewart and Dave Bedford. Bedford, the world cross-country champion, had been vocal in his opinion that Prefontaine was a cocky little prick in need of quieting.

The USSR's Nikolai Sviridov and others led, but listlessly, and the pack remained a tight, worried clump. Pre remained in the middle of the pack, taking elbows and spikes. Everyone else's racing cowardice (or intelligence, depending on how they finished) was combining to create terrible luck for him. Never happy in a pack at the best of times, it was all he could do to keep his cool. He did so by visualizing how great it would be to be free.

They passed two miles at 8:56.4. It was almost time. On the home stretch, with four to go, he cocked his head, moved out, and took the lead. They had been going 67 pace. He ran the next lap in 62.5 and followed with a 61.2. Only five men were in contention by then: Prefontaine, Viren, Puttemans, Gammoudi, and Stewart.

With 800 to go, Viren passed Pre, perhaps as a psychological blow against the kid, who had to be feeling his blazing previous half-mile. Puttemans went by, too, as if he felt Pre was shot and was going to now fall back. Pre responded on the backstretch by charging past them and retaking the lead with 600 to go, just where Dellinger had led in Tokyo. He finished that lap with a 60.3.

At the bell with a lap to go, Viren passed him again, and Bowerman said later that he thought the Finn was sprinting too soon, that if Pre could tuck in and draft on his back, he could run him down late. But Pre wasn't hanging anywhere. As soon as they hit the backstretch with 300 to go, he moved out to pass Viren. But Gammoudi, who had done this to Billy Mills in the Tokyo 10,000, sprinted by, hit Pre so hard he drove him inside, and made his own charge to seize the lead. Pre was third with 250 to go. Again, Bowerman felt that if he gathered and waited, he could catch them in the stretch. Again, Pre refused to wait. With 200 to go he went wide and got to Viren's shoulder. He gave a tremendous effort, his head going side to side, but couldn't get past before the turn. Gammoudi cut him off again and went back into second. The top three men ran the last turn a yard apart praying that after all these moves and countermoves they would have something left in the stretch.

Only Viren did. He drew gracefully away to win in 13:26.4. Gammoudi was seven yards back in 13:27.4. Prefontaine died. At the line he was staggering. The madly sprinting Ian Stewart just caught him to steal the bronze in 13:27.6. Pre was clocked in 13:28.3. He had run his last mile in 4:04. Viren had run 4:02.

In the stands, Pre's girlfriend, Mary Marckx (now Mary Creel), didn't know what to do. "I didn't know how to reach Steve through the bowels of the stadium, so I started running up to the top of the stands. I was alone, crying. I couldn't imagine what he'd do. Would he kill himself? He'd been completely shut out, even of the 'horrible bronze' he'd disparaged."

At the top of the stadium there was a broad concourse. "There were Bill and Barbara Bowerman," Mary would recall. "I said, 'I don't know if he can take this. I don't know if I can help him.' Bill patted my arm and said it was a heroic effort, he couldn't have done any better. 'He's young,' Bill said. 'He's got a lot of races ahead. He'll be fine. Believe me, he'll be fine.'"

Mary knew her man. This was not going to be easy. Mortification did not sit well with Steve Prefontaine.

WHAT'S NEXT?

ON HIS RETURN FROM MUNICH, Pre never questioned Bowerman's race plan. He complained to friends or coaches only of the slow pace and of Gammoudi's spikes and punches. "If it had been 8:40 for the first two miles," he told *Track & Field News*, "I would have had gold or silver. It would have put crap in their legs. It was set up for Gammoudi and Viren." After watching the tape 50 times, I disagreed. I came to feel that if he'd let Viren lead the last 800 and made a single, all-out sprint with 250 to go, he'd have been second even as the race was run. His wild abandon was the reason he had been staggering blind before the line.

Still, Dellinger and Bowerman saw Pre wasn't bouncing back. He was moody, hopping from emotion to emotion. Creel, who would call Munich "a turning point" in Pre's life, saw that, too. Pre began partying and drinking much more than he used to, Creel would say, and seemed to take running less seriously. It may have begun to occur to him, on some level, that he might need to consider making a living at something beyond track.

Tough as it was for Prefontaine to regain his former eagerness, it was tougher for Bowerman. The man who had been such a rock for everyone in Munich came home exhausted and discouraged. He felt that "all the guff he had taken from the Olympic officials," Barbara would say, "defeated what he had tried to do there." He put up a good front for the sake of team and family, hoping the ancient rhythms of timing workouts and making shoes would restore his vigor.

Before those rhythms could take effect, the city of Eugene's fire marshal informed the university that Hayward Field's west grandstand along the homestretch was no longer patchable. The 5,000-seat structure, built in 1919, would have to be torn down after the 1973 season. New stands would have to be built in order for the facility to host future Olympic Trials.

Neither the athletic department nor the university had funds for this, and raising money for it would be an enormous task. "It was impossible," Bill said later, "to do justice to my coaching and to a big construction project at the same time. And we didn't have much time." So, without a word of warning, he retired. After 25 years as successor to Bill Hayward (Oregon's legendary coach from 1904–47), Bowerman, at the age of 62, announced that he was leaving to do the greatest good for the greatest number, by chairing a drive to restore the facility. Dellinger was soon appointed as Bill's successor.

Early in the planning phase for the new stands, pledges were about $25,000 short of what was needed to pay for bulldozing the old structure and for architects' fees. Someone hatched an idea to hold a restoration track meet that, according to Bill Landers, an Oregon administrator, would have "as its big hook our wonder child Steve Prefontaine racing Dave Wottle in a mile." Pre had scheduled a stint in Europe with the U.S. national team, as well as a slate of Scandinavian races. He'd planned to leave a week before the June 20th fund-raising meet, but his loyalty to Bowerman and Oregon prevailed, and he agreed to the race. He also called Wottle. "Come to Eugene before we go to Scandinavia," Pre said to Wottle, "and we'll try for a new world record mile. I'll lead and you'll get a great time." Wottle, a wait-and-kick miler and no fool, accepted that rare gift: a respected opponent setting a hard pace.

A crowd of 12,000 witnessed the Hayward Field Restoration Mile, double what attendance would have been without this duel. Prefontaine took over after the half and hit an eye-opening 2:56.0 for three-quarters. Wottle shot out to a

10-yard lead in the backstretch and held it to the end, which he reached in 3:53.3 to Pre's 3:54.6, both lifetime bests. Wottle had missed Ryun's record but was now the second-fastest American ever. Bowerman exulted that Pre was fully, emotionally back. "He ran a great race," he said. "If Wottle had drifted five yards off, he'd have gotten whipped!"

The meet cleared $23,204. "How many world-class guys," Landers would say of Pre, "would agree to a race they knew they were going to lose?" Afterward, Norv Ritchey, Oregon's athletic director, congratulated Pre for his magnificent gesture. "Well, Pre," Ritchey said, "this is a great thing you're doing, and it will repay every bit of grant-in-aid you ever received." Pre looked Ritchey right in the eye and said, "I did that the first race I ever ran at Hayward Field."

Once Prefontaine graduated, he faced a reality that would be unbelievable to later national champions: penury. To run his best, he needed the freedom to train and travel. A full-time, entry-level job in his major field of communications—lugging equipment at a TV station—wasn't compatible with that. So the bulk of his income came illegally, or at least in violation of the amateur code. He would run bursts of European races, where promoters would pay in cash or fungible airline tickets. And he tended bar at the Paddock, his own favorite haunt. The Pad always did great business when Pre was drawing the pitchers.

Bowerman heard about this and sat Pre down for an unscheduled goal-setting session. He knew his man by now, knew to lead with the irrefutable. "No one in Oregon," Bill said, "can influence kids the way you can."

Once Prefontaine had nodded in prideful agreement, the discussion was essentially over. However free Pre might feel to lead his own life, said Bowerman, he wasn't free to set an example that, if followed by the youngest of his people, would do them harm. "You're right, Bill," Pre said on very little reflection. "I'll quit. You're right."

Bowerman said later that he and Prefontaine seldom engaged in lengthy talks. "But there wasn't a picture of them," Barbara would observe, "where they weren't looking at each other and saying, 'Hey, who's boss here?'" Each operated by laying out a position and presuming the other would respect it.

On April 27, 1974, Pre ran his first serious race of the year, a 10,000 at the Twilight Meet, in rain and wind. It would be a lonely race. The west stands had been bulldozed, and although 7,000 people were in attendance, they were all huddled in the remaining seats on the far side. Lap after lap, Prefontaine ran 67s, but he ran them by sprinting 32s with the wind in front of the crowd and muscling 35s against the wind on that lonely backstretch.

As he came by on the backstretch, eyes rolled back, mouth agape, moaning, he seemed to be running into oblivion. Yet when he came past the crowd and it stood up and thundered, he showed that he heard. The rest of us would hear the crowd, be moved to hang on, and try to lift a grateful arm afterward, but Pre always acknowledged his crowd in the moment. He cocked his head then, surged for them then—and they thundered all the more. He won them by stripping himself naked, unembarrassed at revealing his need and his agony. He ran an American record 27:43.6 that day, only five seconds slower than Viren's world record in Munich. "I think," he said later, subdued, "this indicates I'm ready."

Early in 1975, Pre was offered a $200,000 contract, the largest in the short history of the International Track Association. Pre had little of the traditional distance man's feeling for austerity. "I like to be able to go out to dinner once in a while," he'd say. "I like to drive my MGB up the McKenzie on a weekday afternoon. I like to be able to pay my bills on time." But he turned the contract down. Until the Europeans were well and truly thrashed, he said, "What would I do with all that money?" He had abstained, of course, for one reason—to keep his eligibility to take on Viren in the 1976 Olympics in Montreal.

From Tragedy...

AT 7 A.M. ON MAY 30, 1975, we awoke to the shock of our lives: Steve Prefontaine had been killed in a one-car accident on Skyline Drive, no more than a minute after dropping Frank Shorter off at my house. We walked down through neighbors' yards to the scene. The car had been removed by then, but there was broken glass on the street. We saw the accident report and learned he'd struck a natural outcropping of black basalt. He hadn't been wearing his seatbelt. The car had flipped over, coming to rest on that great chest. He had not broken a bone. It was simply the weight of his beloved butterscotch MGB pressing the life out of him. If anyone had found Pre then, in the first five minutes, he might have saved him with a two-by-four and a brick.

Pre had to have left this world with a fine regard for its absurdities, one being that he was dying on a road he loved to run, on a hill where he made others suffer. His last moments surely recapitulated his finest races, his blacksmith-bellows gasping, his fighting down panic, his approaching death's door, his needing the crowd to call him back.

The effect of all this was to make us wild to cling to Pre's legacy, to define and protect it. He hadn't left a will, but he might as well have. "I did not want to waste or squander any effort Pre put forward," Shorter would remember. "I felt if you could keep momentum going on something he cared about, then you should."

Our leader in much of this was Bowerman. Earlier that year, when Hayward Field's new west stands were completed, the annual restoration meet had been renamed the Bowerman Classic. Bill now scotched that. "He was the driving force in the two restoration meets," Bowerman wrote in a press release. "Our Oregon Track Club Board concurs that in living memorial to Pre—his inspiration, his ambition—the meet he did so much to make successful should bear his name. Next Saturday you may attend the Steve Prefontaine Classic, a first step in a parade of opportunities to share directly in the dreams of Prefontaine."

Bowerman got a note that week from university president Robert Clark. "Your gesture in naming Saturday's event for him was magnanimous," Clark wrote. "We owe much to Steve, but we owe even more to you for your years of service and for the quality in you that brought Steve Prefontaine and others to us."

The Pre Classic would grow into the finest invitational meet in the country. And a living memorial it is, coming at the season he left us, when the roses and peonies are most potent, the season that blends the opposites that warred in him, the voluptuary and the ascetic.

TRUE
ORIGINALS

THE RETURN OF BOSTON BILLY

BY STEVE RUSHIN

Nearly 30 years have passed since Bill Rodgers
won his fourth and final Boston Marathon. Those memorable
victories—along with an endearing, flaky manner—made him
the most popular American marathoner ever. Now,
after battling cancer, he's ready to run Boston again and
prove once more why he is the People's Champion.

MAY 2009

FOR SIX YEARS BILL RODGERS DOMINATED the Boston and New York City marathons like no man before or since, winning each race four times between 1975 and 1980, a run of excellence that ended—inevitably—in a hastily found bathroom in Hopkinton, Massachusetts. He met his Waterloo in a loo 20 minutes before the start of a Boston Marathon sometime in the 1980s. Rodgers cannot recall the precise year, though this much is certain: with 7,600 runners and as many expectations pressing at his back, he felt a sudden and irrepressible need to find a toilet. This was not an uncommon problem for a man of his prodigious dietary indiscretions. "Bill ate a pork chop from the back of his fridge a few days before one Boston, not bothering to notice it was green," says his friend Greg Meyer, the last American to win that race, in 1983.

"As a kid, he put ketchup on brownies, peanut butter on eggs, mayonnaise on everything," says Martha Chuprevich, Rodgers's younger sister.

In his competitive prime, a postrun repast for Rodgers meant sticking a fork in a jar of peanut butter and then plunging it into a bottle of bacon bits.

"I brought a friend to see him after the race one year, and the friend couldn't believe that the guy who had just won the Boston Marathon was spooning mayonnaise onto a pizza," says Amby Burfoot, who won Boston in 1968 while a senior at Wesleyan University, where he and Rodgers were roommates.

"I'm a bit of a scavenger," Rodgers told me one day last fall while eating five-alarm chili from a Styrofoam coffee cup in the cafeteria of the YMCA in Southington, Connecticut. "As a poverty-stricken runner, you'd go to dinner and stick the rolls in your pocket to take home."

All of which is to say this: on that long-ago April day in Hopkinton, Bill Rodgers—"the only man who has ever run 150 miles a week and still had high cholesterol," says Meyer—had to use the bathroom.

Mercifully, Rodgers knew a dentist whose house was under renovation 100 yards from the starting line. He ran there, abruptly did his business, and turned the bathroom doorknob to leave. But the locked doorknob just spun in his hand.

"It was quarter to twelve, and no one knew where Billy was," says Dave McGillivray, who is now the race director of Boston, but at the time was a teammate of Rodgers's on the Greater Boston Track Club.

Rodgers was locked in a bathroom moments before the start of the race that had made him famous—an anxiety dream sprung to life—when a funny thing happened: he was seized by the unexpected calm that comes over people in the latter stages of drowning.

"All of a sudden I was like, 'This is okay,'" Rodgers remembers. "I didn't really care that I was locked in. In fact, it was better that way. I wouldn't have to race. I remember thinking, I don't know if I really want to go out there."

"I did get out and run the race, but it was a sign, mentally, of how I felt about marathons. I think I was just getting worn down and losing my desire. All that time, you know? All that wear and tear."

In the summer of 2008, Rodgers was eight months removed from prostate-cancer surgery and 13 years removed from the last time he had finished Boston when he said to me, haltingly, almost apologetically: "I'm thinking of getting ready to run Boston in 2009." After a pause, he added, "We'll see how I'm feeling. I'll have to decide by December."

April of 2009 marks three decades since he last won Boston and New York in the same year, when his fame peaked and he became an alliterative icon of the Boston sports scene, a bridge between the Splendid Splinter and Larry Legend: Boston Billy.

Back then, to his bafflement, buses would pull up to his curb in suburban Sherborn, Massachusetts, and disgorge Japanese tourists taking pictures of his house. The Japanese baseball slugger Sadaharu Oh once materialized on his lawn and posed for a picture with the bewildered homeowner.

Elite runners from around the world asked to run the streets of Boston with him. Meyer often joined Rodgers on those runs and remembers the pride that blue-collar Bostonians felt for one of their own: "Heads would literally pop out of manhole covers and yell, 'Kick their asses, Billy!'"

At 61, Rodgers says—if he ends up running—he has no intention of kicking any asses this year. His friends hope that he's telling the truth. "I think it would be the greatest thing in the world if he'd allow himself to run Boston slowly," says Burfoot. "Nobody would care, except for the six blowhards who would say, 'I beat Bill Rodgers.'" This is common among Rodgers's friends and family, the wish that he would slow down.

As a boy, Rodgers chased butterflies with a homemade net in a field near his house in Newington, Connecticut. "He was an expert," says his 85-year-old father, Charles, a retired mechanical engineer. "He mounted them on a board and could tell you the name of every one of them. And that's how he began running—by running after butterflies."

"I was a fanatic, a lepidopterist, like Vladimir Nabokov," Rodgers explained to me while discoursing on the pleasures of the elusive tiger swallowtail. "At 12 years old, I'd just run through the fields sweating."

A moment earlier, he had repeated his desire to run Boston in '09, but at a stately pace that might prove as beautiful, in its own way, as his 2:09:27 of 30 years earlier.

Nabokov was nearly as renowned as a butterfly expert as he was as a writer. But it was another novelist, Rodgers's fellow New Englander, Nathaniel Hawthorne, who wrote: "Happiness is a butterfly which, when pursued, is always just beyond your grasp, but which, if you will sit down quietly, may alight upon you."

HE HAS NEVER BEEN ABLE TO SIT DOWN quietly. In a chair, Rodgers calls to mind a live butterfly pinned to a board. He thinks he has attention deficit/hyperactivity disorder—one of his two grown daughters has been diagnosed with ADHD. His father says, "I wish he would slow down. He's always flying somewhere."

When I arrange to meet Rodgers for the first time, at his 32-year-old shoe and apparel store in Boston, he has not yet arrived from Logan Airport. "Bill's running late, as usual," says his older brother, Charlie, who presides over the Bill Rodgers Running Center with an air of Eastern mysticism. His white beard—cultivated over four decades—is two feet long and hangs in twin braids that resemble the tasseled tiebacks on theater curtains. "Relax," Charlie tells me. "Relax. Relaxation is the key."

To expedite that effort, he graciously asks if he can get me anything: "Coffee? Scotch?" It is 3:20 in the afternoon. Meyer worked in the store 25 years ago and says of that era: "It was basically a welfare program for runners Bill liked." (When I told Meyer later on the phone that I'd just met Charlie, the first thing he said was, "Did he offer you hard liquor?")

As I wait, a woman comes into the store and asks Charlie if he is Bill Rodgers. Charlie sighs and says, "No. Short legs."

"Charlie got the short legs and the long torso," says his sister, Martha. "Bill got the long legs and the short torso." Their father, who is 6'4" with the posture of a utility pole, got the long legs and long torso.

And so I wait for Rodgers. It is possible, though he's lived in Massachusetts for nearly 40 years now, that he has gotten lost on the way from the airport to his own store. On more than one occasion, McGillivray has gotten a call on his cell phone as some running-related dinner got under way only to hear Rodgers, lost and running late, asking for directions. "He's a very lucky man," says McGillivray. "The Boston Marathon course only has five turns. Any more than that, he'd have no victories."

Martha recalls riding shotgun as Bill got lost for what seemed like hours on the Silas Deane Highway near their hometown.

But Rodgers eventually arrives at his store, 30 minutes late, still wearing the giveaway T-shirt from a race he'd run in Pittsburgh the night before, the kind of race he makes his living appearing at 42 weeks a year. He hadn't gotten lost. "We have those GPS things these days," he says. And so Bill Rodgers slipped into the Bill Rodgers Running Center unrecognized. At the baggage claim at Logan, a priest had asked him if he was John Rodgers. Says Rodgers, happily: "Nobody knows who I am."

We sit in Charlie's office, a brick-walled phone booth filled with shoes and apparel. There are two office chairs, a desk, and a filing cabinet that looks rather more like a defiling cabinet, supporting as it does 30 bottles of single-malt Scotch. "Charlie's a connoisseur," Bill says with a laugh. The Rodgers are Scotch-Irish, tracing their paternal history to a 17th-century bagpiper from Crieff named Patrick Rogie.

Every year after the Boston Marathon, in a tradition that dates back three decades, 45 or more people—Africans, Kazakhs, Japanese, you name the origin—gather in this office that comfortably holds three and drink expensive Scotch from Dixie cups while raising a toast to the race just run. "I can't stand the stuff," Rodgers says of the Scotch. "I'm not much of a drinker. Maybe a gin and tonic after a race, or a rum and Coke, or a Baileys."

And yet, for a lightweight drinker, Rodgers is at the center of many fine stories involving bars and bartenders. As an undergraduate at Wesleyan, Burfoot would go to bed at 9:30 on Saturday nights and run 25 miles on Sunday mornings. He remembers Rodgers as "a normally talented runner" who would stay out "at bars and discos until 2 or 3" on Saturday nights and join him for the last 10 miles of his Sunday runs.

As roommates, Burfoot and Rodgers were Felix and Oscar. "I remember visiting and seeing Amby's change stacked neatly on his dresser," says Bill's father, Charles. "Bill had a mattress on the floor."

"And a candle-lamp made from a red-wine bottle," says Bill, fairly blushing.

When Burfoot won the Boston Marathon, the victory had no visible effect on his roomie, who notes that the race wasn't even televised 110 miles from Boston, in Middletown, Connecticut. "I don't remember Bill going gaga or asking me a hundred questions," says Burfoot. "There was no such thing as a fawning distance runner in those days. We were all just weirdos."

"People ask, 'Did you know he'd be Bill Rodgers?' The answer is no. How could anyone? What I did recognize was a smooth, relaxed runner, and while I was faster in college, he was perhaps running on a lower percentage of potential than I was."

That percentage of potential would get much lower before it got higher. After graduating from Wesleyan in 1970, Rodgers stopped running and started smoking two packs of Winstons a day and hanging out in the manifold bars of Boston, where he got around town on a used Triumph 650 motorcycle he had bought with $1,000 borrowed from his best friend.

That friend, Jason Kehoe, works at the Bill Rodgers Running Center and recalls leaving a bar with Rodgers one night "after a few beers" and the two running the final 100 yards of the Boston Marathon course—in street clothes.

For three years, Rodgers would ride his Triumph to the finish line on marathon day and stand there smoking as the racers ran by. "I think watching that had a strange, subtle effect on me," he says now.

One night Rodgers came out of a bar to discover his Triumph had been stolen. He would be forced to rely on his own locomotive powers to get to Brigham and Women's Hospital, where Rodgers—a conscientious objector to the war in Vietnam—worked as a special education teacher. Within a month, he saw a stranger riding his Triumph past the hospital. "I was never a speed guy," says Rodgers, explaining why he didn't give chase. "And I think I recognized it was the best thing that happened to me."

It forced him to start walking, and then running, at first on a track, and then around the city. In 1973, after running for six months, Rodgers found himself in Hopkinton, at the start of the 30-kilometer Silver Lake Dodge road race. Burfoot—who had largely lost touch with him since college—was surprised to see Rodgers on the starting line, and not merely because he was dressed like a hobo. "He was in tattered khakis, a tattered shirt full of holes, looking like a bum, like a street person," says Burfoot. "I go up to him, he's this happy puppy dog, his tail wagging, and say, 'It's great to see you're jogging. You've stopped smoking. I'm so happy for you. I'll see you at the finish line.'"

Yet 10 miles and 49 minutes into the race, Rodgers and Burfoot were still linked at the elbows like paper dolls. Burfoot looked over at his former roommate in disbelief. Rodgers was a golden retriever giddily running alongside a station wagon. Running in slacks.

"I used to run a lot in blue jeans," Rodgers recalls, before going on the defensive and saying over my laughter: "Hey, they didn't have the good gear back then! Gore-Tex hadn't been invented yet!" But he remembers the race, largely because the Silver Lake Dodge dealership donated the prize: A set of four tires. Or maybe it was just two tires. "That was road racing," Rodgers says with a laugh. "And I still love that about our sport."

For all the prize money he won, he never prized money. When his apparel business was liquidated in 1988, Rodgers sold his house in Sherborn to the Bank of Boston to pay his debts.

And while he's a good debtor, he's a lousy creditor. When Greg Meyer and his wife had a baby, Rodgers lent his friend $2,000. Three months later, after "winning some races he probably threw me," Meyer tried to repay him.

"What's this?" Rodgers said of the check.

"I owe you money," said Meyer. "You lent it to me."

"Really?" said Rodgers, whose wardrobe then, as now, consisted principally of giveaway T-shirts.

"I've seen him in a tie more in recent years," says Meyer. "He used to always wear his running shoes and a pair of shorts, and carry a shoulder bag for his racing shoes and extra T-shirts."

His eccentricities of dress and laissez-faire approach to organization still give Rodgers the air of an absentminded professor. In November 2008, he signed on to run an 8-K in Philadelphia. "The race just went on and on," he recalls. After six miles—9.6 kilometers—he realized he'd joined the wrong starting queue and was actually in the half-marathon. "Really disturbing," Rodgers says, though he ought to be used to it by now.

"He's always lost or in the wrong place," says his friend Bart Yasso.

"It's a miracle he could remember to run 20 miles on a given day, much less the day before or the day after," says Burfoot. Indeed, his father, Charles, is an absentminded professor. "He's a mechanical engineer whose mind is always off in quasar land," Charlie Rodgers says of Charles Rodgers.

Likewise, there is a whiff of genius about Bill, who behaves the way Einstein might have if Einstein had been a runner. Thirty minutes after I met him for the first time, Rodgers was removing his shoe midsentence to show me his new orthotics. He rifled his pockets for a quote he'd just torn from *USA Today*, about the psychological benefits of running outdoors versus running indoors. His pockets were filled with bits torn from newspapers, each the size of a fortune-cookie slip. He reminded me of the comedian Rip Taylor, pulling confetti from his coat pockets.

All of this has not merely endeared Rodgers to other runners and to the public at large; it has worked to his competitive advantage. "Part of me always felt he was dumb as a fox, and I say that in the most complimentary way," says McGillivray. "He is so approachable and so friendly, and that just wiped away his aura. He's not this guy on a pedestal, and that worked in his favor. Other runners got sucked into this idea of, 'We're all here to run this thing together.' And he was right there in the back of the pack. Then all of a sudden, it's time to go and Bill just went and nobody could go with him. From a strategic perspective, he was a genius."

"No!" says Rodgers, when I put this theory to him. "No, no, no! That was never a part of a strategy. You can't really do that. Most runners get along really good. You might have one or two archrivals—Frank Shorter was a rival, but I didn't dislike him. I had no reason to. It's just a footrace, a sport, with a whole ethic of saluting the other guy if you get beat. You just run your best."

And so Rodgers—in jeans and khakis, in that benighted era before Gore-Tex—entered more races.

His bartender friend, Tommy Leonard, founded the Falmouth Road Race, which Rodgers considers the greatest road race in America. "My bartender friend Tommy Leonard got me to come down in 1974 by promising me that girls in bikinis handed out water on the course," says Rodgers, who refers to Leonard on every reference as My Bartender Friend Tommy Leonard, as if it were a formal title: Her Majesty Queen Elizabeth II. "It was a lie. I got there, and there were no girls in bikinis. But I did get my car towed."

Still, Rodgers beat Marty Liquori at Falmouth that year and won a Waring blender for the effort. He ran the New York City Marathon when it was four loops in Central Park because he loved the Olympics and first prize was a ticket to Athens on Olympic Airways. He didn't win, but those early, uncelebrated New York marathons were their own reward: he was ducking Frisbees and dodging pedestrians and helping to create an event that now annually draws 39,000 runners.

In 1975—two years after running the Silver Lake Dodge in khakis—Rodgers won the Boston Marathon. "One of the things that made him so great was his ability to lock down and focus for months at a time," says Greg Meyer. "Then during the race itself, he was just a freak, with incredible concentration. It goes back to that single-mindedness. When Billy charts a path, it's hard to get him to deviate from it."

"I've read that Michael Phelps is wired like that," says Rodgers. "You follow what you want. You can't always follow other things, but you can focus on what you like. I was lucky to finally find the marathon. It gave me something to sink my teeth into."

Even he struggles to comprehend his two natures: laid-back Bill and laser-focused Bill. "I became intense about the marathon," Rodgers says. "But I am nowhere near that intense in the rest of my life. In fact, I think running is the only way in which I'm competitive. I have a need to run and sometimes I love it. It's probably because I wasn't really good at anything else."

"Billy really didn't have other things to fall back on," says Meyer, who met Rodgers at the IAAF World Cross-Country Championships in Glasgow in 1978. "And I'm guessing that created anxiety at times. Most people hedge their bets with something. Billy never did."

Even Rodgers must be joking when he says Bob Kempainen threw away a promising career in distance running for a misspent life as a physician: "We had this great marathoner, but he wanted to become a doctor! He shouldn't have done that." When I suggest to Rodgers that most people broaden their interests as they grow older, he puts his hands to his eyes to simulate blinders and says: "Not me. I'm very much like this."

It's hard now to fathom how improbable his 1975 Boston victory was. Jason Kehoe, who had drunk-jogged the final yards of the marathon course with Rodgers in 1972, says, "Three years after that night, I'm watching him run the same stretch, but he's winning the Boston Marathon for real. It was unbelievable."

The victory was no more believable to those closest to him. His sister, one year younger, was watching the TV news in Hartford that evening. "They kept saying the name 'Bill Rodgers' and showing all these police motorcycles," says Martha, who could be forgiven for wondering if perhaps he had robbed a bank.

His father was handing out exams that day at Hartford State Technical College, where he was a professor of mechanical engineering. He told his students, in a tone of mild exasperation, "My son is running in that crazy Boston Marathon today." He thought it was a goofy and perhaps dangerous thing to do.

Rodgers stopped four times for water that day and a fifth time to tie his shoe at the base of Heartbreak Hill. Still, he ran 2:09:55, a time he himself did not believe when he found out afterward. "I can't run that fast," he protested.

But he could. In the first five-borough New York City Marathon, in 1976,

Rodgers was surprised to see, as he ran up Manhattan's East side a set of stairs he had to climb. "We didn't care," he says. "We were running the course blind." He won the race.

In the next five years, Rodgers won four straight New Yorks, three more Bostons, and three times was ranked the world's top marathoner, a streak book-ended by Boston pedestals: the wooden platform for the winner at the finish line in '75, and that porcelain plinth of the dentist's toilet near the starting line the next decade.

For 15 straight years, Rodgers never missed more than two consecutive days of running. But in 2003, on an eight-mile training run on Nantucket the day after His Bartender Friend Tommy Leonard's race, Rodgers's right tibia snapped. He fell like a gunshot victim at the side of the road. He hitchhiked from a seated position—a sweat-soaked, grimacing spectacle with his butt on the ground and his thumb in the air. A teenager in a Jeep finally stopped for him.

"I just get in that mode: keep goin'," says Rodgers. "Runners are like that, and I think swimmers are, too." He is fascinated by Michael Phelps, his fellow ADHD sufferer. "But I think swimmers mellow," says Rodgers. "Runners don't. Runners just keep going until they expire."

Aside from the broken leg at 55 and a bout of plantar fasciitis at age 40, Rodgers hadn't a single health problem in his adult life. He was in Barbados for a 10-K in December 2007 when his doctor called with grave news: Rodgers had prostate cancer. "I was with a couple of friends, and we were having a lot of fun," he recalls. "And as soon as I got that call, I was like, 'What now?' You don't know what the hell to do."

So what did he do?

"I ran the 10-K," Rodgers says. "That's what you do."

HE HAD SURGERY A MONTH LATER, and Rodgers is now trying to raise awareness and money for prostate-cancer research, much as the Susan G. Komen for the Cure foundation has done for breast-cancer research through its race series. But he is realistic in this pursuit. "Women are better organizers than men," he says. "Men are reluctant to talk about these things. We like to hunker down in our caves. I sort of have this gut feeling that we"—he means men—"are doomed to failure."

Still, if anyone can rally runners to a cause, it is Rodgers, who remains by some measures the most popular road racer of all time. Meyer calls him "the Arnold Palmer of our sport," a populist icon who still makes his living at it long after his competitive twilight. "Billy fakes it so well," says Meyer. "Someone will say, 'Bill, I met you four years ago in Des Moines,' and Billy will have that person believing that he remembers meeting him four years ago in Des Moines."

At the Southington (Connecticut) Apple Harvest Festival Road Race last fall, Rodgers ran the five-miler and then spent two hours afterward handing out trophies, thanking sponsors, signing autographs, and posing for photos. When the last supplicant retreated, 92-year-old Frank Kosko approached and said that his son used to run against Rodgers. Bill insisted Frank join us for lunch at the Y. On our way there, Rodgers signed a high schooler's bib, and the three of them stood there for a moment in their various postures—the 92-year-old, the 61-year-old, and the fresh-legged 16-year-old—looking, in sequence, like one of those evolution-of-man posters.

Burfoot calls Rodgers "the people's champion" and says, "Frank Shorter was the Olympic champion, a little more distant and imperial than Bill, but Bill was the champion of races that the people themselves ran in—Boston and New York and Falmouth. He literally reached out and touched people, like God on Michelangelo's Sistine Chapel, and that was a big part of the spark that created the running boom."

If Bill Rodgers is best remembered for the Boston Marathon, well, the Boston Marathon might be best remembered for Bill Rodgers, too. "Everyone likes the local product," says McGillivray, the marathon's race director. "It's just human nature to get more engaged and more revved up by them. With all due respect to the athletes winning all the races now, as incredible as they are, it's just—from a fan perspective—not the same as it is when the people up front are those you personally know or have seen around town."

"It's not any worse or better now," says McGillivray. "It's just different. I was part of one of the most amazing, incredible, inspiring experiences I've ever had in road racing when Joanie [Benoit Samuelson] ran the [2008 Olympic] Trials here in Boston. She was three-quarters of the way back, but to hear the crowd, it was like the Pope was coming through. It reminded me of a World Series victory parade: runners were running by, and you'd hear footsteps, then quiet, footsteps, then quiet. Then this continuous roar starts building and here comes Joanie. And that's the way it is with Billy in Boston."

Rodgers is a Red Sox fan who was sorry to see Manny Ramirez get traded. "He just looks like he's having fun," he says of the Sox former left fielder. "He's rich, he's damn good at what he does, and he's a free spirit of a guy."

Remove the rich part, and that's a fair description of Rodgers, who loves the potent cocktail of Patriots' Day: one part Boston Red Sox, three parts Boston Marathon.

"My Bartender Friend Tommy Leonard always says it's Christmas, Thanksgiving, Halloween, and St. Patrick's Day rolled into one," says Rodgers. "It's fun, it's pure fun."

We are interrupted, in the Old Curiosity Shop that is the back office of the Bill Rodgers Running Center, by Charlie, who pops his head in and asks Bill to hand him a Steve Prefontaine poster from the box behind him. The box is full of posters, all of Prefontaine, and I think: Pre is the subject of two feature films and Rodgers is the subject of none? Bill grabs a poster and passes it to his brother as if it were a baton.

"I just love this sport," he continues. "Yesterday, outside Pittsburgh, I'm at a race with 700 people, and we all go over to the race director's house afterward and have ice cream and cake in his front yard. What could be better than that? Then six or eight of us went into the guy's house. His name is Mark Courtney. And he's got a little finished basement with the Boston Marathon finish-line logo. He's a family guy with a 4-year-old daughter, and he has a business and works a lot of hours. But somehow or other he still runs at a high level. There was a wide range of us down there: one guy was more of a track athlete, one guy was a lot older. And we had our beer. And look at this." Rodgers pulls the wrinkles out of the T-shirt he's wearing and reads the front for me: "It was called Courtney's Ice Cream Race."

He gets a faraway look, a 26.2-mile stare. "Seven hundred people in Grove City, Pennsylvania, on a Wednesday night to run a 5-K. A 79-year-old lady who came close to an American record. An 80-year-old former minister who has run 2,500 races. And 200 high school kids." Rodgers is beaming. "It was fantastic. Then we all go to Mark's house and eat cake and ice cream. It's the ultimate community event. That's what running is. We're really like baseball. We're ultimately grassroots. We really are. And we were 100 years ago, at the turn of the century. You look at our sport all the way back, there were all these county fairs, and they all had foot races. So running goes back to our ancient roots as people—the cavemen were running—but it also goes back to our American historical roots."

Running is embedded in our DNA. Just ask the boy with the butterfly net. "You only get cheered in running," says Rodgers. "Every other sport, you get booed."

Greg Meyer told me, "Bill finds it genuinely funny that he gets paid to do this." He gets paid to do what he can't help but do, what he still does every day, for 40 to 50 miles a week: run.

BILL RODGERS HAS STOPPED chasing butterflies. Four years ago, when he last moved houses, he threw away the 50-year-old board on which he'd pasted his Nabokovian collection. Still, happiness has alighted on him.

Rodgers, twice divorced, remains close to his two daughters, both from his second marriage: 18-year-old Erika and 23-year-old Elise, with whom he would like to run a race someday. "I love being a family man," he says while walking—not running—on a trail near his house in Boxborough, Massachusetts. "I love being a dad."

It's a new year, a year in which he has promised to slow down. Over the preceding months, Rodgers became more circumspect about his plans to run Boston in '09. As the weather got colder and his training necessarily curtailed—"I hate running indoors"—he decided not to run. "My health is good as far as I know," he says.

"And I'm running a lot of half-marathons. I was running one in Melbourne, Florida—February's USA Master's Half-Marathon, where he finished fourth in his age group, in 1:34:16—"and during the race I was thinking, This is pretty hard. I'm content just to do halves right now."

So the butterfly catcher really has slowed down.

Or has he? One minute after uttering the statement above, Rodgers is talking, in his store, about the glorious 60-degree morning which he spent driving the Boston Marathon course with a photographer. "It really got the memories and the competitive part of me going," he says in that faraway dreamer's voice. He pauses, sighs, continues: "I still might change my mind about Boston."

Either way, he can't go wrong. If he runs, he knows he'll be carried along by the crowd. "I hear everything people say," he acknowledges. "A lot of people recognize me on the course, and cheer for me—'You're doing great, you're doing great'—and it lifts me up when I'm feeling terrible. And it's a huge advantage. A huge advantage."

And if he doesn't run—well that doesn't mean he's forsaken winning all the spoils. On the contrary. When I left him at the Y in Southington that day last fall, he was the center of a quintessentially Bill Rodgers–esque tableau: seated between a 92-year-old lunch companion he had just met and an elfin plastic trophy on a faux marble base for the winner of the 60-to-64 age group. In front of Rodgers was a five-pound spackler's bucket of chili from the El Sombrero Mexican restaurant that race officials had given to him to take home.

In that moment, he looked as content as any man can be. When I suggested as much, he looked at me over the chili bucket, raised his plastic trophy, and said, smiling: "Victory is sweet."

A LONG,
STRANGE TRIP

BY STEPHEN RODRICK

> He was hanged by his thumbs in Iran for
> wearing the wrong T-shirt. He rode his bike across
> six continents. He spent four months in INS
> custody for illegally crossing the U.S.-Mexican border.
> And now Reza Baluchi is about to finish running
> across America. It's weirder than you think.

OCTOBER 2003

JUST OUTSIDE OF HICKS JUNCTION, Arkansas, kid-filled, DVD-laden SUVs and long-range 18-wheelers jockey for position on I-40. Inside a 1994 Ford Dutchman RV, a CB radio hums with warnings about wobbly U-Hauls, hooter jokes, and guesstimates about the distance to the closest Waffle House. The accents twang and ping in a scratchy Tower of Babel. Then the chatter turns serious.

"Break 1-9, be aware there's a guy running on the Interstate, east-bound side. Damn fool."

"10-4. He's being followed by an RV. Says he's running across America for unity."

Pause. "What the hell is unity?"

Longer pause. "That's when we all stop mussing with each other."

Longest pause. "Where the hell is the fun in that?"

Much laughter. A driver clears his throat and launches into an exaggerated honey-dripping drawl of a certain well-known simpleton: "Uh, life is like a box of chocolates."

Two drivers at once. "Run, Forrest, run!"

Up ahead, a blissfully unaware Reza Baluchi plods on. Some 1,300 miles down, 1,700 to go. He's almost halfway through his journey from Hollywood to

Ground Zero, which is a walk in the proverbial park when you consider that Reza's odyssey started in Rasht, Iran, and has included stopovers in Morocco, Ecuador, and a place called Burkina Faso. All in the name of peace.

If this were the pre–politically correct 1970s, Baluchi would warrant a sit-com. Why did he wear a Michael Jackson T-shirt and leather pants in rural Iran when he knew the local mullahs would be coming after him? That's Reza! Why did he bicycle across 56 countries, fleeing a lion, contracting malaria, and accumulating girlfriends? And as an Iranian national in a post-9/11 world, why did he cross the Arizona-Mexico border illegally and camp out in the desert, earning himself several months in an Immigration and Naturalization Service detention center? Yes. That's Reza!

And now he is running across the country with the help of a 47-year-old unemployed entrepreneur named Dave. Sure, dozens have made the transcontinental run before: Ultramarathoners, midlife-crisis guys, and multiple every-mans running for various charities. But never before has there been Reza Baluchi, an irrepressible, salsa-music-loving peacenik who's hoping to score both a movie deal and a place in the record books. The man is one part humanitarian, one part superhero, and one part the Ego That Ate Tehran.

Now's the time to get on the Reza Express, because he's due in New York City on September 11. So bring along some air freshener, a hanky, and some extra Ragu for dinner. Reza Baluchi will make you laugh, cry, and, occasionally, want to bounce a water bottle off his sweaty, balding head.

Oh, and you might want to get a stretch in. Reza runs between 30 and 40 miles a day.

That's Reza!

HE IS 30 YEARS OLD, about 5'7", and 130 pounds, with sharp brown eyes, and an odd balding pattern—a tuft of black hair at the top of his head exists on an island all its own—that squares perfectly with his personality. His running routine is not one that Jim Fixx would have endorsed. Nutritionally, Reza acts like he still lives in his birthplace, Rasht, a province in northern Iran where going hungry was as natural as the sunrise.

He rises most mornings around 5:30, without the benefit of an alarm clock. Sometimes, he eats a bowl of corn flakes and a banana before beginning his run. Sometimes, if Dave Hyslop (Reza's driver, publicist, and guy Friday) is still sleeping, he skips it. In restaurants, he watches Americans pack their pie holes, and it disgusts him. "American, eat way, way too much," Reza says in his unpolished English.

Despite the massive trucks and endless white noise, he logs the majority of his miles on superhighways. Although this is technically illegal, Dave says he has obtained permission from state police. "The local roads have no shoulder and too many curves," reasons Dave. "He was going to break an ankle or get hit by a car."

After running 15 to 20 miles, at about a 12-minute-per-mile pace, Reza usually takes a short break. He may eat another banana before he gets moving again. Once he hits 40 miles, Reza stops for the day. Then Dave makes him a mega-calorie shake with ice cream, milk, and fruit. His only real meal is consumed around 7 or 8 in the evening: two big bowls of spaghetti made with Ragu tomato sauce.

Gear-wise, Reza isn't picky, but he is a little vain. He wore donated Nikes at the beginning of the trip because he loved the way they looked. But they were too narrow for his size seven EEEE feet, so he switched to New Balance. Every 300 miles, he slips into a new pair. Reza never stretches and apparently never gets tired. "If I not running, I get angry," he says. "I run, I happy. Very happy." But things weren't always so simple.

Fresh from another 40 miles and his first shower in days, Reza brings out a couple of battered binders and begins to tell his story. Dave has parked the RV—his and Reza's home for the past two months—off Exit 42 in Stanton, Tennessee, cozily between a truck stop and the gravely misnamed Countryside Inn. Conversing with Reza is tricky, as he speaks Farsi but very little English. Fortunately we have a translator. Just like Dave, Afsaneh Fathi has become swept up in Reza mania. A high-level financial analyst in Los Angeles, the Farsi-speaking Afsaneh saw Reza off in California, has kept tabs on him ever since, and has flown out to Tennessee for a few days.

The Iran that Reza was born into, in 1972, was a different Iran from the one he grew up in. While the last years of the Shah's reign were marked by corruption, it was a rapidly Westernizing country open to ideas. After Ayatollah Khomeni's ascension to power in 1979, Iran became an unrecognizable place, a theocracy with an extensive cultural and moral police force.

Reza, the son of a rice farmer, is one of eight children. The searing memory of his childhood is his oldest brother, Saddam, returning from the fruitless Iran-Iraq War. "He couldn't work, he couldn't do anything," recalls Reza in Farsi. "The littlest thing would make him hysterical and violent."

At the age of 9, Reza left his family and went to the nearby city of Shiraz, a much more cosmopolitan place. He lived with an aunt and made $3 a week as a helper in a mechanic's shop. As Reza grew into his teens, he fell in love with girls and what passed for Iranian haute couture. This did not sit well with the local clergy. One evening, Reza hit the town in leather pants and long hair. The mullahs grabbed him, he says, shaved his head, and confiscated the pants. Caught eating a sandwich during the holy days of Ramadan, when food and water are prohibited during daylight hours, he was whipped in the city square. At 16, he was caught alone with a girl. They were both whipped.

By his early 20s, Reza was widely known as one of Shiraz's bad boys. One evening, he was caught wearing a Michael Jackson T-shirt. He also possessed a video of a banned Iranian film. When Reza refused to disclose where he got the contraband, he was hung by his thumbs for 24 hours and was later thrown in jail for 18 months for associating with "counterrevolutionaries."

Reza pulls off his shirt to show an unnatural knot in his shoulder. He explains that the police would handcuff him by pushing one arm back over his head and then linking it to his other arm. When I asked him why he would take such risks, Reza smiles and shrugs.

"I like Michael Jackson. He help Africa. He help kids. Michael Jackson good man."

It's heartbreaking to hear a man talk about being hanged by his thumbs for idolizing Wacko Jacko. But Reza's jail time didn't dampen his spirits. Throughout his youth, he had participated in cycling contests, and upon his release from prison, in 1996, Reza bribed an Iranian sports official, scoring a precious exit visa under the pretext that he was a world-class cyclist pedaling across Europe, spreading good news about Iran. Apparently, Reza felt compelled to make the pretext a reality. He flew to Germany, where visa problems stalled him for three years. He entered cycling races, he says, and worked as a mechanic to survive.

And then Reza's story becomes a nonfiction fable. From Germany, he cycled to Turkey. From there, he flew to Pakistan and began cycling east, through India, China, and eventually Singapore. From there, he flew to Australia and cycled down the coast. Then he headed back to Europe. The afternoon of September 11, 2001, found Reza spending time in a hotel in Paris. He was watching television in the lobby.

"I see big fire," Reza says in his limited English. "I think it really good movie. Turn channel, same movie. Then, I understand."

On that day, Reza decided he would bike across the United States. "I show America I like peace," Reza says. "Not all Iranians terrorists." Of course, this being Reza, there was a slight detour. He decided first to pedal from Morocco to Johannesburg. After recovering from malaria and winning a stand-off with a lion in Zimbabwe, Reza flew across the Indian Ocean and began cycling through South America, beginning in Argentina.

Reza's accounts of his journey are largely unverifiable, but his scrapbook provides enough snapshots, plus the occasional newspaper article, to support at least the basic facts. However, what Reza can't explain is why. I ask him the question through Afsaneh several times. "He doesn't like war," she explains. "He wants people of all religions to get along and live freely. He thinks we all need to compromise."

Perhaps because of his prison time, Reza has grown a bit paranoid. He fears that Afsaneh is not properly translating his answers. He repeats over and over, "I like peace. I no like war. I like freedom."

Late last year, after surviving the sinking of a ferry off the coast of Panama, Reza made it to Mexico. He settled for a while in Monterrey, where he met a girl, fell in love, and worked in an Iranian-run pizza shop. He applied for a visa to enter America. However, after 9/11, visa applications for transcontinental cyclists from Iran were moving very, very slowly. Impatient, Reza rode up to the border to make a plea in person. He camped out in the desert, close to the Arizona border—apparently, too close. He woke up one morning to the sound of helicopters. A flashlight tapped him awake.

"Do you know where you are?" asked a border-patrol officer.

"Mexico," replied Reza. "I wait for visa."

"No, you're 15 miles into Arizona," replied the guard. Reza spent the next four months in the INS compound in Florence, Arizona. To bide his time, he ran around the compound's tiny yard in street shoes. Somewhere along the way, Reza decided cycling across America was not a grand enough gesture. If freed, he would run across America instead.

IF REZA DOESN'T RATE a sitcom of his own, how about *The Odd Couple*, starring Reza and Dave?

It's a little after 7 on a humid and damp morning, a few miles outside Memphis. Almost two hours earlier, Reza popped out of bed and began running Highway 70. Dave slept for another hour before driving after him, heading east, as usual. After seven or eight miles, he starts checking convenience stores.

"Have you seen a short, Iranian man in jogging shorts?" asks Dave, a lanky man with salt-and-pepper hair and the patience of Job on his best day.

"Sure, with a little black dog?" responds the clerk. "He's probably two, three miles up the road."

"A black dog." Dave repeats the phrase, not quite comprehending, then climbs back into the RV. Sure enough, about three clicks up on the right, there's Reza, wearing his reflective vest with the Iranian and American flags sewn on the front.

His gait is gimpish, if clock-settingly regular. His left arm swings like a machete in a Hong Kong action flick, the right arm hanging close to his side as if he's guarding some bauble in his running shorts. His back is stained in blood. No, it turns out to be PowerAde leaking from his hydration pack. Nipping at his heels is a malnourished black puppy that is missing a hefty chunk of flesh near his right eye. The dog pants so violently his ribs threaten to burst through his mangy fur.

"Hey Reza, whose dog?" Dave asks. There's trepidation in his voice.

"Rocky Balboa. He follow Reza seven miles," Reza answers. "I keep him. I call him Rocky Balboa."

Reza grins and hoofs on down the road. Dave smiles wearily. He places Rocky inside the RV, gives him some water, and stares at a plague-like skin condition on the dog's back. "Man, we have to find this boy a vet. I better check for ticks tonight," he says. "We'll see what happens the first time Rocky pees on Reza's bed." He brightens a bit. "But this should cheer him up, after what happened last night."

Last night was indeed disappointing. To promote Reza's "Run 4 Peace," Dave arranged a pot-luck supper with a local peace group in Memphis. The media was alerted. Reza had dreams of TV trucks dancing in his head. In many towns, supporters had joined Reza for meals or short runs. But alas, after a mad-dash, red-light running RV romp through the belly of Memphis, we arrived to an empty church basement. No TV cameras, no fellow peaceniks, and no pot-luck supper. Reza sank into a funk. His mood only darkened when the highfalutin restaurant where we ended up brought Reza's ravioli.

Reza, who loves pasta, was hungry. But his plate held just four ravioli. He went silent for the rest of the night.

"He wants to run," says Dave. "When he stops, he wants it to be for a good reason. I think he blames me."

While Reza may run, it is Dave who carries the weight. Raised in Omaha, Nebraska, he is the child of an alcoholic father who passed away when Dave was 16. After graduating from high school, Dave moved to California and spent much of the past two decades working in a television-facilities business in Los Angeles. But he never gained any traction in his career, and at the beginning of 2003, he was 46, underemployed, and deep in credit-card debt.

Then, on the morning of February 1, 2003, he opened the door of his studio apartment and picked up the *New York Times*. Over a cup of coffee, he read about Reza's incredible odyssey for the first time. Almost immediately after reading the article, Dave wrote to Reza at the detention center in Arizona and gave him his phone number.

"He seemed so brave and alone," Dave says as he feeds bologna to Rocky. "Here was one guy with a message of peace just trying to do his little thing to make people understand each other better without fighting."

Over the next two months, the two talked often, although Reza's English made significant communication nearly impossible. Still, Dave made Reza a promise: When you're released, you have a place to stay in California. After a judge granted Reza political asylum, he set off on his Centurion bike for Dave and the Pacific Coast, with a few dollars in his pocket provided by the Iranian-American community of Arizona. Along the way, a strong gust blew Reza over and he tore his groin. Still, he pedaled on.

When he finally arrived, he and Dave plotted Reza's run across America. Reza spent 11 days sleeping at the foot of Dave's bed. Dave helped him plan his route and coordinated his send-off. Dave's television work provided him with many contacts in ethnic broadcasting, including one with Parvis Afshar, a talk-show host who's considered the Johnny Carson of the Iranian ex-pat community in Los Angeles. Afshar started hosting Reza on TV Tapesh every week, trumpeting the friendship between him and Dave as a sign of American-Iranian unity. It struck a chord with the Iranian community. Since President Bush lumped Iran in with North Korea and Iraq—their sworn enemy—in his "axis of evil," Iranian Americans were desperate for a symbol to show that they valued peace as much as their neighbors did. For them, Reza was a gift from heaven. Throw in an American sidekick, and they were ecstatic.

On Mother's Day, Reza was off with a pack on his back, holding a small tent, some walnuts, a cell phone, and a camcorder. Dave went home. He and his long-time business partner prepared to take a lucrative and much-needed job. But when he got home, he started crying.

"It seemed like I was abandoning the guy," says Dave. He tries to hold them back, but the tears come again. He flips his silver hair out of his face and wipes his eyes. To demonstrate his point, Dave fishes out a videocassette. (Part of the RV has been turned into a multimedia center. There's a desktop computer, a printer, a VCR, and a color television.) Dave pops in the tape, which Reza made and sent to him after day four of his run.

Reza's footage is more *The Manchurian Candidate* than home movie. He had made his way through the Angeles mountain range, reaching an altitude of 7,000 feet, before descending into the seedy crossroads town of Barstow, California. In a motel room that an Iranian truck driver rented for him, Reza places the camera a few feet away from himself. A television drones in the background. Reza starts shooting close-up video of his toes, which are covered in blood blisters. Speaking in Farsi, he rambles monotonously about his aching feet. Then he pops the blisters with his fingers and watches the blood trickle into a Kleenex. "That's better," he says. He sits quietly for a few minutes, his gaunt face staring into the camera. Then, apropos of nothing, his face lights up. He speaks rapidly and with great vigor. All I understand is the word Guinness.

"He's saying that he wants to talk to me about whether his trip qualifies him for the *Guinness Book of World Records*," says Dave. "That would make him very happy."

Shortly after that footage was shot, friends in the L.A. Iranian community arranged for a podiatrist to treat Reza's feet. Operating in the backseat of his car, the doctor treated the blisters and cut out an ingrown toenail. The same group raised enough money to rent the RV to accompany Reza on his trip. The driver was going to be an Iranian American chef. Dave didn't think that was such a good idea.

"I could just picture the two of them walking into some small town, not having shaved for a couple of days," says Dave. "The way John Ashcroft has everyone so paranoid you could see somebody thinking they were there to blow up a school."

Dave decided to catch up with Reza and see him to New York. First, he had to tell his business partner that he wouldn't be taking the new job they had worked so hard to land. "You're throwing over your partner of 10 years for a guy who you've known for a month?" asked Dave's pal.

"Yes," answered Dave, "I am."

"My partner was always a temperamental guy," Dave tells me. "I was always the one following up with our clients and telling them he didn't really mean what he said. I got that from growing up with an alcoholic. That way of always trying to make things appear perfectly normal when there's all this chaos. I guess you could say I'm an enabler."

Alas, Dave may have jumped from the psychological frying pan into the fire. The penultimate line in the *New York Times* story he read about Reza would prove prophetic: "For some, glory is like sea water. The more one drinks, the thirstier one grows."

Reza has grown mighty thirsty.

SINCE LEAVING L.A. TO JOIN REZA, Dave has kept a journal of their travels. Many of his jottings are picayune details of people met and supplies bought. Some, however, suggest that Reza can be a handful.

June 11: He shows me the bottle of baby oil I used to massage him this morning. He wants to put it on his legs, no doubt so they will glisten a bit for the TV cameras. [A crew from Oklahoma City was on hand.] No I say, "the sun hits them, it will burn." He said, "I like" and proceeds to slather all over his legs. When he finishes he looks approvingly. "This good." He leaves a half-hour early, then returns thinking maybe it would be a good idea for him to shave his legs.

June 26: Reza almost got hit by a car this evening. He called twice and the phone didn't ring. I got to him at 8:30, and he'd peed his pants he was so scared.

Later, while driving on I-40 just outside Memphis in a rented Volvo station wagon, I get a firsthand glimpse at what caused Reza to lose the contents of his bladder. (Dave, fearful their permission to run on the highway will be revoked, doesn't allow anyone to run with Reza on the interstate.) Even in the comfort of a solid Volvo, each passing semi leaves me jonesing for a Valium. At one point, Reza needs to cross four lanes of traffic as the highway merges with another. It proves difficult enough in a car. I look back expecting to see poor Reza planted on the grill of a Cadillac Escalade. But he bides his time and scoots safely across.

Dave sighs when he recalls Reza's near miss. "I went up ahead to send some e-mails to the media in the next town. When I reached him, he told me, 'Reza runs 40 miles a day, Dave spend all day on the Internet, writing to newspapers. Dave go back to L.A., and Reza write newspapers.' But after an hour, he forgot all about it." Dave is able to forgive Reza for these lapses partly because of his own enabling personality and partly because of Reza's innate likability. For every tantrum he throws, there is an act of kindness—and not all of them involve puppies. Early in his trip, Reza found a $100 bill on the side of the road. He had Dave take him to the nearest hospital, where he bought flowers for sick children. And when Afsaneh will need to fly back to L.A., Reza will insist that we drive her to the airport in Nashville, a 400-mile round trip. At the end of the day, Reza makes sure Dave knows he's the one man in the world Reza can count on. "Dave good to me," Reza says. "Dave only one I always trust."

And so Dave remains loyal. On the RV's dashboard is a CD he made for Reza. The tunes include Elton John's "Your Song," the Rolling Stones' "Waiting on a Friend," and the Bee Gees' "How Can You Mend a Broken Heart." "I wanted songs that reflect the loneliness of running and the courage of his journey," explains Dave. He shrugs and laughs. "I don't think he likes it. Ever since he was in Mexico, he loves salsa music."

So far, despite Dave's PR efforts, Reza's journey hasn't exactly penetrated the American media. There's been some local TV coverage and newspaper stories, but none of the national shows have bitten. Still, Reza remains undaunted. Dave plays for me some promotional videos targeted to the morning shows. One captures Reza at dawn, about to embark on a run. "Good Morning America, from Reza." Another is pitched toward NBC: "Good morning, Katie, I am Reza." One evening after looking at slides of Reza's travels, I jokingly ask him to tell me about the groupies he must have left in his wake. Reza smiles and says, "Steve, I not tell you everything. Reza save for book and movie." Everyone laughs. Reza already knows who is going to play him. "Tom Cruise," he says definitively. "Only Tom Cruise."

IN THE PARKING LOT of a Super-8 Motel, the Midnight Riders of East St. Louis, a group of African American bikers, shine up their choppers. Into their midst arrives Reza. It's noon, and he's already run 25 miles. When he comes to a stop, there's no panting, no sign of distress. "I rest a minute and run 20 more," says Reza. As usual, he is constantly smiling through jumbled teeth. After a few minutes, two bikers wander over.

"That dude is running across the country?" asks one, who calls himself Half-Pint. "That is too much."

Reza shakes a couple of hands and smiles again. "I like peace, I no like terrorism, I want all people to like each other."

"That's cool," says Half-Pint. "I'm for that." He signs his name on the side of the RV, adding it to well-wishers from across the country.

Reza's message of peace doesn't go much deeper than that. It's not as if he has a doctorate in peace studies. One day, I join him for a few miles as he runs through downtown Memphis. We pass the Lorraine Motel, where Martin Luther King Jr. was shot. It's now a civil rights museum. I tell Reza that King is an American hero who worked for peace. He looks at me quizzically and then smiles. "I not know Martin Luther King." He runs another few strides and then pronounces: "Reza want to be American hero."

It's one of the contradictions of Reza's journey. His English is minimal, so he is limited to a few platitudes. In a way, that's not a bad thing. It allows the people he meets to project what they want onto him. There's no *Crossfire*-like quibbling about border disputes, puppet dictatorships, or American imperialism. People leave their encounters with him feeling good about themselves no matter their ideological stripes.

But there are still those who have the other reaction. On a Saturday afternoon, we set out to find a vet to look over Rocky Balboa. Dave eventually locates one in Memphis, next to a tattoo parlor. Reza stays with Rocky as the vet examines him. "Qué pasa, Rocky?" asks Reza in a loving voice. He strokes his snout and Rocky sighs. Dave explains to the doctor Reza's story of running across America. The vet stares at Reza as if he's a Vulcan. "Mmm," he mutters. For the rest of Rocky's exam, he watches Reza out of one eye. For him, there appears to be a direct corollary between running 3,000 miles and spontaneous psychotic behavior.

As the sun falls, we make a pilgrimage to Graceland. Unfortunately, tours are over for the day, even for men running across the country. However, Reza borrows a pen. He walks over to a portion of the wall surrounding Elvis's home that is covered with messages from visitors. In very careful penmanship, he writes a long and elaborate note in Farsi. When he's finished, I ask Afsaneh what it says.

"It's a beautiful Iranian saying," she says. "He wrote, 'Life is very, very hard. We struggle. Only one thing is certain. In the end, we must all die.'" It's the closest I see Reza come to connecting his own suffering with his cross-country run for peace.

We head over to a nearby souvenir shop. Reza dons big gold glasses and mugs for photos with a Vegas-era cardboard Elvis. He then has an idea: Why not buy a T-shirt with Elvis's picture to run through downtown Memphis tomorrow? He grabs one and disappears into the changing room. In a minute, a sheepish Reza emerges. The garment is skin-tight and could serve as wardrobe for the next Village People revival. He looks in the mirror and shakes his head. "Reza give this to girlfriend," Reza says. "This shirt make Reza look gay." Then Reza grabs my arm. "You not write Reza is gay, okay? Reza not gay."

Wait a second. Reza, a man of peace, has a sliver of prejudice in him. How could this be? After his travels across the world? After his own struggles? I think about it for awhile, and although it may be odious, it makes Reza seem more like real flesh and blood. To the humanitarian/superhero/egomaniac trifecta, add human being.

But even that doesn't capture Reza. He surely cares about peace, but that's not all this trip is about. If it were, Reza would have learned more than a few clichés—whether in Farsi, English, or Esperanto—to say on the subject, and he'd definitely be able to ID Martin Luther King Jr. No, Reza is a wanderer. As much as it is about peace or his ambitions to become a star, that's what this trip is about. And Reza is at home in America, because from the Sooners waiting for the signal on the Oklahoma border to the bicoastal commuters of the new century, this is a country of roamers. In the land of the rootless, Reza Baluchi is king.

Reza says that when he completes his journey, he wants to go back to school and study engineering. It's depressing to picture him in a short-sleeved shirt with a pocket protector, commuting to a suburban office park in a Hyundai, and running spread sheets. Reza realizes this. There's already talk of him running back to L.A. via Canada. I get the feeling Dave would be on board, too. "I finally feel like I'm doing something with my life," he says.

On my last day, Dave asks me to drive ahead in my rental car and give Reza some cold water. It's only 10 a.m., but Dave estimates that Reza is about 15 miles down the road. Later, I'll find out Reza has already had an eventful morning. A Tennessee state trooper pulled in front of him and told Reza that running on the highway was forbidden.

"It's okay," Reza replied. "I talk to big police boss, he says okay."

Amazingly, the trooper moved on. However, as I head up I-40, Reza is nowhere to be found. I pull off an exit to begin retracing my steps. Then, my cell phone rings. It's Reza. He's not pleased.

"Steve, I run 20 miles. No water. What Steve do?"

Good point. When I find him—he had ducked into a gas station—Reza is no longer mad. He gulps water and smiles. I ask him if he wants to take a break. He's only had a banana to eat. "No," he says, "I must run." With that, Reza Baluchi trots over to the on-ramp, merging onto the highway between a pickup truck and a Chili's 18-wheeler. Destination: New York City. Dave is busy, too. He's sending a video of Reza to David Letterman.

Everyone's fingers are crossed.

A 6-MINUTE DIFFERENCE

BY CYNTHIA GORNEY

> *Ever wonder how much faster (or slower)*
> *you'd run if you were the opposite sex?*
> *Janet Furman Bowman may be the only runner*
> *in America who knows.*

JUNE 2005

BEFORE THE RACE, in her warmups, Janet Furman Bowman is noticeable from across the parking lot only because she's the tallest woman, and the best dressed. Her pants are black and stretchy and look good on her. The jacket matches. Her blond hair is pulled back in a ponytail. She's wearing small dangly earrings, red lipstick, and a silver pendant on a slender chain. Her socks are rainbow-striped around the ankles.

Is there anyone here who doesn't know? Janet looks around, surveys the gathering runners, smiles. George has arrived, and Hans, and Dave, who's going to do the 5-K pushing his 2-year-old in a stroller. The sky is overcast. Mount Tamalpais, the great woods-covered peak visible from almost anywhere in the eastern half of Marin County, California, looms out beyond the high school driveway where volunteers are collecting entrance fees and marking out the starting line. Men and women trot by, loosening up. Nobody looks at Janet curiously anymore—no sidling glances, no startled double takes.

Morning, Janet.

Hey, Janet.

"Here I am," she says. "Running. With a hundred friends."

She makes it sound like a simple thing.

At 8:45, 15 minutes before race time, she takes off her warmups. She's wearing black shorts and a red cross-back tank top, the same color as her ponytail

217

holder. Janet is lean and long-limbed, like a pole-vaulter, and as she stands in the pack at the starting line, she tips her body forward slightly and tenses up. A whistle blows. For a minute Janet vanishes within the surge of runners angling for position, and then the pack begins to separate: one lap around the parking lot, they've been instructed, and then out across the grass to the trail outside the high school. By the end of the parking lot lap, Janet is in her stride, body upright, both hands closed into fists. The men are already pulling away—not all the men, but a good-sized swarm of them, Hans and George and the teenager Jason and even Dave, with the stroller.

This is the part she hates.

She can't help it. She just does. There is so much to be grateful for, after all that has happened; extraordinary graces, she revisits them every day. But when Janet sprints across the finish line—Pull it in, Janet! Way to go, Janet!—and checks her watch for her time, 23:27, she knows instantly how it compares to her PR for the 5-K: six minutes, 25 seconds slower, or more than two minutes per mile. She used to be able to run 5:30s. Now she can't. She trains, she pushes herself, she uses everything she has; it doesn't matter. On the weekend-morning group runs, when serious Marin runners gather near trailheads to pace each other up the dirt roads that climb Tamalpais, Janet starts with the pack, as she has nearly every Saturday and Sunday for 25 years. "Usually there are a lot of guys," she says. "They start slow. I stay with them for the first mile. Then I start falling away. They're chatting. They don't even notice."

When she was Jim Furman, a 5'11", 148-pound middle-aged man in excellent physical shape, she kept up.

As Janet Furman Bowman, a 5'11", 148-pound middle-aged woman in excellent physical shape, she's too slow.

That, to her astonishment and irritation and unceasing soft regret, is the permanent price she has paid.

MARIN COUNTY IS a famously unconstrained part of Northern California, made fun of on occasion for its receptiveness to every form of spiritual and behavioral experimentation. (From San Francisco, the shortest route to Marin requires driving across the Golden Gate Bridge and into a tunnel entrance framed by a massive painted rainbow.) But six years ago, when only a few people in the Tamalpa Runners Club understood what was happening to Jim Furman, the bewilderment and discomfort were palpable every time the runners convened for a race or a party or a Sunday-morning trail run. The club has more than 800 active members, and its gatherings are central to one strand of social life in the affluent towns around Mount Tam, as the mountain is affectionately called. The biggest running event in the county, the brutal up-and-over-Mount-Tam seven-mile June trail race called the Dipsea, highlights the season for some of the area's best competitors; spring in Marin is prep time for the Dipsea, and at the big road-side Dipsea Café, framed photographs of past years' winners line the walls.

Jim Furman had been one of the club's organizational stalwarts since the early 1980s, when he joined the Tamalpa Runners as a young New Yorker newly settled in Marin. He had been club president, had edited the newsletter, had run the Dipsea and scores of other local races every year for more than two decades. "President for Life, that's what we called him," says Eve Pell, a writer and Tamalpa member who became one of Jim's good friends. "He was reelected every year. He was this shy, slightly hesitant, very smart guy, who I knew, oddly enough, had been a roadie with the Grateful Dead."

The Grateful Dead story was true—Jim had grown up in Manhattan and Long Island, trained as an electrical engineer, and after a stint as a traveling rock-concert recording specialist, had founded a successful Marin County company that made audio products. Most of his friends were Marin runners, and they knew Jim Furman as a quiet, diplomatic, impressively well-read man with a bumpy if unexceptional personal history: two marriages, two divorces. One son, from a third relationship, who lived out of town, but whom Jim was helping support and would see three or four times a year. Girlfriends, sometimes serious, sometimes not. "We'd talk running, girls, politics, history," recalls George Frazier, a business consultant who was Jim's best friend and regular running partner. "You know—what each of us is reading. Jim would always have these stacks of books on science and math and the universe and music. I knew nothing about these things. So it was a way to sponge it all up without having to read about it in the first place."

They ran together every weekend with their Tamalpa friends, on the Mount Tam trails or the paved roads at the mountain's base. The group runs were fast and hard—8 to 15 miles, weather no deterrent, the pace at the head of the pack quickening to 6:30 or faster when somebody decided to push it. "People would, in my parlance, 'bop heads,'" Frazier says. "You know. Somebody would just say: 'Let's go.' It's as natural as a bunch of thoroughbreds in a field, racing with each other."

It was not a men-only clique, the cluster of head-boppers out in front, but only a handful of the toughest Marin women, including a couple of national record holders, were able to match pace when the men were really moving. More cart ponies than thoroughbreds, Frazier would say in self-deprecation, as the hotshots in their thirties turned forty and kept running, but their competition stayed jovial and strong. Jim Furman was never the fastest, but his intensity and tenacity kept him respectably high in the regional standings. By the mid-1990s he had run a 5:05 mile and a 3:01 marathon; he'd done many ultras, too, finishing one 50-mile race in under eight hours. He had short, curly hair that flared out in a wild corona around his temples when he was running and had a beloved collection of faded race T-shirts. At one point he had a good-looking dark beard. He was a downhill skier. He gave elaborate parties, where everybody came in black tie and had a wild time. His business was a big success. He played bass in a rock band.

George Frazier thought he was a terrific guy.

"I never noticed anything," Frazier says.

So one afternoon in 1996 Frazier stopped by Jim's house, which was up on a wild, steep hillside, with a long view of the wooded trails out back. Jim's Jeep was in the driveway, which Frazier knew meant he must be home. Frazier hadn't phoned to say he was coming, but he knocked on the door and called Jim's name. Nobody answered. Frazier banged on the door harder. Finally he started yelling. "Furman! Hey! You in there?"

Inside the kitchen, Jim Furman, who was wearing women's blue jeans, a women's tank top, and a bra, stood for a long time without moving, and listened to Frazier yell.

SHE KNEW, JANET SAYS NOW, when she was five years old. She was a boy then, but something was wrong about that. "The idea was there," she says. "At that young age, I wasn't sure exactly what it meant. I didn't necessarily want to play with dolls—but I was drawn to what my sister was. And I don't really know why. That's the essential mystery. I was intrigued by it. And I did know that I wasn't supposed to be too interested. I remember that as a teenager, my sister subscribed to *Seventeen* magazine, and my mother *McCall's*, or something like that. I remember staying up late and thumbing through those magazines like they were forbidden fruit. I was just trying to fantasize about being female. I didn't really know what I was looking for—I just had the sense that it was a terrible secret, that I couldn't let anybody know I was interested in this. I had to look at those magazines after everybody went to bed."

There are men, both gay and straight, who like wearing women's clothes sometimes and nonetheless have no interest in changing gender permanently. But Jim knew into adulthood that although the anguished secret of his childhood was his furtive forays into his sister's clothes and makeup, he didn't really want to be a cross-dresser. He wanted to be a woman. He had no question about his sexual orientation; he was physically attracted to women, and because he worked so fervently and for so many years to repress the conviction that he was supposed to be one, Jim made it to his late forties persuaded that he had tucked his identity problem off into the most private corners of an otherwise satisfying life. No one knew he kept a collection of women's clothing in a suitcase at the back of his closet. No one knew the clothes were the reason he sometimes stayed home alone in the evenings, in the house on the hillside, where no windows were visible from the street. No one knew that the first time Jim ever tried out an Internet search engine, the word he typed in was transsexual.

"And what came back was just a flood of information," Janet says, "which I just devoured."

In the gratifying anonymity of the Internet, Jim—for there was no Janet yet—began his serious introduction to gender dysphoria, which is the diagnostic name for the psychological distress caused by the conviction that one's gender is not what the rest of the world is seeing. The more he learned about it, the clearer it became to Jim that he had found a way to understand himself, and in e-mails he disclosed things he had never said to anyone. Strangers wrote back with encouragement and stories of their own. He sought out a therapist. He commenced a romance with a woman named Heidi McGuire, a Tamalpa runner he knew, and after a while McGuire's gentle open-mindedness made Jim think it might be all right to start telling her.

McGuire was bewildered but compassionate ("I took it as a big compliment that he trusted me enough to confide something so huge," McGuire says now), and she helped him throw a Halloween party, which Jim hosted in full drag. Janet, remembering: "There was another guy in drag. But he looked like a caricature woman. He had balloons. And they got popped before long. He had a silly fright wig. I had this $200 wig, and this nice cocktail dress, perfectly accessorized, and shoes that fit, and professionally applied makeup. They were all knocked out by how I looked. I was eating it up. I told everybody I was Jamie. And the only thing wrong with that evening was that it ended."

Jim saw that he was going to have to do this now, not as a flamboyant party host in Halloween costume, but outside, seriously, among people who wouldn't assume he was joking. The first time he tried, wearing the clothing, all he did was sit behind the steering wheel of his car, unable to make himself turn on the engine and back out of the garage.

The second time, he drove onto the street and down into town. But he kept the windows rolled up, and never got out of the car.

Once he went out at midnight, in a mail-order dress and a women's overcoat and women's sensible shoes, and drove a couple of towns away, where there's a street that curves alongside San Francisco Bay. He walked up and down the deserted waterfront, in the darkness, and drove home.

Finally, Jim found a local transgender support group in San Francisco. They met in the back of a restaurant. On his initial visit the restaurant host took one look at Jim and said, "The people you want are back there," but when Jim saw them he was startled; they were big, but they looked like women. They said hello and made room right away, and the person who had been Jim Furman sat down and introduced herself: Janet. "When I was leaving for that evening, I had said, 'I need a name.' Heidi said: 'Jamie?' But I said, 'No. That's too ambiguous. I need something definite.'"

And for a while after that, it was as though the house on the hillside contained congenial roommates on opposite shifts. Every morning Jim Furman, the Tamalpas runner and business entrepreneur, got into his black Jeep Grand Cherokee with eqalizr vanity plates and drove to the office, or races, or trail workouts. Janet Furman Bowman—the new surname was invented, a cross between the last names of Jim's parents—went out at night, headed for San Francisco, driving a lilac Taurus that was otherwise kept out of sight inside the garage. The only person who had been formally introduced to both of them, besides the therapist, was Heidi McGuire. When the electrolysis started, Jim leaning back in a salon chair week after week while each hair of his beard was individually and painfully zapped off, he told the electrolysist.

But George Frazier still didn't know, and after a few months the person who was legally James Furman, which was to say Jim some of the time and Janet the rest of the time, could see that it was less like housemates and more like a bad spy novel in which some disastrous collision loomed. By the afternoon of the 1996 door-pounding incident, the transformation from Jim to Janet and back again was practiced enough that no elaborate effort with clothing or makeup was necessarily involved—but the passage was still too daunting to manage with the best guy friend standing outside the house and shouting for Jim. "I couldn't switch gears in a flash," Janet says. "It wasn't like stepping into a phone booth."

In the therapy sessions, the therapist listened as her patient, who was after all a practical businessperson and a disciplined runner, began inventorying the consequences of the hormonal and surgical treatments that would eventually make Jim Furman disappear. "I made a list of all the wreckage that would happen in my life," Janet says. "The people around me. My work. But even more than that, what I really wanted to know was: Could I pull it off? Could I be a woman, and be accepted as a woman? I didn't want to be a guy in a dress and have people turn around and stare at me. I'd had enough of that in San Francisco. I didn't want to have a life being fodder for tourists to sneer at. I wanted to be accepted. To be happy."

At last, after several failed-nerve false starts and then a "stay there I'm coming over right now I have something to say to you" telephone call, Jim told Frazier. Frazier did not take it well.

Let me make sure I understand this, Frazier said—this other persona, this Janet you're talking about, she means you have to get rid of Jim? Why? Why can't you just keep going to San Francisco in a dress? "I tried every argument I could think of," Frazier says. "None of them made much sense. I had a loyalty to Jim that I had a difficult time letting go of." For a while Frazier went around feeling distraught and sad, tangled up in a weird kind of anticipatory grief, until a gay friend in whom he had confided sat him down and told him to stop feeling sorry for himself. "He said, 'By the time you have heard about Janet, Jim is dead,'" Frazier says. "He said: 'You cannot undo this. This is done. Janet has won. And Jim is gone. Get right with Janet.'"

The hormonal treatments started. George Frazier, like Heidi McGuire, Eve Pell, and the handful of other close friends Jim Furman had decided to tell, began working to get right with Janet. Neither Janet nor Jim—or what was left of him—made it easy for them at first. The friends were sworn to secrecy, and because the runner who showed up at Tamalpas events was still Jim Furman, Frazier found himself improvising when other runners sidled up to him and inquired about Jim's hair, which was growing out into a distinctly ladylike ponytail; or his fingernails, which were suddenly manicured in colors. Well, he's in a band, Frazier would say airily, you know how rock stars are. Frazier had no idea how many people were buying it; not many, he guessed. He was also not sure what was going to happen in the competitive rankings once Janet Bowman decided to make her debut appearance among the Tamalpas, but the whole prospect interested him enormously. "I assumed that when Janet started running," Frazier says, "she was going to kick ass."

THE PHYSICAL CHANGES that make up "transition," which is what transsexuals call the definitive crossover from one gender to the other, usually take place on two separate tracks. There are surgeries to change the appearance of the body: breast augmentation, facial alterations, hair transplants, genital reconstructions that create functional male or female sex organs. These are costly procedures, generally not covered by insurance, and a person who wants to switch genders—who wants the outside world's label to match what the person feels like inside—may opt for some surgery, or a lot, or none at all.

But anybody who's seriously en route from male to female, or vice versa, takes hormones. Under the most widely accepted standards of care for trans-sexuals, in fact, a patient is not supposed to undergo genital reconstruction sur-gery until after an extended period of living publicly as the intended gender while taking hormones. Biological women aiming for masculinity (or FTMs, as in female to male) take testosterone. MTFs, biological men headed the other way, take estrogen, and sometimes progesterone, along with an agent called an andro-gen blocker, which curtails the production and effects of testosterone.

It was about 40 years ago that an American endocrinologist named Harry Benjamin published the first extensive studies of transsexuals and the medical protocols for helping them switch gender, and by now there's quite a bit of infor-mation about the effects hormones and other substances have on the human body. Here's what the available literature had to say, for example, when Janet Bowman set out to see what she might expect from the pills prescribed for her, a combination of estrogen and an androgen blocker called spironolactone: Breast development. Smaller testes and prostate. Finer body hair, and less of it. Reduc-tion of any hereditary male-pattern baldness. Drop in libido. Softer skin. Mood changes. Increased emotional sensitivity. Migration of fat onto the lower abdo-men, thighs, and buttocks.

She found no information at all, though, about what was likely to happen to a distance runner's endurance and speed. What extra testosterone does to both male and female athletes is common knowledge by now, particularly in light of continuing attention to illicit steroid use. The word steroid refers to a group of organic compounds that includes sex hormones, and by the time Janet began her hormones research, doping scandal news stories were regularly describing the effects of pumped-up testosterone: muscle bulk, power, sprint strength, aggres-siveness. But losing testosterone and adding estrogen—not many athletes were closely studied for that, as it turned out. The famous 1977 lawsuit of Renée Rich-ards, the tennis player barred from the U.S. Open women's division after her male-to-female transition, ended satisfactorily for Richards but without a great deal of useful information for a person in Janet's situation; a federal court ruled that Richards was legally female and must be allowed to compete, which she did, playing neither memorably well nor memorably poorly, for several more years.

"I thought I'd lose something in my sprint ability," Janet says. "I expected some effect. But actually, I was concerned about being too good." Renée Richards spent the remainder of her tennis career saddled with the transsexual athlete label, a prospect Janet found dispiriting, but more to the point, Janet was 51 when the hormone therapy began. She knew Jim Furman's over-50 times were good, for a man: under 40 minutes for the 10-K, for example. But a woman running those times in the 50-59 age group would be national class—an immediate threat, in fact, to U.S. masters champion Shirley Matson, who at 64 holds many American records, lives in Marin County, and runs for the Tamalpas. And although there was a certain thrill about the idea of suddenly rocketing into the national rankings, Janet went directly to Matson, who was a friend, for advice. Would it be legitimate to race in the women's divisions, Janet asked, once her transition was complete? Would other running clubs accuse the Tamalpas of harboring cheaters? Should she give up racing? Matson's response was an e-mail so pithy and emphatic that Janet saved it to show around: Of course she should race. And she was going to be a woman. Nothing complicated about that at all. "I just had to applaud her," Matson says. "Fine, there's another woman out there competing, that's the way it goes. I admired her conviction. And doing it at home, in front of all of us. If I were going to do something like that, I'd go to Timbuktu. I would not have had the courage."

Eight months later, October 1998, in San Francisco's Golden Gate Park: Janet Furman Bowman's first registered entry in a formal race. It was a flat 5-K, a distance she had run many times as Jim. Here was the grand entrance George Frazier had been anticipating, and halfway through, Janet was sure she was hammering it. As Jim, she had never run slower than 20 minutes in a 5-K, and now as Janet she kicked hard through the finish and thought, with satisfaction, *nineteen flat.* Then she looked at her watch.

"I WAS JUST FLABBERGASTED," she says. Janet Bowman's race time, three quarters of a year into the feminizing hormone therapy, was 22:43. Except for some cosmetic facial surgery and hair transplants, she was still a pre-op, anatomically male transsexual; nothing below the neck had been surgically altered. Her training had diminished as she'd gotten older—around 25 miles a week now, compared to the 40 she had been running a decade earlier—but since January there'd been no real slide. During the weekend trail runs she'd seen that something new was happening, Frazier and the other men making an obvious effort to hold back as Janet pushed hard to try to stay with them, but all runners wax and wane, and nobody had paid particular attention.

So what on earth? Same daily diet. Same leg length. Same narrow hips, long torso, and wiry build; if there had been any "migration of fat," it wasn't visible from a glance at Janet Bowman in running shorts. Same heart, literally, and, as far as Janet could tell from inside her own morphing self, metaphorically as well. Janet wanted to run just as ardently as Jim had wanted to run—as far, as often, as fast. It was true that Janet wept at movies, something Jim had never done in his life, and it was true that Janet's estrogen-stimulated chest was as tender and sore as a 12-year-old girl's. The proposition that there might be some actual linkage between movie-weeping and breast development and speed, that the very process of turning into a woman could slow down a fast racer, sounds like something cooked up to start a bar fight among runners. But that 22:43 race was the fastest 5-K Janet was ever going to run. "Now I look back," she says, sounding wistful, "and that was the last time I broke 23."

At one point, before the hormones, the future Janet had been so worried about obliterating the competition that she called the Indianapolis headquarters of USA Track & Field, anonymously, to ask about the policy on transsexual runners. She was told there was no blanket policy, which was true at the time; since 1991 the organization has maintained a transgender task force, convened after the complaint of a female racer who was irritated about being bested on occasion by one transsexual woman in her region. That complaint was eventually resolved by a finding that the transsexual was legally a woman and could continue racing as one. Longtime task force member C. Harmon Brown, a San Francisco–area endocrinologist, says since then the group has been asked perhaps once a year to advise on similar situations. It was just in February 2005 that USATF's national board finally approved the approach adopted the year before by the International Olympic Committee: Athletic competition, the Olympic guidelines say, should be open to any transsexual whose genital reconstruction surgery has been completed, whose legal status has been changed (driver's license and so on), and whose hormonal therapy has been under way "for a sufficient length of time to minimize gender-related advantages."

The gender-to-performance linkage, in other words, is real. What happened to Janet should come as no surprise to anybody who understands what sex hormones do, Brown says; among their many other tasks inside the body, estrogen stimulates the storage of body fat, and testosterone stimulates both the building of muscle and the production of hemoglobin, which carries oxygen to the lungs and muscles, and so increases endurance. For any athlete who requires endurance, along with muscle strength and speed, being hormonally female appears to be a genuine biological handicap. "Even though she looks the same, and maybe weighs the same, the composition is not likely to be the same," Brown says. "You lose muscle, so you're losing power, and you're gaining fat, which you have to carry around. And you're carrying a male skeleton." Bigger than a female skeleton, that is, and heavier to haul up the trail—but with internal chemistry suddenly inadequate to the task. Says Georgia State University exercise physiologist David Martin, who also serves on the USATF task force, "The transgender athlete probably has a disadvantage, rather than an advantage."

YES, JANET SAYS, THE TRADEOFF was worth it. If anyone had explained in advance that this might happen—had warned Jim Furman exactly what he was preparing to lose—it would have made no difference, Janet says: "Nothing was going to stop me."

She means the transition, but she might as well be talking about running, too. There were multiple surgeries before Janet was finished turning Jim's body into that of a recognizable woman, and each time the recuperation period was over, she returned immediately to running, which for 20 years had been Jim's solace and anchor through difficult times, and without question would be Janet's as well. The fact that running is also simultaneously now the source of her greatest disappointment—that she will never again run stride for stride with the head-bopper men—is simply a complication she's learning to accept. "I can't keep up with all my friends on my Sunday-morning runs," Janet says. "It's the one regret I have."

She keeps track of her PRs now separately, one set for Jim and one for Janet. She recently turned 58, and her times are not shabby for a woman in her age group—a 6:55 mile, a 48:07 10-K. In fact, Janet has studied the World Association of Veteran Athletes' age-grading tables—the standards that calibrate athletic performance according to gender and age—and when she compared her recent race times to Jim's race times, she found something interesting. As a man, advancing through the age ranks, Jim fit in steadily around the 75 percent level—not national class for men of his age, but quite a bit faster than local class. As a woman, working now off a different set of statistical tables, Janet still hits around 75 percent, even as the active competition in her class dwindles. "And as it turns out, I'm quite content to get a medal, or a plaque, that says I was first or second in my age group in a local race," Janet says. "I hardly ever got any hardware when I was a man."

Janet's voice takes a moment's getting used to; masculine timbre is one of the things female hormones don't change, and she had to practice at the muted, slightly breathy contralto with which she now answers the phone. She lives in the same hillside house she bought as Jim, although it's been redone, with sky-lights and rich colors and a new sunroom that looks out toward the running trails. She has a partner who lives there with her, a woman she met through an online dating service. The business has been sold, leaving Janet in a comfortable semiretirement that she fills with running, race organization, business consult-ing, and her beloved rock band, which used to have a dark-haired bass player named Jim and now in his place has a blond bass player with hazel eyes and great legs. She still throws the black-tie New Year's Eve party, which she hosted this last time wearing a pink silk scarf over a spaghetti-strap little black dress; the guest list was pretty much the same as always, and included her son, Matt, who is now a 22-year-old university student with one parent he calls Mom and one parent he calls Janet. Matt is a psychology major. One of his recent courses used a textbook called *Sex Differences: Developmental and Evolutionary Strategies.*

"Honestly, in a strange way, it's brought us closer," Matt says. He was 15 when Jim told him what was coming; until that point, Matt says, his long-distance relationship with his father had been careful, awkward, and somewhat formal. "So this was like a big hammer into the ice," Matt says. "We started talk-ing about something important."

Which is not to suggest that it was easy, either for Matt or for the adults who loved Jim Furman. Janet's widowed 90-year-old mother, who lives in a resi-dential facility in New York, can't bring herself to explain to her fellow residents her relationship to the athletic-looking woman who sometimes comes to visit. ("I just can't do it. I'm not brave enough. I say: 'This is a friend from California.'") Janet's sister, who is also a widow, says she sometimes finds herself mourning her brother along with her father and her husband. Heidi McGuire, reminiscing one day last winter, was asked at one point what exactly she thought had become of Jim, who vanished without dying in the conventional sense, and the stricken look on McGuire's face made it clear that she suddenly wanted to weep.

"Huh," she said. "Well. Jim is just . . . somewhere else. Jim is another time." Then her eyes brimmed. "I've learned to . . . I care about Janet," McGuire said. "I have a lot of fun with Janet. I love Janet a lot. But I miss Jim."

Heidi and Janet run together now, every Thursday morning, on the Tamal-pais trails. They'll go four or five miles, at a relaxed nine-minute pace; at least once a week Janet still makes a point of pushing herself, in a race or the group weekend runs, and this spring she began adding on hills and coached track workouts to train for the Dipsea. By St. Patrick's Day she was in particularly fine spirits, having just edged out three of her strongest local rivals in a tough five-mile race—"I got about two-thirds of the way through and thought, Wow, I am ahead of these people, what am I doing here?"—and she was weighing possibilities for upcoming weekends: a 12-K race, in which the Tamalpas wanted Janet to round out the senior women's team; or George Frazier's annual pre-Dipsea training run, which leads a big klatch of serious runners up and down one steep, wildflower-filled Marin County mountainside, seven miles each way for the ones who go all the way to the summit.

"I used to go to the summit," Janet says. Before, she means. When she was Jim.

And as Janet? "Once," she says. "But all the people who got to the summit got there ahead of me. By the time I got there, everybody had left."

Since then, Janet has run the curtailed option instead, ensuring the steady company of others with similar pace and mileage targets. "The short version is eight miles, and that is plenty," she says. She thought for a while about whether Jim would have felt the same way—choosing companionship on the trail, that is, over the lonely achievement of an arbitrary distance goal—finally she says that yes, she is pretty sure he would. "I've always been in this for the social benefits," she says. "I'd rather run with people than say, 'I went to the summit, and came back alone.'"

THE MAN WHO TAUGHT ME EVERYTHING

BY AMBY BURFOOT

[
Marathon legend, Boston winner,
and cross-country coach John J. Kelley has inspired
everyone who's known him. And no one
has known him like I have.
]

MAY 2007

IF YOU ARE LUCKY in life, you might meet someone who changes everything forever. If you are very lucky, you might meet this person when you are young and lacking direction. If you are very, very lucky, this person might remain an influence for decades to come—a touchstone you can revisit for counsel and wisdom. I was very, very lucky. But I sure didn't see it coming.

It's September 1962, and I've just finished my first high school cross-country race. I'm losing the struggle to keep my lunch—hot dogs and chocolate milk—so I've ducked under the football bleachers, hoping no one can see me. I've already decided that I'll never run again.

But Mr. Kelley spots me and jogs over. He's an English teacher at my school, and the cross-country coach. I figure he'll turn back when he notes my distress, but he keeps coming, like someone who's seen this sort of thing before. Kelley rises up on tiptoes—I'm six inches taller than he is—grabs me by the shoulders, and turns me toward him. We're face to face, his bright blue eyes ablaze. "Amby, that was a great race," he says. "You've got real potential in this sport. If you stick with it, there's no telling how far you might go."

No way. I've finished ninth or something pitiful like that. Coaches don't talk to losers like me. Only winners get praised. This Kelley's a strange one. I'm dubious, but people say he won the Boston Marathon a few years back. He must know running. At home that night, I decide to massage my sore legs. Maybe I'll try them again tomorrow.

Three years pass. I'm running a five-mile road race in Rhode Island when I notice something unusual. There's a mile to go, and I'm gaining on the leader. The leader is Kelley. This has never happened—by now I've finished well behind Kelley in dozens of races—and I don't know what to do. I slow down for a moment. I can't imagine passing the master; I am a mere student.

If not for my oxygen debt, I might have realized that Kelley had been preparing me for this moment. I'd heard him muse so often on the nature of things—the big bang, planetary orbits, tectonic plates, ocean currents, seasons, evolution, the miracle of the sprouting seed—and yet I had never considered how similar forces apply to the aging runner and the young aspirant. I feel a tightness in my throat, but I pass him with a half mile to go and break the tape. It's my first road-race victory. After finishing, I stumble over to a shade tree to catch my breath. I can't quell a creeping sense of shame for the act I have committed.

Kelley crosses the line, sees me, and runs straight toward me, a big smile on his face. He reaches out a hand, grabs mine, pumps furiously. "Great race, Amby," he says. "You timed that one perfectly. When you caught me, I had nothing left."

Two Aprils later, in 1968, we are running side by side in the Boston Marathon. Kelley's time has come and gone, but he's still a fierce competitor, and he hangs with the leaders for 13 miles. My tide is rising. I make a move, and Kelley falls back. An hour later, I cross the Boston finish line as the first American champion since he won in 1957. Someone puts a laurel wreath on my head, a medal around my neck. I hear cameras popping on all sides. I am surrounded by mayors and governors and newspaper reporters.

But I only want to talk to one person—the one who made it all possible. He finishes 15 minutes later and fights off his fatigue to find me. I've never seen anyone look so happy after a bad marathon. "Amby, you did it," Kelley says, wrapping me in a big hug. "I knew you could. I knew this was going to be your day."

JOHN JOSEPH KELLEY, NOW 76, was the first truly modern American road runner, the first fast American marathoner, and a Renaissance runner for the ages. In addition to his 1957 Boston Marathon victory, Kelley has second-place finishes in five other Bostons, including 1956, when he ran the equivalent of a 2:18:10. "Kelley led the generation of young, track-trained college men who changed the marathon from a pure endurance grind to an event of speed and tactics," says Boston Marathon historian Tom Derderian.

(Despite what many assume, John J. "The Younger" Kelley is no relation to "Old John" A. Kelley, who completed Boston 58 times, won twice, and died at age 97, in 2004. The two did, however, form a strong friendship through their many years of New England road racing.)

Kelley also won eight straight USA National Marathon Championships, a mark that will never be equaled. He took the gold medal in the 1959 Pan American Games Marathon in Chicago, and twice competed in the Olympic Marathon. He was the first trail runner I ever met, a mountain runner (setting the course record at the Mount Washington Road Race in 1961), a vegetarian, an organic gardener, a run-to-work practitioner, a lover of great literature, an ardent environmentalist, and a truly pathetic triathlete. In the late 1970s, I watched Kelley get fished from Long Island Sound. He was swimming backward in a triathlon at the time, his crawl no match for an unexpected current.

You think I'm stretching the truth with that Renaissance-man bit? Consider this: In Utica, New York, at the 2002 National Distance Running Hall of Fame induction ceremony, Kelley is being honored along with Bill Bowerman, Doris Brown Heritage, and Browning Ross. There has been much speechifying about shoes, waffle irons, pioneering runners, and early running magazines. More is expected as the diminutive, stoop-shouldered Kelley shambles to the microphone. Only he wants to talk about Copernicus and poetry.

"As you know, Copernicus advanced the heliocentric theory—the then heretical principle of the sun being the center of the universe, rather than the Earth," Kelley begins, looking down at his sickly wife, Jacintha, in the front row. They have been married for 49 years; she will pass away the next spring. The crowd in Utica's glorious Stanley Theater stirs. What's this guy talking about?

It seems that Kelley had strolled around Utica the previous afternoon and happened upon a Copernicus statue. This got him thinking about man's place in the firmament, one of his favorite topics. "It occurred to me that when we're young, we naturally think of ourselves as the center of our universe, and we hope to eventually establish a niche in some hall of fame. But in the development of the individual, the humbling effects of a larger universe take their toll, so by the time an honor such as this comes along, we hedge a little about accepting it."

He's saying, in part at least, that he's uncomfortable being singled out and presented with awards. Kelley is one of those people who always gives credit to others but wants none for himself. He doesn't want the stage for long either. His acceptance speech lasts three minutes and concludes with a poetry reading. He evokes Charles Hamilton Sorley, author of "The Song of the Ungirt Runners." The poem expresses, Kelley says, "the feeling of oneness and humble place" that he has always found in running. The last stanza:

> The rain is on our lips,
> We do not run for prize.
> But the storm the water whips
> And the wave howls to the skies.
> The winds arise and strike it
> And scatter it like sand,
> And we run because we like it
> Through the broad bright land.

Kelley concludes by telling us that Sorley was 20 in the summer of 1915, when he wrote these words. Three months later, he died in World War I. The remarks are pure Kelley—from Copernicus to running through wind and rain to life's sad, ironic twists—dense and tangled, but always inspiring.

KELLEY TAUGHT ME EVERYTHING I would ever need to know about running and most of what I have found to be true in life. I learned that consistency is everything, that long runs increase endurance, that hills build character, and that speedwork is good, but only on a limited basis. He taught that running comes easy on some days, is tough on others. That you can win many races if you have talent, train hard, stay healthy, and run your guts out. But you'd better learn humility, too, because no one wins every race. And the crushing defeats might ultimately outnumber the eased-up victories.

Most of all, he showed by example that running should be wild, adventurous, deeply personal, and soul satisfying. While other high schoolers ran endless laps on a track, Kelley led us on romps through thick woods, nature preserves, and abandoned apple orchards, where we ate green fruit and got sick. We splashed through streams and marshes and the lapping waves of Long Island Sound, ruining countless shoes.

The tougher the terrain, the worse the weather, the more he liked it. To this day, I can sit out a perfect spring or fall afternoon. But if a blizzard roars in or the mercury skids below zero or blasts past 100, I can't wait to lace up my running shoes, open the front door, and confront the elements.

Oh, the trails we ran! Almost every Sunday, we finished our 14-miler in the bramble, rocks, fallen trees, and rushing rivulets of Pequot Woods. I floundered as his light, springy stride carried him into the distance. By the time I reached his backyard, he had already stripped off his running shirt, showered with the outdoor hose, and begun digging in his garden. The first time I saw his steamy compost heap with its thousands of fat, squirming earthworms, I cringed and turned away.

Kelley knew every off-road jaunt within 25 miles of his home. Two days after Thanksgiving 1964, he led Jeff Galloway and me on a 20-mile run on the blue-stripe Narragansett Indian Trail in North Stonington, Connecticut, today the site of the immense Foxwoods Resort Casino. I was too young and frail to match the marathon veterans. Kelley and Galloway, a future Olympian, dropped me after the turnaround, and I had moments when I wondered if I would ever escape from the gnarly forest, moss-covered valleys, and high, rocky ledges. When I did, a good 30 minutes behind the other two, I felt beaten and yet staunchly determined. I vowed to match them the next time. And I did.

The run I remember best took place in a pelting January rainstorm—a nor'easter that turned treacherous when the temperature dropped to the mid-20s. Kelley and I had emerged from the woods for a brief roadside run before ducking back onto a trail. At that moment, a state trooper drove by. Even after slowing to 10 miles per hour, he could barely control his car, which slip-slided on the black ice. He rolled down his window and yelled at us: "Get off the roads, you crazy idiots."

We responded in kind, perhaps adding a Sicilian accent, and maybe even a certain hand gesture. I don't remember for sure. I only remember the way we roared with laughter. This guy had badges, a uniform, and authority to spare, but we knew there was no chance he could maneuver his vehicle to chase after us. Who was crazy to be out in this weather? We laughed until we forgot the frozen cotton sweat suits plastered to our skin, and the nine miles still to go, and the diamond-sharp sleet ripping our faces.

After runs like this, we repaired to the Kelley kitchen, tiptoeing around the latest litter of kittens. We drank big pots of tea and honey that Jess prepared for us, and talked about anything and everything. Or rather, Kelley talked. I simply listened, entranced. I've never met anyone who has read more widely than he has. He loved the transcendentalists, particularly Thoreau, and would quote endlessly from such works as "Walking," "Civil Disobedience," and, of course, Walden.

How many times did I hear Kelley recite: "I wish to speak a word for Nature, for absolute Freedom and Wildness"? Kelley was the first person I knew to read Silent Spring and the first to condemn the automobile, which he called "the infernal internal combustion machine." He's never stopped being angry about environmental insults. "If you're a runner and you love getting out into the natural world," he says, "then it's inevitable that you'll feel yourself pitted against 'prog-ress' and the 'establishment,' because they are always taking our trails away and turning them into highways, subdivisions, or business parks—a grotesque oxy-moron if I've ever heard one."

The individual struggle, the individual quest, the individual achieve-ment—these have been the cornerstones of Kelley's life. Follow your heart, he always told me, it's the one thing you can count on. Let your passion ignite bon-fires, and feed the flames every day. "The things we do should consume us," he says. "If they don't, our lives won't have any meaning."

THE SON OF AN IRISH IMMIGRANT, Kelley grew up in New London, Connecticut, a former whaling city on the deep-water Thames River. He played hooky for most of his junior-high years, spending long hours in the public library, where he devoured James Joyce, Hemingway, and other great works of classical and contemporary English literature. "I found reading shortly before running and threw myself into it with the same sort of fervor," he says. "I was especially drawn to the writers fixated on explorations of idealism."

He probably would have skipped high school, too, except that another stu-dent cajoled him into attending a cross-country practice. The coach had only one workout in his repertoire: a daily time-trial over a 2.3-mile course. And so Kelley gave chase to the team star, George Terry, two years his senior. "I felt this fire in my gut, a cutting pain," he says. "I didn't know you could experience pain that sharp except from a knife wound or gun shot."

He stuck with the sport nonetheless, and kept chasing Terry all the way to the 1949 Boston Marathon. Terry had graduated from high school by then; Kel-ley was a 17-year-old junior. He had a badly swollen knee and a high school coach who had forbidden the ludicrous marathon escapade. That was all Kelley needed; his impetuousness and rebellious streak provided the rest. The knee forced him out at 13 miles, and the angry coach made him run a dual-meet mile the next day ("the most excruciating experience of my life"), but Kelley couldn't shake the Boston memories. "The field was small by today's standards, but it seemed to us the whole world was there," he recalls. "You had the sunny April day, the blooming forsythia in Hopkinton, the smell of liniment permeating the air, the crowds on the sidewalks. It was such a thrill."

The next spring he ran the year's fastest high school mile, 4:21.8, and earned a scholarship to Boston University, where he was expected to run many more fast miles. But the marathon had grabbed his heart. He read (of course!)

everything about Boston's history, befriended Jock Semple—a Boston Athletic Association (BAA) official—and the BAA road runners, and searched out information about a Scandinavian forest-running method called fartlek and an amazing Czech named Emil Zatopek, who trained harder than anyone, while seeming to enjoy it more.

From these shards, he stitched together a training program that matched his expansive spirit. "I wanted to make running fun, to do more long, rhythmic runs, and to explore my surroundings," he says. "I tried new ways of training that fit my basic instincts. I felt so much freer when I was running by myself on the roads or trails, away from the hegemony of a coach."

Kelley kept racing for BU but by 1953 could no longer resist the Boston Marathon. He ran 2:28 that year and the next, then skipped 1955 to focus everything on the 1956 Boston Marathon and Melbourne Olympic Games. He was living a life that no current elite marathoner could fathom, student teaching in the mornings and working 30 hours a week in the late afternoons as a jewelry-store stockboy. The days went like this: wake up at 4:15 a.m.; run 16 miles along the banks of the Charles River; dress hurriedly, drive to school, teach until early afternoon; return home to the tiny Boston apartment without stove or refrigerator that he shared with Jess; jog two miles to the downtown jewelry store ("I never counted this in my training log, because I wasn't in running gear, but it gave me a few more miles in the confidence basket"); work until 8 p.m.; jog two miles home; and wolf down a quick dinner with a half quart of milk. "I'd go to bed at 9:30 every night and start the whole thing over again the next morning at 4:15," he says. "There wasn't a moment of leisure time in my day. But I had a great plan—to see how much I could get out of my body and how fast I could ultimately run the marathon."

On Saturdays, he'd do a warmup mile across the Charles to the MIT track, run 40 x 440 yards in 75 seconds with a 440 recovery jog, and do a cooldown mile back to the apartment. On Sundays he'd run a steady 20-miler. Monday was a rest day.

The 1956 Boston Marathon brought cool, cloudy conditions, perfect for a fierce attack, and Kelley and Finnish marathoner Antii Viskari raced the Boston course as no one had before. They ran side-by-side for 25 miles before Viskari opened a gap. He broke the tape in 2:14:24, a Boston record by more than four minutes. Kelley was just 75 yards behind in 2:14:33, far faster than any American had ever run at Boston or anywhere. "It was a pitched battle all the way, and I never cracked," he says. "Viskari just had more speed than me the last mile. I was extremely happy because the race vindicated my training theories and methods." Disappointment followed when the course was remeasured and found to be 1,183 yards short, as it apparently had been since 1951. This still gave Kelley an equivalent time of 2:18:10 for a full-distance marathon.

That November, as a member of the U.S. Olympic team, he met the great Zatopek at the Melbourne Games. In fact, the two trained together many afternoons. One of Kelley's teammates refused to join them, declaring it a sacrilege to run with an immortal like Zatopek, who had won three gold medals—the 5000, 10,000, and marathon—in the 1952 Helsinki Olympics. But Kelley, ever inquisitive, couldn't be held back, and he found the Czech little different from most other runners. "Zatopek was recovering from a hernia operation, so he ran with a little limp, but he was a wonderful, affable fellow," he says. "He put me at ease instantly, and I marveled at all the languages he spoke. We exchanged cards for years after, and Jess and I gave our first daughter the middle name Emily after Emil. He sent us a beautiful cut-glass bowl when she was born."

Melbourne's marathon day turned ugly, with a blazing sun and temperatures that reached the mid-80s. Kelley believed he could run with the best and did so for 12 miles. Then the heat crushed him. He walked and jogged the last eight miles to finish 21st. "Melbourne was a fantastic experience, but I was perhaps naïve to think I could run with the leaders," he says. "At the end, I was parched with this overwhelming thirst. I was burning up. It was a terrible denouement to my Olympic dream."

Worse than the Olympic outcome was his dread of facing people back home. "I was so thin-skinned, and I hated that damn question, 'What happened?'" he says. "Americans only understood winning. Even second was considered a disgrace. They couldn't figure out why anyone would run 26 miles for no money and then lose to Europeans and Asians."

He threatened to quit running, but Jess and Semple wouldn't let him. Semple pointed out that the 1957 Boston Marathon was only four months off. "This is going to be your year, Johnny," Semple kept saying. "It's your turn to win." No member of the BAA had ever won the club's great sporting masterpiece, and Semple desperately wanted Kelley to be the first.

By early 1957, Kelley was training full-tilt again, now in Groton, Connecticut, where he has lived ever since. When he won several premarathon tune-up races around Boston, the papers began beating a drumroll: KELLEY ONLY AMERICAN HOPE IN THIS YEAR'S BOSTON MARATHON. Each new story threw him into a panic. "I was haunted by the specter of losing," he says. "I'd run every race a thousand times in my sleep and get so spooked that I'd lose any enjoyment of the race before I even got to the starting line."

The night before the 1957 Boston Marathon, he stayed with his namesake,

"Old John" A. Kelley, who played sentry. "No, he's not here, and I don't know where he is," Old John barked to every news guy who called. Young John slept well that night. The favorite in 1957 was another Finn, Veikko Karvonen, who had scored a stunning upset win three years earlier at Boston when he destroyed British world record holder Jim Peters on the famous Newton hills. Karvonen figured to try the same strategy again. Kelley was ready for him.

The race itself was surprisingly easy, "one of the few enjoyable marathons I've ever run," Kelley says. He felt comfortable the whole way, gave Semple the thumbs-up sign whenever the press bus thundered past, and gained confidence by watching the thick beads of sweat on Karvonen's neck. On that pleasant spring day, the crowds were thick and boisterous, waving American flags and cheering lustily for the little guy with the wavy blond hair and the blue unicorn on his singlet. The hills came, and Karvonen showed nothing, so Kelley scampered away, building a big lead. He won by nearly four minutes, in 2:20:05. "The race was more tactical than the year before, and I ran well within myself, to make sure I didn't foul up," Kelley recalls. "The tremendous crowds were a big boost. I felt carried along by their cheering for the American up front."

Running past Fenway Park, into Kenmore Square, down Commonwealth Avenue, and onto Boylston Street, Kelley tried to treasure every moment. "I was euphoric, of course, and I wanted to savor it, even as I was still driving for the finish and wondering if I might break 2:20," he says. "I considered Jock the embodiment of road running, and the heart and soul of the marathon. I wanted to win it for Jock."

IT'S A COLD, GRAY AFTERNOON in mid-January of this year, and I'm sitting on a rickety wooden stool next to the cash register at Kelley's Pace, in Mystic, Connecticut. It's a specialty running store, and Kelley works here full-time. His name's on the store but not, after several business reversals, on the ownership papers. That makes Kelley possibly the oldest wage-slave in a U.S. running store, and for sure the only former Boston Marathon winner.

While Marcus, his 11-year-old golden retriever, rearranges himself in a nearby corner, Kelley phones several customers whose special-order shoes have arrived. The wall above Marcus holds a mishmash of running photos, newspaper clips, memorabilia, and road-race entry forms. The biggest and most striking photograph shows a smooth-striding Kelley as he hits the Boston finish line in 1957, while Jock Semple awaits, mother-like, with a wool blanket.

Kelley arrived at the store after 20 years of public-school teaching, 20 years driving a late-night cab for his brother-in-law's taxi company (and bicycling the

10 miles home at 4 a.m.), and a long assortment of freelance writing gigs. In 1981, with Tom Murphy, he co-authored the Jock Semple biography *Just Call Me Jock*. It contains many vivid, first-person accounts by Kelley, rare chronicles of those forgotten days of New England road running. Kelley's three daughters live nearby, and he has eight grandchildren, one of whom, Jacob Edwards, is a talented young college runner.

Kelley ran many Bostons into the early 1990s—including a 2:34:11 at age 44 in 1975 and a 3:01:40 in 1986 at age 55—but then lost interest in the grind. These days, he doesn't race. He has never been drawn into age-group competition. "I genuinely envy those runners who can get excited about masters racing, but it's not for me," he says. "It never was. In my day, I put everything I had into my training and racing. When I look back, my intense sense of purpose seems almost insane. Now I feel no pull to race."

After my high school and college years, I lived in the Mystic area for 20 years and visited the Kelley household as often as I could. My mother died when I was 18, my father a few years later, and Kelley's house became a second home. The place was always chaotic, incredibly welcoming, and full of intense discussion. Whenever I faced major life decisions—marriages, job changes, and the like—I hurried over to the Kelleys'.

During the 1960s and 1970s, I would stop at the Kelleys' after every weekend road race. I needed someone to hear my stories—the wins, the losses, the outright heartbreaks—and, of course, there were few sympathetic ears in that era. But if you had Kelley's attention, you didn't need anyone else's. He could understand, respect, and respond to every high and low. After all, he had lived them himself.

Since moving to Pennsylvania 20 years ago, I see less of Kelley and enjoy each reunion more. On this particular visit, I am surprised by two things: First, he's really good in the store. His natural warmth, conversational gift, and extreme politeness—no one says more thank-yous than Kelley—encourage many repeat customer visits. "I really like these shoes, and I think they'll be great for you," he tells an 80-year-old female walker. "But what you think is more important than what I think, isn't it? So take a couple of laps around the store and see how they feel."

Second, I'm impressed that Kelley seems little changed, in many ways, from the staunch nonconformist. He's carelessly dressed in a baggy fleece jacket, a T-shirt hanging over his belt, light hiking boots on his feet. The blue eyes still sparkle. He's still got that lock of wavy hair spilling onto his forehead, though the color has gone from blond to gray. The face is thicker, with a bit of a jowl. He probably doesn't hear many people tell him that he looks like Bobby Kennedy, or even James Dean, as he did in the old days.

Most important, he's still hewing his own path. In the 1950s, Kelley aspired to marathon greatness despite the scorn and objections all around him. His coach wanted him to focus on the mile. His mother wanted him to make money, not blisters. Many Boston sportswriters referred to marathoners as "the saps who come out to run in the spring." Kelley paid them no heed, choosing instead to search, like Holden Caulfield, for his own truth.

Kelley's peers, the other educated young men of that time (he went on to obtain a master's degree at Boston University), were beginning their careers at GE, IBM, AT&T. Forty years later, they would retire with bulging stock and pension plans and second-home condos next to a golf course in Scottsdale. Kelley would be working retail, tallying the day's receipts. "The only thing I hate worse than counting other people's money is counting my own lack of it," he says, adding up a small pile of bills and checks.

But Kelley harbors no bitterness. He's at ease with who he is, where he is, and all the miles he has covered. No great marathoner has ever shunned attention more than Kelley, the polar opposite, he points out, to Boston's other, more famous Kelley. "Old Kel was an actor looking for the limelight, and he found his stage in the Boston Marathon," Kelley says. "He loved every minute he was playing that role. I've always been more the solitary type, happiest running or walking alone in the woods, lost in my own thoughts."

Kelley eats Saturday-night dinners with his daughters, bashes out various freelance assignments, and reads everything that calls to him. Recently I caught him deep into I, Goldstein: My Screwed Life, by Al Goldstein, publisher, pornographer, and five-time husband. I wagged a scolding finger. "No, Amby, it's really good," he retorted earnestly. "This guy was screwed in so many ways. There's a lot in here that any of us can relate to."

In place of daily training runs, Kelley's inviolate ritual has become his walk with Marcus, through Pequot Woods or along the Mystic River. On weekends, they take longer hikes in different natural areas of southeastern Connecticut. Over the past 50 years, no one has spent more time in these retreats than Kelley. "I love my life just the way it is," he says. "I still love to go out for a run or walk. I still love the act of moving my limbs through nature. It's just that the reasons are different now."

FOR MORE THAN FOUR DECADES, Christmas Eve was the big event of the year at Kelley's—the night that he'd fall asleep on the living-room floor. He's a Christmas Eve baby (1930), and each new December brought a gaggle of friends, season's revelers, and birthday well-wishers to the tiny Kelley house on Pequot Avenue. You can't miss the house; it's the one with the evergreen forest for a front yard, the result of all the living Christmas trees Kelley planted and nurtured over 50 years.

On Christmas Eve, runners came in droves, but the house also filled with poets, writers, folk singers, jazz musicians, artists of all stripes, hippie radicals, vegans, cyclists, sailors, animal lovers—in general, with any who felt disenfranchised. "We all have something different to say—the artist, the writer, the marathoner, the tightrope walker," he says. "It's important to find your voice, even if you don't understand where the impulse comes from. All we truly know is that we feel this compelling urge to express ourselves."

In the kitchen, Jess brewed endless pots of tea and served towering platters of sweet stuff. The apple pies were her favorite. "Apple pie without cheese is like a kiss without a squeeze," she'd squeal with delight, blushing at her own words.

A few feet away, Kelley would embrace each new guest with a firm handshake and shoulder slap. The conversation often led to a Kelley tirade against the day's latest atrocities—DDT, Vietnam, Watergate, Reaganomics, oil spills, excessive highways, Monicagate, Iraq, global warming, rolling farmlands turned into suburban sprawl. By 10 p.m., Kelley would be hitting the wall. Just as the party was picking up steam, with 50 or 60 people jostling about, Kelley would sag to the floor, curl up in a fetal position, and rest his head against one shaggy dog or another. We'd have to step over his inert body to get back to Jess's refueling table in the kitchen.

By 11 p.m. I'd be ready to leave, and I'd step gingerly over his torso. But a hand would reach up and grab my ankle. I'd hear Kelley say in a thick, sleepy voice, "Don't go, Amby. Stay a little longer. I'm just taking a short..." His thought would be interrupted by the wailing voice from the phonograph (then tape player, then CD). It was Bob Dylan, a perennial Kelley favorite. Kelley would catch a phrase or two, then go silent as he pondered its full meaning.

> *I saw ten thousand talkers whose tongues were all broken.*
> *I saw guns and sharp swords in the hands of young children...*
> *And it's a hard rain's a-gonna fall.*

Now, fully absorbed in the song lyrics, he'd forget the wrestling match with my ankle. He'd stare off into some faraway place. "You sing it, Bobby, you sing it," he'd say. "I only wish more people could hear you."

AT THIS YEAR'S BOSTON MARATHON, on April 16, Kelley will serve as the official Grand Marshal, riding the Saturn pace car just ahead of the elite women.

Through Hopkinton, Ashland, Framingham, and Natick, he'll wave to the gathering crowds. As the Saturn hums past the coeds at Wellesley, Kelley will stand taller and wave more vigorously. Who wouldn't?

On Heartbreak Hill, where families gather generation after generation, he might remember how strong he felt in 1957. Most of these spectators will be under 50, not born yet when Kelley won his Boston. But a few will grasp a grandchild's hand and point at the gnomish figure with the unkempt hair. "I remember watching Kelley win back in 1957," they'll say with a certain pride. "He was the big local favorite, and we were all rooting for him. It was a great day for Boston when he won, like the day three years later when Ted Williams hit a home run in his last at bat."

In downtown Boston, Kelley will be growing weary of the car time. He'll be wishing he could hop out, find Marcus, and take a solitary walk along the Charles River. A hundred yards from the Boston Marathon finish line, Kelley will be liberated at last and free to move under his own power. He'll be wearing BAA colors, as he did in 1957; he's still the only BAA runner to have won at Boston. He'll prance, with that springy stride, past the Lenox Hotel and alongside the Boston Public Library.

The thick grandstand crowds will respond with booming applause, not because they appreciate all Kelley has meant to American distance running, but because they have been waiting too long for something to happen. Kelley understands this; it doesn't trouble him. He has never sought recognition or acclaim, a podium or an audience. He has simply followed his own chosen arc. He has run far, struggled hard, and collected few tangible rewards. Still, he knows he has lived deeply and well. "We runners are all a little nutty, but we're good people who just want to enjoy our healthy, primitive challenge," he says. "Others may not understand running, but we do, and we cherish it. That's our only message."

At a little before noon, Kelley will cross the Boston Marathon finish line, ahead of the top women and the 20,000-plus others still running through Wellesley and Newton and Boston proper. He will be first again, just as he was 50 years ago—just as he has always been for me and those lucky enough to know him best.

THE RUNNER'S HIGH

FINDING
MY STRIDE

BY BENJAMIN H. CHEEVER

[*Fat and unhappy, the author surprised himself—and his famous father—by transforming himself into a runner.*]

NOVEMBER 2007

PHEIDIPPIDES IS SAID TO HAVE RUN the first marathon. That was in September of 490 B.C. He brought news that the Persians had been defeated. Athens was saved. Civilization was saved. "Rejoice!" he said. "We conquer!"

As Robert Browning would later write, "Like wine through clay/Joy in his blood bursting his heart/He died—the bliss!"

The bliss is what I'm after.

Although mortality is part of it. I was moving in a pack of runners 20-odd years ago on a sidewalk in White Plains, New York, after a half-marathon. Spotting others in singlets and with the distinctive postexertion matted hair, we waved our bony little fists. "Good race!" we shouted.

"Good race!" they shouted right back.

A funeral cortege appeared suddenly on the street beside us. The contrast between this ominous procession and our own towering spirits silenced the pack and made us—for an instant—ashamed. Then one of the runners waved his fist at the hearse. "Good race!" he shouted.

When long-distance running found me 30 years ago, I had begun the transition that I hoped would be my last. I yearned to become an adult male—a full suit with a job, a lawn, and a temper. I'd sold the motorcycle. In an exact reversal of the life cycle of the butterfly, I'd stopped flapping around and had settled down to learn a skill. This done, I was reconciled to a long caterpillar-like phase of dull work capped—I fervently hoped—with solvency.

As a child, I'd felt most myself when I was out of doors. Now I lived on Edgewood Road, but I rarely plunged into the woods from which our development took its name. The only face time I had with Mother Nature was spent weeding the pachysandra or cutting the lawn. I was throat-deep in a marriage that didn't work for anyone, not even the pets. I was employed as the only male on the copy desk at *Reader's Digest*. My idea of exercise was cadging cigarettes from colleagues who had the conviction to buy their own. I was 28 years old and all set for a wooden overcoat.

Then I spent $11 on a tag-sale bicycle. The frame was too big for me and had been sloppily repainted in Creamsicle orange. The machine had 10 speeds, though. I'd never owned a bicycle with 10 speeds. "I'll ride it to work," I said, justifying the expense. We had only one reliable car. "Maybe I'll lose some weight." I got a two-piece outfit in lime green with a zipper down the front and zippers at the ankles. Like tuxedo pants, the bottoms had a stripe of darker material down the outer seam. I liked the look, but clearly these "warmups" were from the bathrobe/pajamas family, the material sheer, the zippers frail. The label said DRY CLEAN ONLY.

I drove a suit, shoes, and neckties to the office one day and left them in the closet. There was a shower in the basement at *Reader's Digest*. The next morning I stuffed a fresh shirt, socks, and underwear into a backpack along with my papers.

On that first day I made the left turn out of Edgewood Road and onto Route 133. This was the big road, and I could hear the big cars on it. I was frightened, and I was right to be. I hadn't bicycled since I was a child. I was slow and I wobbled. The shoulder—when there was a shoulder—was pocked with holes and littered with broken Heineken bottles.

A couple of miles out, I caught the left leg of my warmups in the chain. This stopped all forward motion and I fell slowly, gracefully, into a gap in the middle of a lane of traffic. Scrabbling out of the way, I heard brakes and then a horn. Who is this asshole? they must have wondered. I wondered, too.

I made it, though. There were a lot of downhill stretches on the way from Ossining, New York, to *Reader's Digest*. The ascents were gradual, almost forgiving. I took my shower and found my post at work. That afternoon I hung my suit in my office closet and climbed back into my warmups. I dreaded the ride home. The machine had 10 speeds, all right, but you still had to pedal. At 5'7" I weighed 170 pounds. I couldn't make it even a third of the way up the first hill. I must have looked absurd: a fat man wearing green pajamas and walking an orange bicycle.

I heard the cars driven by colleagues growling up behind me on the first steep ascent above the Saw Mill River Parkway. The road has many curves, and they were forced to wait for a chance to pass. And passing these same people in the hall, I'd see it in their eyes—recognition, a flicker of amusement, and then nothing.

I might have given up the plan immediately if I hadn't already spent $11 on that eyesore of a bicycle. I developed a wicked case of what veteran cyclists call beginner's butt. If it didn't rain in the morning and dampen my shirt before work, then it rained in the afternoon and soaked the proofs I ferried home.

I'd watch the end of the local TV news and base my plans on the beaming meteorologist. I bicycled to work so often in the rain that I took to setting a clock radio and listening to the morning weather report. I still got wet. I kept setting the clock radio, but instead of listening to its buzzing prophecy, I'd step outside and smell the air, peer up at the sky.

Slowly but decisively, my body began to change. A month went by. Maybe two months. Then one afternoon without dismounting I made it up that first hill. Within a week of that triumph, I was looking forward to the commute. Flying down Roaring Brook Road in Chappaqua one day, just after dawn, I was shocked to hear a cry of pleasure, a yodel, really.

That was me.

CRAZY FOR ENDORPHINS, I TRADED stories with the runners I met in the shower at work. Then one Saturday I ran a mile. I was astonished. It must have been winter, because I was wearing a black crewneck sweater from the Army Navy store, blue jeans, and sneakers. I stood in front of the bathroom mirror, my face crimson with the effort, and thought: I ran a mile. Impossible!

My experience was solitary and seemed one of a kind, but this was 1977 and I was being worked on by forces of which I was not entirely cognizant. Kenneth Cooper's *Aerobics* had been published in 1968 and picked up by *Reader's Digest*. Frank Shorter had won a gold medal for the United States in the marathon at the 1972 Olympics.

Turned out that my mile—a circuit of the development I lived in—wasn't quite a mile. Nor were the seven miles I ran within the month a true seven. But here's the thing: I was an adult male—hairy, married, and stolid. I wore a necktie. Running was for children. And yet I'd just run seven miles. I did lose weight.

I wasn't afraid anymore. I mingled with the other runners. Some of these men were way up the masthead. I was painfully aware of the disparity in status and power. Was this reaching? Was I a striver? Did it show? Then one day I got to the basement a little late. Assistant managing editor Jerry Dole gave me a look that might actually have been stern and said, "You're late, Cheever!" Now, Jerry's exquisitely polite. He'd never have said anything if he had actually been angry.

I was delighted. I repeated the exchange over and over in my mind, mimicking the affection I'd caught in Jerry's voice. In the locker room and on the roads we would be equals.

Apparently, my transformation was noticeable, because a *Digest* colleague, Tom Lashnits, wrote a column for the *New York Times*, which began, "It all started for me when my friend Ben began to run. He's the son of a famous writer..."

Since I'd read *Walden* in high school, I had been haunted by Thoreau's charge that when I came to die, I might discover that I had not lived. If I run a marathon, I thought, I will have lived. I also thought I might die. Marathon champion Alberto Salazar once said, "Standing on the starting line, we are all cowards." This was a brave and generous thing for him to say. And it's true. But we also feel like heroes.

That first year I signed up for the 47th annual Yonkers Marathon in New York. It's the second-oldest 26.2-miler in the United States. (The oldest is Boston.) I fell in beside a helpful veteran named Spencer—or Spenser? I never saw it spelled, although we met each other at other races after this. Spenser was planning to break three hours, a good goal for a veteran, but ambitious for a first-timer. "You have to run the New York Marathon," he told me. "The crowd will suck you right up First Avenue."

We stayed together, and I moved quickly and well, until I came down into Tarrytown at about 15 miles. Then it was just as if I were a car and the fan belt had gone, just as if somebody had shattered my engine block with the .44 Magnum Clint Eastwood had introduced to the public in *Dirty Harry*. And no, I didn't feel lucky. This was the wall.

I did finish the race, in three hours and 31 minutes. And although I didn't walk, I was more than half an hour off the time I'd need to qualify for the Boston Marathon. I went to other races and reported the experiences so excitedly that civilians assumed I must be winning. When I explained that I wasn't winning, they didn't get it. Other runners got it. This wasn't about image or fame. The sport had its celebrities, its icons, and we adored them, but we didn't expect to replace them.

On weekends I took long bicycle rides with my father, and we began to repair a friendship that had been damaged and then severed by his drinking and my claustrophobic marriage. "We share an interest in rudimentary forms of transportation," he liked to say.

I spent $18 and change on a pair of Brooks running shoes, which I found marked down at Macy's. *Runner's World* had selected the Brooks Vantage with the "varus wedge" as the shoe of the year. Perfect—but they were a size too small. So I wasn't wearing socks for my first long training run in them. One foot was heavily bandaged when I ran a 2:59:46 in New York and qualified by a whisker for Boston.

I waited in Alice Tully Hall for the results. It was that close. Bill Rodgers won in 2:12:12. Grete Waitz set a women's world marathon record finishing in 2:32:30.

I wore my yellow New York Marathon T-shirt with childish pride. A woman stopped me in the produce section of the Millwood A&P to ask where she could get such a shirt. I paused at first, embarrassed, pondering her question. Then the majesty of my accomplishment dawned on me. "You need to run the New York Marathon," I told her.

"LOT OF SMOKE, NO FIRE, CHEEVER." That's what the wrestling coach used to shout when I groaned noisily in an attempt to escape from the opponent who was powering me around the mat. This was in high school, and it's when I first learned that time stops if you're anxious enough and in pain. I could look up at the clock three times during a 45-second drill.

Poor Coach. I was fat, I was slow, I was uncoordinated, but it was worse than that. I was easily frightened.

Take baseball, for instance, the national pastime. There's a reason they call it hardball. The ball, it's hard. Like a stone. I didn't want to be hit by one of those. I'd as soon have jumped into a wading pool full of hammerhead sharks as step into the batter's box. I was supposed to stand there, all tender parts exposed, while another boy hurled stones down at me from a hill.

If I'd had any chance of hitting the wretched thing, I might have mustered a little courage. There was no chance. Legendary Red Sox slugger Ted Williams is supposed to have been able to see the stitching on a ball screaming across the plate. I rarely saw the ball at all. I wasn't even certain it had been thrown until I heard it *thunk* into the catcher's mitt. The best I could do for my team was to get beaned and walk to first.

When the other team was up, the coach would send me deep into the outfield. Emboldened by distance and isolation, in remotest left field, I found myself wanting to play. Now that I was safely out of the action, I yearned to hustle. But man is—above all else—an adaptive creature. So I adapted. There was nothing for me to do. So I did nothing. I'd put my mitt over my face and look at the world through the V of the glove. I liked the cool leather on my cheeks. I liked the smell of neat's-foot oil. I'd dream. I'd breathe deeply. In, out. In, out. The Zen of baseball.

Bored almost into a coma, I'd squint through the glove at the other players. I'd watch their distant dramas with admirable detachment. Why are they so excited now? I'd wonder. I didn't know there was another Cheever on the team. Why is everyone rushing toward me? Why are their faces crimson? Why are they waving their arms in the air?

In the eighth grade I ran the 880 for Scarborough Country Day School. We had a meet with Peekskill Military Academy. They had a 220-yard track. When my race started, the coach wasn't there.

Now, it happened that three of the runners from PMA were substantially faster than I was. Yet at one stage late in the race, we were neck and neck. What my late-arriving coach didn't realize was that for the runners from PMA this was the fourth and final lap. For me it was the third.

Coach and a few others appeared just as the race became fevered. The four of us were thundering around that final curve. "Hustle!" he shouted. "Hustle, Cheever. Dig it out."

In his hoarse cry, I could hear Coach thinking, What do you know? Maybe I've been wrong about young Cheever.

Then we all crossed the finish. The PMA runners staggered off the course. I made the turn and headed manfully off for my final lap.

Coaches are supposed to have small and weathered hearts, something on the order of a horse chestnut. But this is the sort of performance that breaks even a chestnut heart.

My sporting achievements couldn't have been much good for my father's vitals. The man wanted an athlete as a son.

Freshman year looked like my breakthrough. I made it onto the varsity squad of Scarborough Country Day School's six-man tackle football team. Steve was first-string center. He wasn't all that big, nor was he particularly fast on his feet. Steve had quick hands. The moment the ball was snapped, he'd reach across the line of scrimmage, grab the face guard of the opposing lineman with one hand, and with the other he'd drive the nose he found there back into the face it belonged to.

This happened in games with other schools. It also happened in scrimmages between the first and second team. I was second-string center.

A cobra is supposed to strike so quickly it can't be seen by the naked eye. Steve's hands were that fast. I'd spend the rest of the play staggering slowly around in circles while the tears that had obscured my vision ran down my face.

My father was an unusually articulate and forthright man. He used to like to say that he and I operated "on a basis of absolute candor." And there was something to this, although he didn't tell me about his bisexuality. Nor did I tell him what it was actually like to play second-string for the six-man tackle football team at Scarborough Country Day. He knew that I—a freshman—was on the varsity squad. And it was a fine thing to have won my father's approval. Practice wasn't over until after the last bus had left the school. My father ordinarily hated the chauffeuring part of parenting, but after football practice, he was pleased, he was honored, to pick me up. On the way home, he'd stop and buy me fresh dinner rolls at the Ossining Italian bakery. He had a phrase for me—a mantra really: "My son, the football player."

Fortunately, he never went to a game.

As a sophomore, I went off to boarding school and, yes, I went out for football.

All the varsity and junior varsity football wannabes lined up in front of the cage. ("Cage," for those of you who have not been—as I have—varsity athletes, is the term used for the room or the locker in which sporting equipment is left to gather mold and grow fungi.) A whistle was blown and we rushed the cage. We tore off our street clothes and donned equipment. This was social Darwinism at its purest. The toughest, pushiest boys came up with the best equipment. The shy, uncertain boys made do with what was left.

I managed somehow to secure pants, pads, and a jersey. I was still searching for a helmet when I heard the whistle. We all charged out onto the field. We were divided into squads. We ran a few simple drills. Then we were lined up to scrimmage.

The coach noticed me.

Coach: "Yo."

Me: "Yes."

Coach: "Where's your hat, son?"

Me: "My hat?"

Coach: "You gotta have a hat to play ball."

Me: "A hat?"

Coach: "Go back in and get a hat."

Two days later, I was cut.

Because I was at boarding school, contact with home was limited to letters and the occasional call on the pay phone at the end of the corridor. I considered withholding the information, but the next time I called in, I blurted out the news. "I didn't make the team."

There was a silence on the other end of the line. The subject never came up again. Ever.

THE APRIL AFTER I RAN a qualifying time in the New York Marathon, my father celebrated my acceptance into Boston by taking the whole family to spend the eve of the race at the Ritz Carlton. For breakfast on race day, the Carlton waived the necktie requirement in the Grill Room. My father suggested I write a "casual" for the *New Yorker* about this.

I finished the race in three hours and three minutes. When I came back to the hotel room, nobody was there. The phone rang. It was the Associated Press asking to speak with John Cheever. The phone rang again. It was UPI asking to speak with John Cheever. I drew a bath.

My father came into the hotel room and then into the bathroom. "You finished the marathon?" he asked.

I nodded. "And you won the Pulitzer Prize," I said.

I finished my postrace bath while he spoke with reporters. Walking near the Prudential Center afterward, he noticed all the other runners still conspicuous in their silvery capes. "Nobody knows that either of us did anything," he said.

In a letter to a friend he wrote, "Ben came in gallantly under three hours, which is considered winning, and when I returned to the hotel he was sitting in the bathtub, holding in his teeth a wire from the Pulitzer Prize Committee."

He'd chopped four minutes off my time.

The New Yorker turned down my casual, and although it hurts me to admit it, I expect their judgment was sound. Still, it meant a great deal that my father had suggested I try. Good writing was mistaken for good character in our family.

My father wrote an essay about running, which was rejected by the New York Times but purchased by Reader's Digest. Held for some time, it finally ran in May 1982 and was the last of my father's writing published while he was alive. In the past, he wrote, he'd been heartened when he traveled by the sight of lovers. Now, he was encouraged by the runners he saw everywhere. He saw "five runners crossing in front of the Kremlin in Red Square."

My father seemed delighted by my emergence at last—approaching 30—as the athlete he'd always yearned for in a son. In a television interview shortly after I'd run Boston, he said that I had broken two hours in a marathon. Now he'd chopped an hour and four minutes off my time. And the man hadn't had a drink in years.

JOY CHANGES THE LANDSCAPE. My old life began to loosen around me like somebody else's shell. I felt naked, exposed. I had flashes of ecstasy, but pain was also more available to me. Not just physical pain either. I was swept with waves of remorse. And, alarmingly, I also felt the stirrings of ambition. I'd stumbled into an arena where I could go all-out, holding nothing back, and nobody—nobody—would be injured or even threatened. The smell of 3-in-One oil was as nostalgic for me as the madeleine is fabled to have been for Proust. I bought a new bicycle, a Raleigh Grand Prix with the Alpine gear, and loved the music made by the click of its chain. The Grand Prix was royal blue, and I kept it in the kitchen at home and in my office at work. Life is a miraculous undertaking if you're paying attention.

And there was all this talk, a sort of buzz about how good distance running was for me. I was getting thin and fast, and—the cherry on the sundae—I might live forever.

"Most Americans are in terrible shape," wrote Jim Fixx in his 1977 best-seller, *The Complete Book of Running*. "We smoke and drink too much, weigh too much, exercise too little, and eat too many of the wrong things."

I read somewhere that when you run for longer than an hour, your body begins to adapt in miraculous ways. I couldn't actually have thought that my arteries were growing, but it was like that.

But in the background I could hear the fearsome rumbling of infuriated authority. Having come into my office on other business, one of my superiors spotted the new blue bicycle.

"My wife has the car," I explained.

"Tell your wife," he said, "that you can drive to work or not come to work at all." He laughed when he said this, but it was a mirthless laugh.

I was told I would soon be a couple of inches shorter. That my hips might be damaged, my retina detached. Lots of people saw arthritis in my future, and many expected cancer. "The body isn't designed for that kind of wear." I felt 10 years younger, but a week didn't pass without a perfect stranger wondering out loud about my knees. "And where do you find the time?" One well-educated colleague told me that marathons were once held in Madison Square Garden.

"What happened?" I asked, going for the bait.

"They realized how harmful marathons were for the athletes ... The culture moved on. There was an editorial condemning marathons in the *New York Times*." This I didn't believe, but the tidbit rankled. And I harbored doubts of my own. I was having fun, all right, but fun is not always a good sign. Was this about vanity? Were we narcissists? Did we run because we were afraid to die?

Coming up from an afternoon workout in my shorts and a T-shirt one evening, I found Temple Williams, the editor who was then my best friend, waiting in my office. My calves were suddenly prominent, and my knees had thickened dramatically. There was a new bridge of cartilage running downward from the point of my kneecap.

"You've changed your body type," Temple told me. "You're a different person now. You can't ever go back."

RUNNING SCARED

BY AMBY BURFOOT

> *There's only one thing more powerful
> than the desire to win the Boston Marathon:
> the fear of losing it.*

MAY 2008

EIGHTEEN MILES INTO THE 1968 Boston Marathon, I looked up and didn't see another runner on the road ahead. Not one. I had dreamed every night for years about winning Boston. And now I was almost there. I had just turned the corner at the Newton fire station and begun the run eastward on hilly, serpentine Commonwealth Avenue. Ahead, thick crowds edged onto the road—grandparents and their children and their children's children—shading their eyes and peering at the colorful stream of runners, all 890 of us. Three motorcycle policemen led the moving spectacle, and a photo truck, and a yellow school bus containing the Boston press.

For five years, I had set myself the singular goal of winning Boston. I ran up to 175 miles a week, entered every road race I could find, broke down on occasion, as all runners do, but then resurrected myself and trained even harder. Always with Boston as the focal point. If I could hold on, my name would go into the record book with the likes of Clarence DeMar, Les Pawson, Tarzan Brown, Gerard Cote, "Old John" A. Kelley, and my coach-mentor, "Young John" J. Kelley, the 1957 winner.

Only one thing stood between me and a Boston victory—the shadowy specter that was stalking me. I couldn't hear him, only my own desperate breathing. Couldn't see him, for he was a stride back. But when I glanced down at my feet, I saw two dark shapes—my own, tall and angular. And my pursuer's—shorter, more compact, with arms that pumped more vigorously than mine.

I had come so far. I was so close. I had given so much. I was a 21-year-old senior at Wesleyan University in Middletown, Connecticut, who in four years of college had set new records for dullness. Hit a Saturday night keg party? No way.

I detested beer and, more importantly, had to rouse myself at 6:30 for the ritual Sunday-morning 20-miler. A weekend skiing trip? Not a chance. Skiers twisted their knees and broke their ankles and risked countless other injuries. Go on a simple dinner or movie date? Not those either. I had no time for flirtations or anything that might muck up my marathon ambitions.

As we reached the first of the three hills on Commonwealth, I drove myself harder. Sweat flew from my forehead. My throat was dry and scratchy, the sun having targeted us from the start, producing a perilous dehydration. Like other marathons in those days, Boston offered no water stops. I reached the top in a near swoon, but the extra shadow was still there. Moments later we started up the second hill, and I dug deeper, gritting my teeth with each stride. Nothing changed. The haunt stuck with me—silent, apparently effortless, mocking my furious exertions.

That left only the third and last hill—the storied Heartbreak Hill. It was longer, steeper, and deadlier than the others, peaking at the 21-mile mark— beyond The Wall, beyond the marathoner's last reserves, deep in the zone of zombie running.

In my youthful racing career, I had already lost scores of races at the end, outkicked by others with superior speed. Every time I ran the mile, I led for three laps, then the field sprinted around me. Same thing in the two-mile, only it was worse because I would lead for seven laps before the floodgates opened. I found some solace in road racing with its longer distances—10 miles, 20 kilometers, and beyond. But I lost even those races when another runner tailed me to the final yards before blowing past. This Boston Marathon was feeling far too familiar.

Worse still, I knew my shadowy rival's name, Bill Clark, and he knew mine, and we both knew he would beat me. Clark, 24, was one of those distance runners I envied for their speed. He could run a 4:06 mile—much faster than my best—and had marathon endurance as well. I was in deep trouble.

My day hadn't begun well either. After passing the "physical exam" in the Hopkinton High School gym and picking up my race number (17), I headed for the locker room patrolled by de facto race director Jock Semple. I had changed there the year before, thanks to my friendship with John J. Kelley, Semple's protégé. It was the year before that Semple gained worldwide infamy for attempting to bulldoze Kathrine Switzer off the course.

That was the very same Semple I encountered as I swung open the locker-room door. With head down, he charged me: "Oh, fer Chrissakes, will you git the hell outta my locker rhume." At the last second, he looked up. "Oh, Ammmby, Ammmby. It's okay, Ammmby. C'mon in."

I was still rattled when the race began at noon. But once in motion, I calmed down, happy that we had finally begun the journey to Boston. I drifted into the front pack, the miles passing quickly, almost silkily, that's how smooth I felt. Near the 10-mile mark in Natick, I decided to make a full race assessment. I edged to the side of the road and turned for a wide-angle scan of our lead pack. It included a Finn, three Mexicans, and a half dozen Americans. Bill Clark lolled a few yards back. I audited myself most closely of all. Breathing? Blisters? Leg pains? Overheating? The answers came back one by one and led to a rare conclusion: Nothing hurt. Everything felt great. I was having a dream day—one in a million.

At 14 miles, I mounted a little surge—the most middling of accelerations—to stretch my legs and gauge how the others would react. I shortened my stride, veered from the group, and broke into a quicker, more flowing rhythm. There was more air around me now, and it felt invigorating. When I slowed again after about 200 yards, I expected the whole gang to circle around me.

Instead, there was only Clark. I looked back in disbelief. In shock. The others had drifted 20 yards behind. They were struggling. Just two of us remained. This was terrible, the last thing I wanted. No more comforting cocoon. Now it was a race. Man against man. A winner, a loser. With 12 daunting miles to go.

What to do? It was too soon to begin a charge for the finish, yet I didn't dare slow and let the others regain contact. For certain, I needed a plan that would save me from getting outkicked again. An insistent voice in my head said: Maintain for now. Wait for the hills, wait for the hills, wait for the hills. Then run your guts out. At the bottom of Heartbreak, Clark's shadow still taunted me. With every stride, my chances of winning grew slimmer.

IN MY TENTH GRADE BIOLOGY CLASS, I was enjoying a peaceful post-lunch nap when the public address box startled me awake. "Harrumphhhh"—the despised sound of our principal clearing his throat. "We've just received the first radio update from the Boston Marathon, and our own Mr. Kelley is running with the leaders after six miles." A sports report sure beat another lesson on cell division. And I had actually seen this Kelley in the high school hallways. He was the short one with the suit jackets that dwarfed his thin torso.

The principal returned with several more updates in the next 90 minutes. Kelley fell back, but he still finished fourth that year, 1962. Five months later, I joined the cross-country team he coached at Robert E. Fitch High School, high atop Fort Hill in Groton, Connecticut, and competed in my first distance races.

I had been a baseball fanatic, but running gave broader compass to my obsessive personality. I had a stern, Germanic mother, and from her I learned self-discipline. It required no particular effort to run 35 miles a week during my senior year at Fitch or to double that to 70 my first year at Wesleyan. I believed that whereas success in other sports depended on raw physicality—your height in basketball or your weight and strength in football—distance running rewarded those who trained the hardest.

On our Sunday-morning runs, Kelley filled me with alluring tales of Boston's improbable history. The pull was irresistible. One April morning in 1965, my father drove me to Hopkinton to run the marathon for the first time. A light dusting of snow covered the colonial rooftops and a few hardy forsythia blossoms. On the town green, five Japanese runners warmed up in spotless white sweats. I also caught a glimpse of "Old John" Kelley in a crimson Harvard sweatshirt. I had never seen so many runners in one place—358 that year—and I couldn't wait to join them.

I remember passing through Framingham at six miles and spotting the first of the Boston Athletic Association's bright orange checkpoint signs in the road. It said B.A.A. MARATHON: 193/8 MILES TO GO. How puzzling, I thought, and then: Too bad I've never run that far in my life. This frightened me enough that I kept a conservative pace, and with every passing mile caught one or two struggling runners. At the crest of a modest slope near Boston College, I yelled out to the crowd, "How much farther to Heartbreak Hill?"

The response came quickly: "You just reached the top."

In the last five miles, I passed clumps of spent runners and continued running strongly to my 25th-place finish in 2:34:09. Two days later, I had to run the mile and two-mile in a track meet against Brown. I was outkicked in both races.

Every year after that, I tried to train longer and faster. One crisp October day in 1966, my cross-country teammate Jeff Galloway, a precocious young marathoner, proposed a stunning workout: 40 x 440 yards in 75 seconds with a 110 jog. We ran barefoot on the grassy field surrounding Wesleyan's cinder track and adjacent football field—Jeff with his muscular chest and shoulders and his light forefoot prance, me tall and skinny with my shuffling heel-strike. When we finally finished the 40th 440, the sun had set behind the hulking Wesleyan Library, my feet were freezing, and we still needed to jog a two-mile cooldown to complete the nearly 17-mile workout. Of course, I had already run seven miles that morning. And would again the next morning.

The winter of my senior year, I ran a series of uninspired indoor track races, except for a two-mile in 8:45 that far outstripped my wildest expectations. In mid-March my Wesleyan track team took a spring training trip to Quantico, Virginia. With Boston just a month away, I wanted to pile on the miles. The first morning, I was up early for a 17-miler. That afternoon I talked my teammate Bill

Rodgers (yes, that Bill Rodgers) into joining me for what I promised to be a relaxed 12-mile run. And it was, until we got totally lost in the twisting trails of Prince William Forest Park. After two hours in low-80s heat, we walked a couple of times, then started up again, and eventually emerged to some roads. The run took three hours. I wrote it down in my log as 22 miles. That gave me 39 for the day, a good beginning.

Over the next two weeks, I averaged 25 miles a day, hitting 350 miles for the 14 days. After a few days of recovery, I noticed that I was running fresher than ever. Even when jogging, I skimmed along at six minutes per mile. This had never happened before. It has never happened since. But in April 1968, I was in the "flow," to use a term psychologist Mihaly Csikszentmihalyi wouldn't coin until 1990. I was totally focused on the upcoming Boston Marathon and totally energized by the process.

In the late '60s, we knew nothing about visualization or positive self-talk. No one talked himself up; that would be presumptuous bragging. I did tell my brother Gary and one trusted training partner that I thought I could win. Then I swore them to secrecy.

WHEN CLARK AND I reached Heartbreak Hill, I closed my eyes, groaned loudly, and ran for my life. This was it—now-or-never time. If I didn't drop him here, he would outsprint me later. But I was a good hill climber. I had won many races on hilly courses, my low shuffle chopping the hills down to size. I still had a chance.

Out of the corner of my eye, I saw a young boy, perhaps 7 or 8, rushing my way with a slice of orange. I wanted it badly—any liquid, any calories, any jolt. But I couldn't spare the effort to reach out for it. I had only one mission: to run to the edge. I saw the child turn away, chagrined, and retreat to his parents. I felt guilty for rebuffing him.

I was pumping, pumping, pumping to drop the shadow. Halfway up Heartbreak, no luck. I had nothing left to give. Zilch. My breathing rose to a wail. I remembered what my former coach Kelley once told me about Roger Bannister's 1954 breakthrough in the mile. Kelley believed that Bannister and others of his era were impeded by a primal fear. Many prominent doctors and academics argued that four minutes was an actual physical barrier. The human body wasn't designed to run that fast, they contended, and the man who dared a sub-four would risk death. The heart might explode, the lungs burst, or the arteries rupture.

Bannister proved the naysayers wrong, but now I wondered if it was the brevity of the mile that saved him. The marathon—that surely wasn't a distance intended for human recreation. I didn't imagine that I might die, but I figured that my body might simply stop functioning at any moment. I was imploring it to go faster. What if it had other plans?

One hundred yards to the top of Heartbreak Hill, and my vision closed to a narrow slit. There were no more sidewalks, lawns, trees, or houses. No more cheering spectators. No more blue sky overhead. No sound, no colors. Just driving arms, leaden legs, stinging salt, a thin patch of asphalt dead ahead. And two shadows. I gave a final big heave.

It didn't work. I hit the top of Heartbreak, and my tormentor was still there. I almost stopped on the spot. What was the point? I felt my body sag, deflated and depressed. I stumbled briefly, but caught myself and staggered on. We were heading downhill now, beyond the Boston College spires and toward Evergreen Cemetery on our right. I knew it was only a matter of time before Clark stormed past.

And then the shadow was gone. I blinked a couple of times and rubbed my eyes. This made no sense. I was a lousy downhill runner, Clark a fast finisher. Where was he? In 1968, I didn't know this stretch of the course was named Cemetery Mile because it had buried the hopes of many Boston runners. Here the stiff downhill slope forces the quadriceps muscles to contract eccentrically, opposite to the concentric work demanded by Heartbreak Hill. The abrupt change often induces muscle cramping, and that's exactly what happened to Clark. His spirit, heart, and lungs were willing—perhaps more willing than mine—but his legs were not.

Suddenly the press bus zoomed past with Jock Semple hanging from the front door. "Give it hell on the downhills, Ammmby," he bellowed at me. "Give it hell on the downhills." In the big rear window, I saw "Old John" Kelley brandishing his fists for me. Kelley had recently had hernia surgery; this was one of the few Bostons he didn't run, among his 58 finishes.

I would have loved to seize the moment and press my advantage, but I had nothing. I had completely spent myself on the hills. Even as my small lead grew inch by inch, I knew my pace was slowing. The race had become a survival of the least defeated. Crossing the trolley tracks at the bottom of Cleveland Circle near 23 miles, where the course joins Beacon Street, I felt a stabbing pain in my left side.

Ahead, a throng of spectators gathered in the street, literally filling it. The downtown crowds were immense and police control almost nonexistent on this warm Friday afternoon in April. As I approached, the spectators would move aside at the last moment and then close behind me. Yes, I felt a little like Moses parting the Red Sea. But I was also filled with torturous doubts about the army of marathoners behind me. What if Clark regained his rhythm? What if someone had paced the race better than I had and was now gaining fast? I was fading, no doubt about it.

When you're alone at the front of the Boston Marathon, surrounded by thunderous crowds, a burning sun overhead, your body's sugar supply depleted . . . this is not a good time for an aptitude test. I grew faint and confused. Where was I on Beacon Street? I couldn't tell; all the blocks looked the same. Why wasn't I making any progress toward the damn Fenway Park light towers? Time nearly stopped. I was going nowhere, running with an awkward tilt—bent over, trying to knead out that side stitch—at what seemed like a 10-minute pace. I had never been so parched in my life. Two hours earlier, David Costill, a Ph.D. studying sports drinks, had weighed me in the gym at Hopkinton: 138 pounds. At the finish, I would barely top 128.

I must have looked back a hundred times in the last several miles. The first time he saw this, Clark thought, Aha, I've got him now! I couldn't imagine anything worse than losing the Boston Marathon at this late stage, and yet it seemed certain to happen. How could I win Boston when I was falling apart like this?

I reached Fenway and lurched into Kenmore Square, twice as crowded, twice as tumultuous as anything before. I felt so small, so vulnerable. A half mile later, turning onto Hereford Street and seeing no one on my heels, I finally started to believe. On Mayflower Hill, 170 miles to the north, high above Colby College in Maine, my brother Gary sat with a small transistor radio jammed against his ear. "One of the runners has broken away," he heard. "It's Burfoot." He jumped to his feet and danced a little jig. At a track meet in Storrs, Connecticut, the news spread quickly, reaching Bill Rodgers. "It was hard to comprehend," he says today. "To me then, a marathon was like a race from another planet." Jeff Galloway, on a Navy ship off the coast of Vietnam, heard nothing for two weeks. But after he reached the Philippines and caught up on the news, he wrote me a letter. It said: "After I heard about your 8:45 two-mile, I knew you were going to have a great year."

I've seen video of my last 100 yards in front of the Prudential Center, where we finished in 1968. I don't look at all like a marathon champ. I look more like the tottering Scarecrow in *The Wizard of Oz* after he's lost all his stuffing. When I hit the finish line in 2:22:17, just 32 seconds in front of Clark, I collapsed into Jock Semple's arms. I vividly recall how weak I felt, how utterly wasted. And how warm he was, how strong and solid.

But even more I remember Jock's words. And his tone. As he held up my full body weight (what was left of it), Jock spoke with a soft lilt I had never heard from him before, not once. He wasn't roaring now. He was purring, and his mouth formed the sweetest words I have ever heard. "You did it, Ammmby," he said. "You won the Boston Marathon."

SOMEONE TO RUN WITH

BY SARA CORBETT

> *A friendship in nine acts*
> *(and who knows how many miles).*

I.

REALLY, THIS IS A SAD STORY. It's about a once-together woman who manages to lose her independence over many, many miles of running and eventually turns into a jealous and out-of-shape shrew who feels like she ought to run a lot more miles just to beat some of the loneliness out of her bones. But she doesn't. She just goes for a short run and then calls up her friend Clare. Clare and I used to have a friendship that was all about running, but now it is mostly about talking. Clare lives in New Mexico, and I live in Maine. The good news is we talk a lot about running. There are days I will go out for a 40-minute run and then call up Clare to tell her, over the course of a 60-minute conversation, that I went running. This is how it works with us. I don't run without calling Clare afterward, and she doesn't run without calling me. Sometimes we call each other to report that we actually won't be running—that we have conferences with our kids' teachers or a deadline at work or our backs are aching or one of us has just accidentally eaten a gigantic bag of M&M's and couldn't possibly think about moving. At which point the other person says, pretty reliably, in a sing-songy voice, "I think you should sneak out for a run anyway. Remember how it makes you feel!"

Every so often I bring my cell phone and talk to Clare while I am running. I know this makes me sound lonely and pathetic, but keep in mind this is supposed to be a sad story. I wear an earpiece headset and narrate the important parts—Hey, my knee isn't hurting! Or, Boy, that was a pretty fast mile!—as we keep up our usual patter about our jobs and kids and husbands, who are awfully sweet but nonetheless require ongoing scrutiny.

Out on a trail around the bay near my house, I pass women pushing baby joggers in the other direction. I pass a couple of older men chugging along. The high school girls cross-country team blows by me just as Clare, in her office in Santa Fe, says something funny about her dog and I burst out laughing. The girls look back at me over their shoulders, startled. "Time to hang up," I say through the headset. "I'm making people nervous."

II.

WHEN I FIRST MET CLARE, I didn't like her so much. This was mostly because she was from California. A lifelong New Englander who just recently had moved west to Santa Fe, I treated Californians with the same sort of suspicion I treated, well, everybody. It was 1995, and Santa Fe was full of transplanted Los Angelinos walking around in sequin-studded cowboy hats and hugging everybody they met. Back east, we were not huggers. Californians, I'd figured out in my six months in Santa Fe, loved both new people and new things—spirulina drinks, past-life rebirthing, high colonics, and so forth. On weekends, I called my mother in Massachusetts and described my new life out west with a mix of horror and intrigue, like a frontierswoman sending dispatches back to the Puritans at home. "They burn sage why?" my mother would say. "Your neighbor is a vegan shaman and he did what?"

Anyway, here was Clare, hugging my friend Andrew, whom she knew from California. Clare worked for a vitamin company and looked the part: She was a narrow-shouldered woman, 30ish, with a golden-girl tan and supermuscular legs. She wore an enormous pair of mirrored wraparound sunglasses. The first thing I remember thinking about Clare is that she looked like the Terminator, if only the Terminator had a perky little ponytail and a freckled nose.

"Clare just did an Ironman," Andrew announced, casually. And then he said something I didn't appreciate.

"Sara's a runner," he told her.

"Recreational runner," I added, but it was too late.

Maybe she was desperate for company, or maybe she found some sort of sick pleasure in the thought of overpowering lesser humans, but behind her Terminator sunglasses, Clare lit up. She gave me a big hungry smile. "Oh, goody," she said. "I really want to do a marathon soon. We should run!"

III.

A FIRST RUN is not unlike a first date. Early one fall morning, I met Clare at a trailside parking lot, where she continued to intimidate me. She wore shiny technical-fiber clothes. She stretched her Ironwoman quads and took long pulls on a bottle of energy drink that the vitamin company sent her for free. Next to her, in my cotton college T-shirt, with my plain-Jane water bottle and underdeveloped, pasty-white legs, I appeared purely amateur. And that was fine, I kept telling myself. Because I'm only doing this once.

We trotted out of the parking lot and along a sandy, sage-dotted trail that built slowly into a mountainside. As a teenager and right through college, I'd run with only one friend—my old best buddy, Sue—and since then, nobody had quite lived up. I'd run with people who were too fast or too slow or too silent for me. But Clare was none of these things—least of all, silent. Over the course of an hour, we rambled through stories about her move from San Francisco, about our respective pets and our respective boyfriends and underwhelming jobs and how someday we were each going to do something spectacular and also have enough money to take beach vacations at least twice a year. I missed the Atlantic and she missed the Pacific, but it was the Caribbean we agreed to pine for. Hammocks and waving palms and rum drinks, and so on. We were, as they say, off and running. We ran up the mountain without a single thought toward slowing down. We ran across switchbacks and up a few steep pitches, with my dog racing alongside through the scrubby pine. Pace never entered the conversation, but I calculated that I was running just faster than I normally ran by myself. This was better, in other words, than being by myself.

Back down at the bottom, Clare gave me a big fat Californian hug. Releasing me, she said, "We should do a marathon."

"Nope, not me, no marathon," I said. I'd run exactly one marathon and I would not be running a second with any hardcore triathlete. "You frighten me," I said, just to make things clear.

"What about just a run then? Up the hill again?" said Clare, climbing in her car to go home to her dogs and horses and her sandy little ranch south of town. "Tomorrow, same time?"

IV.

THE MARATHON went pretty well, thanks for asking. After leisurely chatting her way up and down that mountain in Santa Fe with me nearly every day for four months, Clare had lost some of her triathlete steel and I'd grown a smidge more fit. We were, it turned out, a good athletic match. We'd also taken to getting giant full-fat lattes after our runs, sometimes with pastries, sometimes with waffles. This helped my cause. My mediocrity, we might say, was prevailing over her superhumanity. In the midst of all the talking and all the eating, I had let Clare sign us up for a marathon in Utah. She advertised it as a "downhill marathon," something we could dispense with quickly and painlessly—qualifying for the Boston Marathon while we were at it—and then we could go spend the night at a spa built next to some hot springs.

Clare has a credo. It goes like this, and I am quoting her: "Pamper, pamper, pamper!" Which is to say she doesn't believe in running a marathon if there is not a spa involved on the other side. In Clare's universe, the body performs, the body gets its payback. Over the years, she has marched my conservative New England bones in and out of all manner of bodyworkers' offices. Postrunning, we've had acupuncture, Thai massage, shiatsu, mud baths, IV vitamin drips, and once she took me to have what she called "internal acupuncture," involving wires and electrodes and something called the Quantum Xrroid machine. ("The Quantum what?" my mother practically shouted into the phone from back east. "Really, isn't it time to move home?") In preparation for the Utah marathon, Clare found us a massage therapist named Big Jim. Big Jim was about 6'5" and his particular genius was how he could drive an elbow expertly and with the full force of his body weight into our glutes. We took our glutes to him weekly. We had earned it, after all.

I have learned so much from Clare over the years. I have learned a lot about vitamins and also that it is not so bad to talk to strangers or to spend money on fresh flowers and keep them for yourself. She is a look-on-the-bright-side kind of girl, a devotee of small indulgences, a believer that a gift should be exquisitely wrapped, that a houseguest should be served coffee in bed. She is a horse-loving ranch dweller who walks around caked in manure but not without her toes painted. She lights candles on the dinner table every night of the year.

But still: there is no such thing, really, as a downhill marathon. I learned this halfway up what amounted to a four-mile megahill beginning at mile seven of the Utah marathon. My mind was trying desperately to float away from my body. Next to me was Clare, doing the same agonized shuffle but saying in her chirrupy way, "This isn't so bad. Really, this is not so bad!" To get ourselves over the top, we started fantasizing about waving palm trees and beachy rum drinks, and right to the moment we flopped over the finish line, Clare was still talking about how not bad and not hard it all was.

I do love her for this.

Within hours, we lay starfished on our respective beds in our room at what turned out to be not so much a spa but rather a rustic wilderness retreat that had already basically closed down for the season. We were the only guests. We'd been dreaming about cold postmarathon beers only to have the idea crushed by the discovery that we were in a dry county and that beer was 25 miles back down the road. Even the hot springs were a 10-minute hike from our room, and now that both of us felt like we'd been beaten with a big stick for three hours and thirty minutes (and three seconds, if you care to know), there would be no hiking. Not even to the other side of the room where we had left the Advil marooned on a dresser.

"I'll pay you five dollars to bring me three Advil," Clare said.

"Ha," I said from my spot on the bed.

"Ten dollars," she said. "And I'll give you an extra 200 if you drive back to town and get us a six-pack."

"Ha, ha," I said. But then, feeling suddenly like I owed her a whole lot more than this, I stood up and hobbled across the room to fetch the ibuprofen, free of charge.

V.

"HOW MANY MILES do you think we've run together?" I ask Clare one day on the phone.

"Hundreds," she says. "Definitely. Over a thousand? Two thousand? I don't know."

We mull this over for a minute and then decide it's not worth calculating.

VI.

AFTER A COUPLE OF YEARS in Santa Fe, I moved back east, to a small town in rural Maine, far away from Clare and Big Jim and the Quantum Xrroid machine. Suddenly, I was running alone again, on the empty country roads near where we lived. The silence was daunting. It rained a lot. My seven-mile runs became six-mile runs and then four-mile runs. Back in New Mexico, Clare had taken up yoga.

One fall day, she and her boyfriend arrived for a visit. Clare and I immediately put on our running shoes and headed out the door. It was deer season. I made her wear a blaze-orange cap so she wouldn't be confused for a deer, since in western Maine deer were a lot more common than runners. We started down the long, narrow road that ran ribbonlike through the dense forest near my house. The trees seemed to lean in on us, idly dropping red and golden leaves as we passed under—a scene that might have felt sylvan and magical were it not for the bursts of rifle fire coming from the woods all around us. It took less than a mile for me to understand that Clare and I were both miserable. I was lonely living out in the country, and her relationship was ending, in excruciating slow motion. We talked a little but not a lot. We just ran hard.

A few months later, the boyfriend was gone. Clare and I were on the phone. She was lying on the floor in New Mexico. I had been promising her that someday soon life would be so good that this would all seem trivial, that she'd be thankful it happened, even. I tried to make her bet me money on it, but she wouldn't do it.

"Okay, you have to get up now," I said to her.

"I don't think I can."

"Get up and go outside and go for a run. It will help," I said. "I promise, I promise, I promise."

VII.

ANY FRIENDSHIP that is based on running is, in essence, about accrual—of time, of miles, of intimacy built over a lot of small steps forward. It sneaks up on you that way, I think. It can seem merely enjoyable until you need it for more. One winter day, just after my 30th birthday, my mother was killed in an accident. For weeks, Clare, who had lost her own mother to cancer years earlier, called on the phone and tried to talk me off the floor. Then she flew to New England and sat on the couch with me and let me weep for a good long time. Afterward, she stuffed my feet into my running shoes and pulled me out the door, not needing to say a word about why it was necessary now to go out and breathe.

It would be easy to be sentimental here. Having told you some of the sad parts of my running days with Clare, I could balance them with the joyful ones. I moved out of the boondocks to a small city near the ocean that I cherish and married my steadfast Santa Fe sweetheart. We've gone on to grasp some version of the fat domestic enchilada my mother had wished for me—having three children; buying the house, the minivan, the power mower. All good and fulfilling, but my running, over time, has become less regular, less liberating. Every year Clare and I pick out a race or two we're interested in—the New York City Marathon, a trail run in Colorado, the all-women's marathon in San Francisco, or something on Maui, maybe—but in truth we almost never get past checking out Web sites for spas in those places. Life has grown too full, too frenzied, too loaded with little competitors for our time.

As for Clare, she met her true love. On the day she married him, she and I rose early at her house in Santa Fe and went for a long, meandering run in the sage and scrub, during which I took the opportunity to gloat about how I had been right when I told her things would get better.

I credit Clare with teaching me, over so many miles, to cling to my optimism. Because if you want to see it this way, life is something like a downhill marathon. You have to believe it's easier than it is. Or at least it helps to have a friend who views it that way.

VIII.

THEN LAST YEAR, we pulled it off. Clare rented a house on the beach north of San Francisco and found a massage therapist who made house calls. We signed up to run the half-course version of the Nike Women's Marathon, in San Francisco. I invited my old running friend Sue, with whom I'd run practically every day for four years during college. Sue was my old Clare. Or Clare was my new Sue. In any event, the women's marathon went right through the heart of San Francisco, but according to Clare, who claims to have carefully inspected the elevation map on the race Web site months earlier, it was "really pretty flat," and therefore none of us bothered much with hill training.

You'd think I would've learned by now.

Before the race, Clare and Sue and I gathered at dawn in Union Square where someone announced on a loudspeaker that about 10,000 women would be running the race that day. We huddled in close to one another, joking, telling meaningless stories, waiting for the starting gun. I was happy to see Sue and Clare, who'd never met, gabbing like old friends. It hit me that I have been running since I was 15 years old and that truly all of my dearest female friendships have been built around running. I was thinking how lucky I am, how unique this was, how sustaining. But the sun was coming up and all around us there was a sound starting to mount, a murmuring that seemed to reach across every corner of the city square, ballooning through the open spaces and growing slowly louder. I recognized it then and knew it was something to marvel at—a familiar force that would carry us all once the gun went off and we started to run.

I looked at my friends. "Do you hear that?" I said, a little bit incredulously. "That's the sound of 10,000 women chatting."

IX.

HERE NOW IS THE bitter part of my tale. Clare has a new running friend in Santa Fe. Her name is Laura. Laura is very fast, I'm told, and she runs races all the time without a whole lot of effort. Her son goes to school with Clare's daughter, and so it's all very cozy. I am trying to feel good about Laura. But Laura has helped Clare get faster, which is to say that she is suddenly out—way out—ahead of me. She calls me to tell me she just ran 12 miles. I call her and tell her I ran 3.6 miles, maybe 3.7.

"That's so great!" says Clare.

"Oh, come on."

"No, really."

I am silent, sullen.

"I need someone to run with," I say. "I need a Laura."

Clare and Laura recently went back to California to run a half-marathon. I was feeling spiteful and jealous about this right up until the minute Clare called me up to tell me all about her race, and I found myself whooping congratulations. I can't help it. I've known her too long. It's not that I'm jealous of Laura, exactly; it's that I miss being 28 years old with no dependents and bountiful time for friends and running followed by waffles and massage.

And, by the way, I did get myself a Laura, in the form of a friend who'd just moved back to Maine from Italy. Lily. Lily and I meet on a trail by the ocean regularly and crank out a bunch of miles without pausing one single second in our talking. It's fall again. The trees throw their leaves at our feet. Lily is my Laura. She makes me faster and stronger and happier about life. Or maybe Lily is my Clare, as much as Clare can never be replaced and I still call Clare every time I finish a run. But Clare was once my new Sue, who will always be my first old running pal. And maybe Laura is Clare's Sara. And Clare is Laura's somebody else. Maybe there's really only one thing to say about all of us women who run in tandem or in groups, who configure and reconfigure like kindred constellations moving across the sky. Maybe it's that we're all wrapped up in the same cosmic downhill-but-not-really marathon and more than anything, we just don't feel like doing it alone.

THE INTERVAL WORKOUT

BY JOHN L. PARKER JR.

[*A hard thing to have to know.*]

MAY 2009

AN INTERVAL WORKOUT," CASSIDY once explained to a sportswriter, "is the modern distance runner's equivalent of the once popular iron maiden, a device, as you know, used by ancient truth seekers." Although overdistance laid the foundation, intervals made the runner racing mean. Quenton Cassidy liked them. Others preferred bamboo splinters under their nails.

Cassidy figured that a natural affinity for interval work was the difference between those who liked to race and those who liked to train. And there is a difference. Racers express little enchantment with training for its own sake.

An interval workout is simply a series of fast runs of a specified distance in a specified time with a specified rest. The variables are limited by the imagination of the coach and the physical limitations quickly apparent in his athletes. (It is one thing to write "10 quarters in 58 seconds with a 220 jog" and quite another to carry out those instructions.) While a 10-mile overdistance run might be generally thought of as a pleasant diversion, few of Cassidy's teammates thought of intervals as anything but a grueling ordeal, satisfying at best, horrifying at worst. It was precisely the kind of training, he knew, that tempered the body for racing. Though the distance runner is constantly striving for aerobic efficiency, the race itself is primarily an anaerobic experience. Everyone, the winner in his painful glory as well as the loser many seconds behind in his equally painful anonymity, suffers the physical bankruptcy of total oxygen debt. And since interval training is usually sharp enough to bring the runner to grips with oxygen debt very quickly in the workout, he learns to deal with the debilitating fatigue from the first repetition on. Other sports use an abbreviated form of interval training called "wind sprints," but where football and basketball players run 30 or 40 yards and take several minutes' rest between each, the miler will run 220 yards, 440 yards, a half mile, or even three quarters of a mile at a time. Each second of his minute or two-minute rest period is sweeter than life itself.

It was little wonder Bruce Denton took more interest in Cassidy's interval training than in anything else that made up his 140 miles a week. Denton had begun coming to the cabin on interval days, sometimes spending the night. If such a program had a deleterious effect on his marriage, he never mentioned it to Cassidy.

"I HOPE YOU LISTENED to me and took an easy day yesterday," Denton said as they jogged to the field.

"Consider me psyched out. What's the program?"

"Twenty quarters in sets of five, 110 jog between the quarters, 440 jog between the sets, 62- to 63-second effort but no watch as usual. That's it. For now."

Cassidy was surprised. It was a tough workout, but nothing he hadn't done many times before. Denton had been talking ominously about it for days, and now the runner actually felt a little let down. With Denton he never knew what to expect. When weeks earlier he had instructed Cassidy to let his hair grow and not to shave, Cassidy made it a point not to act surprised. He had his suspicions, but he also knew that Denton wasn't about to tell him any more. If he had wanted Cassidy to know, he would have told him already. Now the sun-bleached curls were around his ears and his chin had sprouted a reddish beard, which Cassidy was now rather fond of. He pictured himself a gaunt Viking.

When they got to the field, Cassidy removed his shoes and joined Denton in some striders to loosen up. It was a gloriously clear, warm day, and soon the shirtless runners were wringing wet with perspiration. Although he knew few runners who did so, Cassidy loved training barefooted. Denton considered it an aberration, but since it seemed to cause no complications, he tolerated the practice.

There had been, in fact, a few world-class runners who competed barefoot on the track and seemed no worse for it; and then there was Abebe Bikila who, incredibly, ran the 26-plus miles of the marathon barefooted at the Rome Olympics, winning easily. There were arguments pro and con about whether it could be helpful in training or racing, but Cassidy just did it because he liked it. It allowed him to be closer to the grass, the soil, closer to the deepest hidden yearning of the runner: to fly naked through the primal forest, to run through the jungle.

They began. The first few always seemed especially bad. Actually that was misleading. They seemed sluggish because the body was shocked by such a sudden demand for sustained speed. The heart rate shot up to the hummingbird levels it would have to maintain for some time. The legs became prematurely heavy, and the central nervous system sent up the message that such punishment could not be endured. But the central nervous system is overridden, of course, the runner knowing far better by now than his own synapses what his body can and cannot be expected to do. The runner deals nearly daily in such absolutes of physical limitation, which the nonrunner confronts only in dire situations. Fleeing from an armed killer or deadly animal, a layman will soon find the frightening limits that even stark terror will not overcome. The runner knows such boundaries like he knows the sidewalks of his own neighborhood.

After the shock of the first several quarters, Cassidy settled into the pleasant, nearly comfortable rhythm of the workout, where each interval, though difficult, felt very much like the one before and the one to follow. After they finished the first set of five, the quarter-mile jog prescribed by Denton seemed almost too luxuriously long. During this time, once he had recovered his breath somewhat, Cassidy made a few remarks and generally tried to engage Denton in conversation; the older runner demurred, jogging on in what Cassidy thought a rather grim manner. They began the second set.

Round and round the field they went, each repetition so much like the one before they had to count out loud lest they forget how many they had done; Denton, the true compulsive, would assume they had done three rather than four and they would take a chance on doing an extra one. Cassidy, therefore, paid close attention to the tally. The only difference between one and the next was the slight increase in lactic acid in the lifting muscles on the top of the thigh that made each a little more difficult and started hurting earlier in the sprint. Otherwise, it was almost as easy to drift into the near-neutral mental state as it was on their long-distance runs. Denton was a perfect training partner; the pace did not vary more than half a second from one to the next.

In the third set Cassidy felt as though Denton was picking up the pace, though it was unlikely. It simply required more effort now to keep up the same speed. A miler, whose pace in a race was quite a bit faster than 63 seconds, could still get a lot out of such a workout. The key was not how fast he could run, but how fast he could run when tired.

Cassidy did not allow himself to think of racing pace, for these 63-second quarters required so much effort it would have been heartbreaking to think how much faster he needed to run in a race. There were too many other factors:

rest, a faster surface, and more important, the incredible psych he would build up prior to the race. Such comparisons were not helpful and were dismissed quickly. In training it was best to think about training. As he circled this little field 12 miles from Kernsville on a Saturday afternoon, racing seemed an exotic and glamorous activity indeed, the "trial" part of his Miles of Trials.

Number 14 was especially poignant. Finishing it, Cassidy rasped: "Eeeow, that one hurt!"

"Little . . . fast." Denton gasped the words. Occasionally during a repetition one of them would let his mind wander to a race, long since run, and as the memories seeped in, the pace would inch up as adrenaline began surging involuntarily through the system. The other would respond and soon they would be flying around the worn path, racing different phantoms from the past. The price for such a lapse was steep. They would begin the next repetition still out of breath.

As bad as he felt at the end of the third set, by the time they finished jogging their quarter, he was recovered. Denton's training called for short recovery periods and Cassidy had been amazed how he responded to the snippets of rest. Recovery was key; the faster one recovered, the faster he could race. "A race," Denton would say, "is all go and no blow. So why practice resting?"

The last set felt very much like the one before and when, at last, they finished number 20, Cassidy let out a whoop. They had been running very hard for an hour. He looked over at Denton, expecting to see the happy relief that follows a hard workout, but Denton jogged on grimly.

"What now?" Cassidy asked cheerfully, thinking they might finish with some striders or a mile warmdown.

"Another 20." Even though Denton said it seriously, Cassidy had to smile. After they did a few strides and Denton did not dispel the grimness of his pronouncement, Cassidy knew he was serious. This, he thought, was a dirty trick.

And they began it all again. In their minds they took up each set separately, as if it were all they had to do. Five little circuits to be conquered, a mile and a quarter of hard running interspersed with those nearly cruel bits of rest, each quarter becoming in its own way a milestone, a feared and adamant obstacle that had to be dominated and put away so that its brother, now looming, could be faced. The sun was soon at tree level, splashing the field with dark cool shadows from the surrounding oaks. But for the desperate nature of their struggle, it would have been a remarkably pleasant scene; to the runners, however, it might just as well have been sleeting, so fierce was their attention to their toil.

Although as they finished the second set his legs were merely numb, Cassidy's arms and shoulders ached. When he slipped out of the trance to look at

Denton, he saw no sign of unusual fatigue. This is how he puts the fear of God into them, he thought; he just keeps going and going like this.

They had both long since stopped speaking except to call out the number of the repetition as they finished, both of them gasping finally: "20!"

The trees were now steeping in the dusty pink-orange glow of sundown, the color of ripe mangoes filling the sky behind dark oaks. They jogged on, saying nothing; their deep gasps echoed across the field. It did not dawn on Cassidy until they were halfway around the field. By this time their breathing was getting back to normal, but they were still in distress. "Bruce, you're not going to . . . I mean, this is . . ." His voice faltered, weak with self-pity and resignation.

"Twenty more, Cass."

They jogged on quietly. Cassidy felt close to tears and wasn't even ashamed about it.

"Bruce. Sixty quarters. Bruce, you can't be serious. Nobody does that kind of stuff anymore. Arthur Lydiard—"

"Screw Lydiard. Quenton, this is where you find out. This is the time and place. All the rest is window dressing."

"I don't know if I can do it."

"Quenton." He smiled for the first time all day. "You can do very nearly anything. Haven't you figured that out?"

"Yeah."

"Look, runners deal in discomfort. After you get past a certain point, that's all there really is. There's no finesse here. I know you can do this thing because I once did it myself and when it was over I knew some very important things."

"That you're a lunatic?"

"Maybe. Maybe we all are. But I expect you'll find out in your own way. That's why I'm going to let you do them by yourself, just the way people do everything that's important. You can slough off if you want, but by God, you'll sure as hell know when you're doing it, won't you?"

"I suppose," he said glumly.

"I'm going back to the cabin. I'll be back about the time you're finishing up."

"Swell."

HE BEGAN THE MELANCHOLY ritual as night was falling. After the first five he was running by the soft glow of a huge, clear moon. Cassidy thought, Bruce thinks of everything.

Then he sought out the mental neutrality that is the refuge, the contained, wan comfort of the runner. He grooved his mind upon the thin platinum rail of his task, a line that stretched out in front of him and disappeared into the gloom, farther than he could contemplate all at once, even if he had the desire to, which he did not. When his trance broke and a word or phrase popped into his mind, his dizzy mind played with it like a seal with a beach ball, in a disturbing, gibberishly mad way, the way your mind acts in the druggy twilight before sleep. In a very controlled, abstract way, he knew how much he was suffering; the slightest break in his concentration allowed self-pity to well up in him instantly.

He was, in a manner of speaking, accustomed to this distress in the same manner that a boxer is "accustomed" to being struck; but the familiarity of experience in no way lessens the blow or mitigates its physiological effects. It merely provides the competitor a backdrop against which his current travail may be played, gives him a certain serenity in the face of otherwise overwhelming stimuli, allows dispassionate insight where otherwise there would be only a rush of panic. In a hail of killing blows, the fighter's quiet center of logic, schooled in brutality, will be calmly theorizing: We are hurt pretty badly. If we do not cover up and take up the slack we will soon be unconscious.

Not that this quiet center of logic fears unconsciousness (indeed, how welcome it might seem at times), but it knows that one can't win while unconscious. Likewise, no highly trained runner slacks off because he fears pain, but because the quiet center of logic says he will win nothing if he runs himself to a standstill.

All of this availed Cassidy not at all. His deeply ingrained conditioning and his mahogany-hard legs merely allowed him to push himself that much more. He had the mental ability to literally run himself right into the ground like Sambo's tiger. He knew that Denton expected him to do exactly that, and, just as each repetition made the next seem more impossible, he knew that without question he would do it. There was no refuge in injury; his body could not be injured in this way. There was no refuge in mercy; there was nothing to forgive, no one to issue dispensation. And at last he saw: there was no refuge in cowardice, because he was not afraid. There was no alternative; it just had to be done.

He finished number seven, running it too hard, which caused him to take deep, painful gasps and to spend a few seconds bent over grasping his knees before beginning his weak jog on to number eight (in his mind number three, and after that only two to go—beyond that he did not think). It was becoming harder to get his breathing anywhere near normal in the 110-yard jog; he was starting the next interval gasping as if he had not stopped at all. Into the next one he charged, down the straight, around the turn, by a pine tree slashed in half by lightning (that to him meant only the halfway point), into the last turn, and then the last 50 yards, legs, arms, shoulders, jawbone, ears, chest, fingers, all battling the strained numb pain of the lactic acid, all striving for that normality of motion that would preserve—should heaven and hell fall into each other in a cosmic swirl—the integrity of the stride. Let others flail; the runner runs truly to the end. He finished and rasped, "Eight . . . you . . . bastard."

But the ninth took special revenge, reduced him to such a level that he had to spend several seconds holding his knees and sucking in sweet but maddeningly unsatisfying air. When he finally trotted on, he looked up at the bright, clear stars and his eyes welled; mixed with the hot sweat of his face, tears ran down to the spittle around his mouth and chin, and he felt quite literally that he was melting, turning to human slush as he jogged along. Only when he started a repetition did he become solid once more.

His mind had now taken up a melody, "Für Elise," and played it constantly without apparent pattern except that as each new quarter mile began, so did his fragment of Beethoven; whereas the stars were cold specks of illuminated space dust to him, those haunting notes reassured that there were at least others in the universe capable of understanding. Each new quarter now began in a kind of physical sorrow and ended in nothing less than spiritual despair. He remembered suddenly the one marathon he had run. On the 23rd mile he had looked around and discovered that everything seemed unfamiliar. Convinced he was lost, he ran on like a forlorn child, blubbering and wailing. When he finished the race, in 2:33, he saw he had been on the right course after all. But he still couldn't keep from weeping; he just didn't know why any longer.

After his 15th quarter he would have had to think for a moment to recall his own name. But now he had his full quarter mile of rest, which he took in mincing little steps, savoring every instant. His mind came out of neutral, reveled in giddiness. He was incredibly thirsty; his tongue was stuck to the roof of his mouth and he no longer had to spit out the thick white fluffs of congealed saliva; there was none. He dared not think of water, or of the first beer. Parched to the marrow, wobbly, near mad, he took his tiny jogging steps and waxed (so he thought) poetic:

> Somewhere they fox-trot madly
> While in lunar shadows sadly
> I keep pace with crickets gladly
> And Moon rises with my bile

Lord Godamighty, he told himself, launching into number 16 (in his mind number one). "Für Elise" cranked up again and he wished it would go away. He hardly felt anything now. He hardly cared. As he was putting 17 away, "Für Elise" degenerated into a steam calliope gone haywire. Misplaced notes made what had been haunting, ugly; what had been precise and logical, mad and horrifying. As if to keep pace with the crumbling music, his form occasionally broke and an elbow would flap out, a knee would catch its brother instead of sliding by. Poor Elise, he thought. Poor everyone.

Eighteen was a shambles. Nineteen required all his effort to keep the pace from slipping to a stumble. It had fallen off badly during the last few sets, but there was nothing to be done about it. When he finished the 19th, he let out a slight, wild, but oddly unjoyous, whoop. He was vaguely aware that Denton had returned, but it quickly slipped his mind. His mind was devoid of any thought save finishing.

On the last he simply sprinted away the life in him. The thin sliver of monorail that had once stretched out to forever now dropped off into a sheer abyss just over the horizon. Once more down the straight, around the far turn, past the pathetic half pine, into the last turn, flailing now a little, and (all slow motion now), feeling each step of the last 50 yards until it was over.

He staggered about, tightly grabbing his knees, eyes clenched shut, painfully, for the tears could not get out, while the sweat seemed to seep in easily. Denton stood beside and held him steady, with a gentleness of a medic treating the newly wounded. And like a casualty, Cassidy seemed not to notice him.

Denton walked him back slowly, talking to him quietly all the way. Cassidy, still deep in his anguish, said nothing. Denton fed him from the blender, let him drink all the liquids he wanted, then gently put him to bed.

"Quenton, you—"

"I know," Cassidy said. His eyes were still moist; he turned away. "But it is a very hard thing to have to know."

Denton nodded, smiled at him as he swatted him once on the fanny (the muscles there were quivering, he thought, just like it was for me), and left. Cassidy was in a deep sleep by the time Denton was out the door.

Cassidy awoke only once during the night, filled the toilet with bloody urine (something Denton told him might happen), and went back to bed. He slept 17 hours altogether, and when he awoke at last, the runner, paragon of fitness and efficient mobility, this runner at least, had trouble getting around. He went back to bed.

LONG TIME GONE

BY JOHN L. PARKER JR.

[
Quenton Cassidy was once a runner—a great one.
Now he was something else. Fortunately, he had always
believed in comebacks and second chances.
]

DECEMBER 2007

THE CABIN SAT BACK off the road in the dripping trees like a part of the forest itself, earthy brown, and plain, with a skin of cedar shakes, organic but for its giveaway straight edges. In the gloomy afternoon downpour the familiar shape seemed the essence of refuge. Could it possibly have been just a year? Yes, and some days. The screened-in front porch wasn't latched, and he had already retrieved the front door key from his shaving kit, where it had been for more than a year. Cassidy backed in, dragging two big canvas equipment bags, disturbing spiders at work, breathing in the familiar scents of raw lumber, mildew, and the pepper and earthy decay of Spanish moss and north Florida piney forest. The place was perpetually unfinished inside, with stacks of building materials lying around and wiring showing in bare stud walls. Bruce wasn't kidding; he hadn't been out in a long time.

He dropped his gear in the chaos of the so-called living room and just stood there with his eyes closed, the echoing scents of an earlier life making him dizzy with nostalgia.

As the rain deflected lightly off the steep sides of the A-frame, it seemed to him that this was the kind of day that seemed to happen in your life when Something Big had just ended. Back before it all happened, during all those long days, nights, weeks, months, and years of training, he thought of the future as a kind of foggy diorama. If everything turned out the way it was supposed to, his later life would be some kind of stroll with a desirable female into the middle distance, a happy American epilogue befitting the narrative line, inspiring music crescendoing into the Warner Bros. logo, a glad coda for a three-act culture.

But he had always kept it nebulous in his head, and now that the time had come, he found that the girl had actually married someone else and gone away and he had not Won the Big Race and he would not grace any cereal boxes. Also, he didn't know how to stroll, and there was no music except for one eerily chipper Gilbert O'Sullivan ditty he could not turn off in his head, something about climbing a tower and launching yourself into the indifferent void. Standing there in the familiar musty half-light of a late-summer thunderstorm, he thought, It's just like the lady always said: no bugles, no drums.

The small television set was where he had left it in the oven, cord wrapped round and round. A bunch of books were still stacked next to the cot in the small bedroom in the back: *A Fan's Notes, The Bushwhacked Piano, Zen and the Art of Motorcycle Maintenance.* He had done a lot of reading out here as he lolled around between workouts, trying to coax his body back to life so he could go out and carefully brutalize it again.

Loll. That was the word for it. Time lolled away, napping, thinking, daydreaming, waiting for his damaged corpuscles to rearrange themselves into a more perfect union.

He went to the plate-glass window at the front of the cabin and, sure enough, down in one corner were the faint dusty outlines of the words he had written in reversed mirror script on the foggy pane one lonely winter afternoon long ago: Help. Imprisoned in February.

I should unpack, he thought. I should make the bed, get this place organized, something. But there it was: no ambition. At all.

So, he did what he had done so many thousands of times before when his life was at loose ends and he didn't have a thought in his head: he pulled on his togs and blew out the front door and was hitting right at six-minute pace before the screen door had even finished double-slamming behind him.

His battered lemon-yellow 914 was still clicking in the cool rain as he splashed down the rutty red-clay drive that always reminded him of North Carolina. He turned at the blacktop, and after a quick half mile, veered off at the familiar trailhead and disappeared into the forest. He had felt so logy that he was surprised his legs loosened up quickly on the carpet of pine needles, and it wasn't long before he fell into a miler's tempo stride and began clipping miles off at not much slower than five-minute pace. It was much too fast for overdistance, he knew, but he wasn't training anymore. He was just running.

The trail went deep into the endless stand of blackjack pine and water oak and up by Otter Springs and then almost all the way down upon the Suwannee River, where, in fact, very few old folks stay. Four miles into the run at the bottom of a gentle rise that he called Blackberry Hill, he was startled to see his own ghostly footprints at the edge of the trail. He remembered the day he had made them, long ago. It was rainy like this and he was skirting a big puddle, trying to keep his shoes dry as long as he could. Strange to think the evidence of his ephemeral passing would still be here, hardened into the earth, partially hidden by encroaching weeds, like poor little Lucy's footprints on that plain in Africa, still there after three million years. Taking the hill with big strides he thought: We never really know what will happen to the scratches we make in this thin dust.

Familiarity, as always, made the trail go by quickly, and he blinked back from a daydream having to do with billfishing in the Gulf Stream to realize he was almost finished. Good thing, too, with the glistening woods now darkening before his eyes. Eight miles and he hadn't seen a living soul. He had seen a herd of deer, a probable wild turkey—at the distance he couldn't be sure—a red-tailed hawk, and several mullet, evading predators or just jumping for joy.

He finished, as usual, going hard down the last perfectly straight row of Sidecar Doobey's pecan grove, the flat grass inviting speed and bringing on the old fantasy of being in the final straight of the Olympic 1500, straining to reach the leader, leaning for the tape, and reminding himself over and over: Go through the tape, go all the way through it, with nothing held back. Just like the old days when he would be out there with Mizner and the guys, running along the sidewalks of Kernsville in pretend slow motion as the half-miler Benny Vaughn did his mock-serious announcer, giving them all funny foreignized names to make them sound more glamorous, doing the play-by-play as they made agonistic faces and leaned histrionically toward the imaginary finish line. Benny had named him Quintus Cassadamius, the famous Greek miler. It struck him for the first time just now—and with a quick flare of pride—that a new generation of dreamy kids might now accord him his own name. In these mock race scenarios Bruce Denton had no glitzed-up fantasy name, a gold medal being about as glamorous as you could get in their little world. Cassidy wondered now if maybe a near miss was worth something, too.

Funny, he thought, I was there in real life, yet running down this lane I go back to the same old fantasy. We few who get to experience both eventually find out that the real thing and the fantasy can coexist in your head. He would love to tell the undergraduates about that. It was the kind of thing they would talk about for hours on training runs. Mize, Nubbins, Burr, Atkinson, Schiller. Old dour Hosford. They were mostly gone now, graduated or otherwise scattered. Off to wars, other schools, wives. Where, oh, where, he wondered, are my light-foot lads? What has become of the old team?

He jogged in from the highway, using the long driveway as a cooldown, and was glad he had left the porch light on, dark as it was getting. He toed off the muddy shoes and left them outside, fetching a dry towel from the bedroom but returning to the porch to continue dripping. It wouldn't do any good to shower yet; he would just start sweating again, so he plopped down in an aluminum lawn chair and watched the rainy night come on. He had been wet so long his fingertips were wrinkled. Steam rose from his skin.

He didn't know if it was bad yet. Bruce said it would get very bad before it got better. That was just part of it. The big buildup and then the really big letdown. Worse than you could ever imagine. Truth be told, though, at this moment he was feeling pretty darn good.

He was through with the Trial of Miles, the quest that had consumed him these past umpteen years. He was wet and hungry and, in a general epistemological sense, adrift. He was sitting on a borrowed porch at the end of the road at the end of the summer at the end of his athletic career, dripping salty rainwater in a perimeter around a cheap aluminum chair. And he was once again staring into the moist gloom of Marjorie's ancient piney flatwoods.

But 27 miles away, back in Kernsville, catty-corner from the campus, was a white-columned, faux Southern mansion that housed the University City Bank, an establishment founded by Sidecar Doobey's old man with the obscene profits he made running rum on shrimp boats from Key West up the west coast of Florida. That bank had been his last stop before heading out to Newberry that afternoon. It contained a safe-deposit box, number 1347, newly opened in the name of Quenton Cassidy and paid for a year in advance, the key now dangling from the fresh-air lever of the beat-up Porsche in the front yard. Box 1347 was in the lower left-hand corner of the far wall of the vault. It was the smallest size offered. The slide-out metal drawer held only one item: a flat oblong leather box.

In that box was an Olympic silver medal.

CASSIDY WAS ALMOST ON TIME as he banked the Vincent Black Shadow into the La Fiesta parking lot on the outskirts of Raleigh. North Carolina State Assistant Professor Bruce Denton, ever the scientist, had given very precise directions.

Within a very few minutes they were holed up in a comfortable booth and equipped with a pitcher of margaritas and a hot, oily basket of chips, Cassidy munching happily, still buzzed from the ride down the interstate.

"You're looking pretty darned fit for a guy can't run," Cassidy said, redundantly salting his chips.

"I bet I haven't gone more than three miles in five years," Denton said, looking chagrined. "It's this thing they call pseudo gout. It's this buildup of calcium pyrophosphate in the joints. Took forever to figure it out. Finally this orthopod whiz at Duke nailed it. It sounds kind of silly, but when I'd try to run, the pain would wake me up at night. They told me I don't behave, pretty soon I'll have titanium hips."

"Seriously?"

"Damn right, seriously. I do the stair machine and this rowing thing that's pretty good. And I eat an amount of food that would barely keep a starling aloft."

"That can't be easy for someone like you. You were a garbage disposal. Remember the all-you-can-eat fried chicken things at Morrison's on Tuesdays and Thursdays? We'd have three or four skinny guys down there..."

"Pile the bones up in a heap in the middle of the table like a bunch of Vikings?"

"People walking by staring. The waiters thought it was hilarious and would keep hauling out these platters..."

"Yeah, the managers were kind of nervous, though. Sure, I remember it. I have dreams about it. All that can change pretty fast. It can catch up with guys don't figure it out quick enough. Stop running and turn into little butterballs."

Cassidy looked at his old friend and decided that he did look pretty good. The still-boyish face was etched a bit by time, but was tan and taut. There were flecks of gray at the temples, but the eyes still shone with amusement and irony.

"So what's it like being a professor?"

"Quenton, I still keep *Mad* magazines under my bed, if that tells you anything. Most of the guys in the department are like that. Once your geek self-image is set at an early age, all the degrees and Olympic medals in the world won't change it."

Cassidy knew there were probably people who had worked with Denton for years before they found out he had been an athlete, much less an Olympic gold medalist.

"You doing much teaching?" Cassidy asked.

"Hardly any. This semester, none. Half my time is research, genetically induced pest resistance, which is the latest rage. The other half I'm out in the field with the growers and other ag specialists. Cotton is king around here, and the boll weevil is my sworn enemy."

"That explains the tan. And you have a pretty good group in the afternoons?"

Bruce brightened, refilling their salt-rimmed glasses. "You'll meet them tomorrow. Yes, when I was still running, they'd just do my stuff, kind of like the old days in Kernsville. Now I'm more of a clipboard kind of guy. I head to the stair machine when they're out on the roads. Sometimes I mountain bike with them just for grins."

They hadn't really seen each other in person in several years, and Cassidy noticed how easily they had fallen into the worn groove of their friendship.

"I haven't even asked about the family unit," Cassidy said, setting his menu aside.

"They're great. Jean does computers in the math department, staff type. Matt's getting to be a bruiser, God help us, maybe a football player. Terry's leaning toward ballerina. Some of the kids from the team are around the house a lot. It can get to be quite a zoo around there. You'll see."

"Looking forward to it."

"So you've been up here for a while? I was sorry to hear about your grandfather, by the way. There was an article in the paper even over here."

"Yeah, thanks. I've been staying in this old house they have up the hill on the farm. It's good and quiet up there. Good place to run. Good place to think. I've been up there for a couple of weeks now." Cassidy idly traced figure eights in the frost of his glass. "For the last few years my grandfather cut less and less of a swath," he said. "One summer when I was in high school, I was sitting with him on the porch one afternoon and one of his old cronies dropped by. Old farmer in bib overalls—over-hauls, they call them—doesn't even shake hands, just pulls up a chair like he's done a thousand times, gets out a red bandanna to wipe his forehead, and he's going 'Lawdy, Mr. Jim, it's a hot one' and all that. Then he says, 'Mr. Jim, how you been gettin' along?'"

"My grandfather looked at him and—I'll never forget this—he looks at the guy and he says: 'Gettin' old!' But I mostly remember the way he said it. He wasn't trying to be ironic. He had this tone of voice that I didn't get for a long time."

"Yeah? What was it?"

"Surprise. My grandfather was surprised."

Denton nodded while the waitress distributed their plates. "Runners are much more in tune with the winding-down process," he said.

"You think?" Cassidy was digging in.

"Oh, yeah. Your average citizen isn't that connected to the physical realm. Builders, farmers, your grandfather probably was more than most. In an older time, with, say, manual agriculture or hunting-gathering, you always knew how much less you could carry than a year ago. Believe me, when dinner depends on running game to the ground, you notice pretty quick when it starts to get harder."

"You've done some thinking about this."

"You will, too. Modern civilian though, things happen too slowly to notice. Jeeminy, when did the basement steps get me wheezing? Am I old or just out of shape? And if you were never in shape, is there any difference?"

"Whereas we can just watch ourselves slowing down like there's a gauge on the dashboard," Cassidy said.

"Yes, the same black-and-white numbers that we used to live and die by, all those landmarks along the way, like the first time you go under 4:10, your first sub-30 10-K, all that. But if you keep at it long enough, you get to play it all back in reverse. I'll never forget the first time it took me more than 32 minutes to finish a 10-K," Denton said, amazement in his eyes.

"People don't realize what it's like to be in a sport where you can compare yourself so easily with guys in Europe, guys in Africa," said Cassidy.

"Or even with guys from a different generation."

"Or with your own younger self."

"Well," said Denton, leaning back and licking salt from the rim of his glass, "at least you can still run on both legs."

"And I don't have the hips of an 80-year-old rodeo clown."

Denton smiled painfully.

"Sorry," Cassidy said.

"No, it's true. It's kind of a karma thing. Payback for our arrogance when we could run a hundred miles and sort of pitied people who couldn't."

"Yeah, I guess."

"You ready?" said Denton.

"Sure, but first tell me something. Do you miss it much?"

Denton paused as he was sliding out of the booth. "Quenton, you'll come to understand this eventually. I had my time, I really did. It was wonderful, no doubt about it. Stood up there blubbering like a schoolboy with my hand on my chest..."

"Bruce..."

"...and that was then. Now I have a wonderful life. Family, career, good health..."

"Bruce..."

Denton laughed. "More than I can tell you," he said, picking up the check and handing it to Cassidy.

DENTON WAS DISPATCHING his minions for the afternoon. Cassidy—pretending to stretch—was lolling around like a sprinter on an expanse of indoor-outdoor carpeting in the NC State field house.

"Okay studs and stud-ettes," Denton said. "Thirteen miles no faster than seven-minute pace. Mile of striders. Mile jog. That's it. Interval miles coming up on Wednesday. And Dick, no collecting." Big laugh for that as they headed to the doors.

"Huh?" said Cassidy, as Denton grabbed his mountain bike and they followed the others.

"Endris," Denton said, situating a foot in the pedal clip. "One I told you about getting his entomology doctorate at Southeastern? He's a fan of mixed metaphors, like you. I told him some of yours one day. 'More fun than a barrel of rotten monkeys, barking up the wrong sleeve,' the ones I could remember. Know what he said?"

"Can't imagine."

"He said, 'It's no skin off my teeth.'"

"Hah! That's pretty good. He has obviously taken to it like a duck out of water. But what's this business about collecting?"

"Oh, on runs Dick occasionally picks up specimens. He puts them in a piece of scrap paper or a flattened Dixie cup and tucks them in his waistband. One Friday before spring break last year he comes across this huge female wolf spider with an egg sac on her back. Dick finds a Dixie cup and scoops her up. Wants to count the babies, he says, maybe keep her as a pet. Back in the locker room he gets gabbing, forgets all about it. He takes off and goes back to Kernsville for the week. Next thing you know everyone's back from break and someone opens a locker and suddenly it's a creature feature in here."

They were crossing the busy campus now, and the sunny afternoon was clouding up quickly. Denton started laughing at his own story, making the bike wobble.

"Remember that scene in the original *Blob*, where at one point this big crowd comes screaming out of the movie theater? It was just like that. Endris's locker was just alive with very active little *Lycosae carolinensis*. Merriment ensued."

"Ah, the high jinks."

"Rollo—the varsity coach—wasn't all that amused."

It had begun to rain, but neither said anything. In their college days they had run so often in downpours that it scarcely rated comment. The heat and humidity of north Florida often made the afternoon thunderstorms the best time to run in the summer. It worked tolerably well, except for the perpetually slimy training shoes.

This rain was chilly, but they generated enough heat to be comfortable, even in T-shirts. On his bike Denton easily kept up with Cassidy, who was putting some effort into it, enjoying the soft trail that snaked around the perimeter of the campus. They would be doing seven miles, and for Cassidy it would be a tempo run.

The rain slacked off to a steady drizzle, and they were soon out far enough to have left the campus traffic behind. They continued in a comfortable silence for stretches at a time, each lost in thought.

"You know, Bruce," Cassidy said finally, "you've given me some pretty good advice at some critical times."

"Can you hold that thought and repeat it later to my wife?"

"I mean it. It was scary how right you were about that time afterward, after the Olympics. It's a good thing I was at least a little bit prepared for it. Going back to Kernsville, the cabin, the routine, it probably saved me."

Denton said nothing.

"But it was still hard."

"I know."

"It was slow going, coming out of it, getting back to an even keel. I heard about some of the other guys who were a mess for a long time. Maybe still are."

"Yeah, I knew some from my time, too. The ones who didn't have a very broad base. You could pick them out, the ones who were going to have a hard time, win or lose," Denton said. Then he added: "Losing's tougher, of course."

"I can vouch for that."

"A silver medal is not losing."

"It is in this country."

"You know better than that. Besides, not even every gold medalist ends up on a Wheaties box."

"I suppose," Cassidy admitted.

"Look at Bob Schul. Only American ever to win a 5000-meter gold medal, and couldn't draw flies at a pig boil," Denton said. "But you came through fine, Quenton. You were as focused as anyone, but you were never one-dimensional. You had a good athletic career, you went to the Olympics and did great. And you came back to the real world reasonably intact. You came through just fine."

"Well, that's just it, Bruce. I don't know how fine I am anymore."

DENTON'S PLAN CALLED FOR a cautious early buildup of mileage, most of it at a very slow pace, with a few well-placed tempo runs thrown in for mostly psychological reasons. Sanity runs, he called them. Otherwise, it was seven-minute miles with some striders at the end. Cassidy also did a 30-minute upper-body routine in the afternoons with some very light stretching. The morning run was only four miles, but he no longer considered it optional. In the afternoons he usually went anywhere from six to 14 miles, with the first several miles at a very slow pace in lieu of a warmup.

It was a lot different from the kind of running Cassidy had been doing for years now, a sort of carefree out-the-door four- or five-miler at close to all-out effort, with liberal days off now and again when work at the office caught up with him or when he had overdone the previous day's run. He found that if he missed two or three days in a row, it did not indicate a major character flaw, destined to snowball into a lifetime of lethargy and decadence. He even found—surprise!—joy in it again.

"That's just running," Denton told him. "It's not the same as training. Training takes discipline and consistency, and it's not nearly as much fun. Also, it won't be easy. It never was before and it won't be now, no matter what you think you remember. I won't be here to slow you down, so I want you to figure out what various paces translate to on your different courses. When the schedule calls for a seven-minute pace, I want a seven-minute pace. You show back up here four minutes early, well, you record it accurately in your log, but just know I'm not going to be happy. When you send your weekly reports, I'm going to bring it up. I'm going to keep on bringing it up until you're sick of hearing about it. When you get sick enough of hearing about it, you'll straighten out just to get me off your back."

Cassidy had indeed forgotten the strange reverse logic of Denton's training system, which called for running hundreds of miles, but many of them at maddeningly slow paces. The advantage they'd had in the old days in Kernsville had been that Denton had been there every step of the way. And since he was by far the most accomplished runner in the group, it would have been not only presumptuous but also risky for one of the pipsqueaks to spit out the bit and head for the hills. It happened on occasion, and when it did, the pipsqueak usually found himself in an all-out race that he could never win.

As one of the milers in the group, Cassidy had been among those who most ached to break out of what felt like a boring and ineffectual jog. Now that his race distance was to be so much longer, Denton's program called for an even bigger buildup of aerobic miles.

The real saving grace of the system at Kernsville was that they were all in it together, the varsity runners who had joined them as well as the graduate students who had journeyed south to train with an Olympic gold medalist. But not a single one of them could believe how slow Denton wanted them to run on that first morning. They thought it was a joke, that they were on some runner's equivalent of a snipe hunt.

Still, they stuck with the program and they learned to distract themselves with chatter to help pass the time. It became a very social little group of raconteurs and jokesters who looked forward to the afternoon workouts.

But the thing that really made it work was simple success. Everyone who stuck did well. The system was no joke, and the performances were no fluke. The miles piled up, but then so did other kinds of running, all nicely integrated into the program and interspersed through the training weeks. Everyone stayed boringly healthy and uninjured, and before long they were running better than they ever had before. Cassidy didn't need to be convinced all over again. He had been through all that, and he knew how tough a grind it could become.

He just needed to find a way to keep from going crazy while he was undertaking this strange and brutal process one more time, to try to make his last Olympic team.

CASSIDY WAS WORKING HARD up the trail from Thunder Lake, slinging sweat with every stride despite the coolish bite in the air on the sundown side of the mountain. The schedule called for 10 miles, with the first three easy, then five at a 90 percent tempo effort, and the final two miles as a cooldown.

Early on he had felt "pretty much like dog-doo" (as he would write in his log) and was dreading the fast part, but then it had gone surprisingly well once he got into the rhythm. Workouts often unspooled like that. Years ago he had come up with what he called the Two-Mile Rule, which said simply that you shouldn't try to figure out how you're feeling until at least two miles into the workout. The phenomenon seemed to apply in the other direction, too: some days he felt great out the door and then fell apart a few minutes later.

Today he had been really fooled. An involuntary afternoon nap went on too long and too hard, with lots of crazy dreaming and the porpoising slumber of continual near wakenings. He finally woke for good late and grumpy to find the autumn sun alarmingly close to the tops of the Blue Ridge Mountains to the west.

Damn it, he thought, all I'm doing up here is running, and if I don't get that done, I'm not doing anything.

He bolted out of his hay-bale bed, pulled damp shoes onto his sockless feet, bolted out the door, and was still wiping sleep from his eyes as he hit seven-minute pace on the uphill through the pasture before plunging into the already darkening woods, there slowing down finally, remembering that he was supposed to be warming up.

But there was no night running out here, and if you didn't do it before sundown you didn't do it. His nap dreams had been vaguely disturbing, but he couldn't for the life of him remember more than scraps. Something to do with dogs, feral dogs, and an old girlfriend he couldn't quite place, a chilly apartment. Something about a pilot light going out. Oh well.

As soon as he hit the long downhill slope toward Thunder Lake, he picked up the pace and knew immediately that it would be a good tempo run. Another mile farther on he was fairly flying down the gentle incline at better-than-five-minute pace, and he could tell it was going to be one of those wonderful days when he would not be able to make himself tired.

It occurred to him that days like this didn't happen as much as they used to, and for that reason he should surely cherish them. He flew around Thunder Lake in the waning light, feeling only the joy of nearly effortless speed, surprised to feel his footstrikes digging in so smartly that he was throwing chunks of gravel out behind him.

He left the lake road and started back up the hill, amazed to find that his pace was hardly affected by the grade. The lower parts of the woods were getting darker now, but at this pace he would break into the light soon enough.

The trail got slightly steeper and the forest lighter as he got closer to the top of the hill, and when he came to the intersection with the Feedrock Trail, he slowed to a trot, the tempo portion over. Then, oddly, he walked. It was getting late, and he didn't have a lot of light left, but the fast run had left him exhilarated.

On the home leg, Cassidy cruised easily along the rocky trail just below the ridge, admiring how the undersides of the taller trees reflected liquid gold down onto the pine-needle forest floor, glowing reddish itself now. When he came to a big spruce by scree scattered across the trail, he coasted to a stop, turned, and jogged back. Why not? he thought. It has turned out to be a wonderful day after all. A day of taking stock.

There was a very steep face of bare rock leading up to a lightly timbered lookout ridge, and he took to the granite face with powerful, lunging strides, feeling his quadriceps burning instantly and his calves stretching as he powered up what seemed like a near-vertical wall. Three-quarters of the way up he gave up the heroics and hiked the remaining few feet to the crest, breathing hard again. A narrow path led into the thin edge of trees and out the other side into the thin, blue air.

He cleared the shadows and stepped out into the sunlight of the ledge, puffing hard from the sudden effort, and stood, hands on hips, taking in the entire Cedar Mountain valley, flecked in the high places with splashes of yellow but mostly suffused now in a smoky, blue-gray haze. An orange plush toy of sun liquefied at the dark edge of the Blue Ridge Parkway, and the miniaturized tableau below was faded but recognizable: there was the tiny volunteer fire station three miles away, Sarah Sneedon's little craft store and some other places along the dark thread of highway, and beyond that his grandmother's house, leaking wood smoke, and beyond that her neighbor Virginia Coldiron's snug little place up in a dark hollow toward Connestee Falls.

He thought, not for the first time: Doing this thing you occasionally get to a rare overlook. He realized that as long as he could remember as a runner he had judged every landscape he encountered as to whether or not he would like to run in it. That was what nature had been to him: somewhere you run. When he passed a lovely grass meadow beside a highway, he would imagine how it would feel to fly barefoot down its gentle slope at four-minute mile pace, to trod its deliciously smooth turf as the world record holder, the fastest human ever. Running was simply how he related to nature, to the aesthetics of the natural world, and thus the most beautiful landscapes to him were those with room to amble: easy passageways or smooth footpaths disappearing into the distance. Lovely flora and fauna, moving waters, azure skies, all were desirable, of course, but good footing was truly essential.

It was difficult for him to imagine that his capacity to move quickly through landscapes meant that within a half hour he would be inside that distant miniature house, sitting at an old applewood kitchen table, eating his grandmother's chicken livers and mashed potatoes and gravy. It seemed contrary to the laws of physics and the plain evidence of his senses.

And yet as he stood there still glistening, breathing deeply, he knew for a fact that failing a broken leg or some act of God, it was true, and it would not even require an unusual effort. It would require only the well-worn routine: jog, shower, dress, and then the quick, chilly motorcycle ride down the hollow.

That mental image of chicken livers made him suddenly woozy with hunger, and he turned from the glowing ledge. Backpedaling his gravity-fed way slowly and carefully down the rock face, he repeatedly jammed already sore toes into the ends of his Tiger Cortez training shoes before hitting the shadowy trail below and starting back into it slowly, allowing his eyes to adjust again to the gloom.

Picking his way carefully along the trail, he thought about something he had read about the great Alpine climbers. As children, they grew up surrounded by a vast landscape of unattainable peaks. As they grew older, stronger, and more skillful, when they looked up, they saw more and more places they had been to and to which they could return at will. That zone of accessibility would grow and grow over the years until the very best of the guides could stand in their village squares and turn full circle, searching the horizon in vain for some tiny, forbidden aerie they had not conquered, some remote crag beyond their powers.

It would have to be a wonderful and prideful thing, to feel so thoroughly at home in such a daunting and beautiful landscape. But as they grew older, the climbers who survived would find that some peaks were difficult again, some climbs strangely taxing, some routes quite impossible. They would realize, to their surprise, that the process was reversible; that it was, in fact, reversing.

You could see them, the aged former heroes sitting sadly in the village square, turning full circle to gaze at a frozen world once again inaccessible to them.

Lit orange now by the last of the sun, Quenton Cassidy cruised down the darkening hillside with languid strides, thinking, I may be older and I may nap too long, but I can still scald dogs down to Thunder Lake and back.

Breaking out into the thin sunlight of the open pasture above his cabin, he thought: I can still have a day like this.

ADVENTURES & INVESTIGATIONS

SECRETS OF THE TARAHUMARA

BY **CHRISTOPHER MCDOUGALL**

They run like no other people in the world,
but as the author discovers,
their ways are worth imitating.
If you can find them.

DECEMBER 2004

UNTIL THAT STRANGE SCENE in 1993, no one had ever taken the Leadville Trail 100 ultramarathon lightly. Leadville forces racers to run and climb 100 high-altitude miles over the scrabbly trails and snowy peaks of the Colorado Rockies. You don't train for Leadville with intervals and striders; you train the way a prison gang handles a rock pile, by constantly banging out lots of slow, steady miles and building the kind of thin-air endurance that lets you grind along at 15 minutes a mile all day long and then continue into the night. The Leadville ultra, you could say, is closer to mountaineering than marathoning.

But there, next to the carefully pulse-monitored and Polarfleeced top seeds at the 1993 starting line, were a half-dozen middle-aged guys in togas, smoking butts and shooting the breeze, deciding whether they should wear some new Rockport cross-trainers they'd been given earlier or the sandals they'd made out of old tires scavenged from a nearby junkyard. Most opted for the sandals. They weren't stretching or warming up or showing the faintest sign that they were about to start one of the most grueling ultramarathons in the world.

They were Tarahumara Indians from the Copper Canyons region of northwestern Mexico. Their curious appearance matched their mysterious legend—that they defy every known rule of physical conditioning and still speed along for hundreds of miles. The Tarahumara (pronounced Spanish-style, "taramara," by swallowing the *hu*) didn't work out, or stretch, or protect their feet. They chain-smoked fierce black tobacco, ate a ton of carbs and barely any meat, and chugged so much cactus moonshine that they were either drunk or hungover an estimated one-third of each year (one day on their backs, that is, for every two on their feet). "Drunkenness is a matter of pride, not of shame," Dick and Mary Lutz wrote in their book *The Running Indians*. And yet, the Lutzes insist, "There is no doubt they are the best runners in the world."

Leadville was sure to test that claim. Once the starting gun sounded, around 4 a.m., a sea of taller heads quickly swallowed the Tarahumara runners, who faded into the middle of the pack behind the world's most scientifically trained ultrarunners. As the sun rose, though, and the course began climbing toward the 12,640-foot peak at Hope Pass, the Tarahumara began easing forward, running so beautifully that one Leadville veteran was left mesmerized. "They seemed to move with the ground," Henry Dupre would later tell the *New York Times*. "Kind of like a cloud or a fog moving across the mountains."

At the first aid station, the Tarahumara who had decided to try the Rockports were now shucking them and pulling on the trash-picked sandals. By the turnaround point, sandaled feet were pattering hard behind the leaders. Not only were the Tarahumara gaining, but they also seemed to be getting stronger; they weren't picking off the faders so much as picking up the pace. Reports from observers at mountaintop stations said the Tarahumara were even smiling as they passed. Joe Vigil, the legendary American track coach, happened to be at the Leadville 100 that year, and he couldn't believe what he was seeing. "Such a sense of joy," Vigil would later say.

As the lead runners came to the finish, the Tarahumara had added reason to be happy. Breaking the tape, in a time of 20:03:33, was 55-year-old Victoriano Churro, a farmer and the oldest of the three Tarahumara. He was followed by Cerrildo Chacarito in second and Manuel Luna in fifth. The three Tarahumara were still bouncing along on their toes as they crossed the line.

Their performance proved to be no fluke. A year later, another Tarahumara runner, Juan Herrera, would win at Leadville, finishing in 17:30:42 and chopping 25 minutes off the course record. Then in 1995, three Tarahumara finished in the top 10 of the rugged Western States 100 in California.

How did they do it? Before anyone could find out, the Tarahumara vanished from the ultrarunning scene in the mid-'90s, retreating to their canyon-bottom homes, and taking their miraculous distance-running secrets with them.

One runner, it was said, set out after them.

HE'S SUPPOSED TO BE as tall as Sasquatch and speak a raucous, gibber-gabber tongue that's neither Spanish, nor English, nor Tarahumara. The Tarahumara call him Caballo Blanco—the White Horse—because every once in a while, the villagers say, he will come galloping down from the hills, stomping his feet and snorting like a runaway stallion. He has an invisible sidekick he's always talking about, an Apache warrior he claims is an even greater runner than the Tarahumara and who he says is called Ramón Chingón (which, if you throw in a certain expletive, means the opposite of "everybody loves Raymond").

He'll be invited to gulp a cup of *piñole*, a traditional Tarahumara dish of ground corn mixed with water, and then bound back up the trail with his quick, billy-goat gait, a parade of kids laughing and trailing behind. "Caballo Blanco és muy amigable," the villagers say, "pero un poco exquisito." The White Horse is a good guy, in other words, if you like 'em goofy. But if any outsider has mastered the Tarahumara secrets of long-distance running, they agree, it's Caballo Blanco.

No one seems to know Caballo Blanco's name, or age, or nationality. Some say he's American; others, German; still others, Dutch. He came to Mexico years ago, the story goes, and wandered deep down into the wild, impenetrable Barrancas del Cobre—the Copper Canyons—to live among the Tarahumara.

For two days I've been searching Mexico's Sierra Madre mountains for the phantom runner, and the search has finally brought me here, to the dark lobby of an old hotel in the dusty town of Creel, hard by a stretch of railroad tracks and hundreds of miles across the desert from Chihuahua, where we started.

"Sí, he's staying here," says the desk clerk.

"Really?" After hearing we'd just missed him so many times, in so many places, I'd started to suspect Caballo Blanco was a ghost story, a Loch Ness *monstruo* dreamed up to yank the crank of gullible gringos.

"And he's always back by 5," she adds.

It's almost too good to be true. Then, I check my watch. "But it's already after 6."

The clerk shrugs. "Maybe he's gone away for a few days."

I slump down on a lumpy sofa. I'm exhausted, and as I doze I can almost hear his voice. Then it hits me: I am hearing it. My eyes pop open, and I see a bony, blond gringo in trail-wrecked Tevas and a floppy jungle hat bantering with the desk clerk.

I erupt from the sofa. "Caballo?" I call out, my throat still sleep-clogged. He turns toward me. "Damn, am I glad to see you!" I explode, scaring the wits out of him. Once I reassure him that I'm not a cop, a con man, or a deadbeat American looking for a handout, Caballo Blanco beams a big, toothy grin.

"Sure," he says. "I'll tell you about the Tarahumara. But first, let's get some beans."

We walk to a tiny, backstreet restaurant, a single room with two rickety tables at arm's reach from an ancient gas stove where a deliciously fragrant pot of frijoles is bubbling. As we stoop through the doorway, we see an old woman with a wooden spoon. Immediately, she calls out, "Hola, Caballo."

"Como está, Mamá?" Caballo Blanco shouts back. He's got *mamás* all over Latin America, he says: motherly women who fill him up with beans and tortillas for only a few centavos, so he doesn't have to worry much about money and can concentrate all his time and energy on running instead.

His name, he says, is Micah True (though he would later tell me he was born Michael Randall Hickman and renamed himself for the Biblical denouncer of decadent living). He lives in a simple shack in the old mining town of Batopilas, close to the hidden canyon homes of his Tarahumara running buddies. He's tall, sandy-blond, and Nordicly toothy, which partly accounts for the confusion about his nationality; that, plus the fact that he's from Nederlands, Colorado, and has an atrociously tin ear—even after 10 years in Mexico, his Spanish would make a Berlitz teacher wince. He's 51, but likes to suggest he's older, probably because he knows he looks it; feats of endurance under an unforgiving sun have left Caballo a little on the skeletal side.

"I came to running late ..." Caballo begins, but suddenly stops, bug-eyed with hunger, as Mamá plops several big bowls in front of us and futzes over them with chopped cilantro, jalapeños, and squirts of lime. Caballo hasn't eaten all day. He'd set out this morning with a friend for a short hike to a natural thermal spring in the woods, but once he spotted an unfamiliar trail through the trees, hike and hot tub were history. He took off running, with no clue where the trail was taking him. "I wasn't even going to run today, but I was loving it," he says. An hour or so later, he found a trail linking back to town, turning what should have been a relaxing soak into a half-marathon.

That's one of the first and most important things he learned from the Tarahumara, Caballo explains between spoonfuls of beans: the ability to break into a run anytime, like kids in the schoolyard. "Look," Caballo says, pointing first to his waist, then to his feet. He's wearing ancient hiking shorts to go along with his dumpster-ready pair of Tevas. "That's all I wear." When he sets out for a 20-mile run, he's no more equipped than any Tarahumara hunter: just shorts, sandals, and a bag of piñole.

"It's a beautiful thing," Caballo says and smiles. "And I'm still just learning." Imagine learning hoops by playing with Bird, Magic, and Jordan every day, he says. That's what it's like running with the Tarahumara. Not even the best Kenyans have figured out what the Tarahumara know, Caballo swears; the Kenyans may be faster over the short haul, but few runners can handle more miles, for more years, than the Tarahumara. In fact, Tarahumara runners have competed for Mexico in the Olympic Marathon twice (in 1928 and 1968) and both times finished deep in the pack. Afterwards, they complained that the race was too short.

"As a culture, they're one of the great unsolved mysteries," chips in Danny Noveck, who has joined us at the table. Noveck is a pal of Caballo's and a University of Chicago anthropologist now researching the Tarahumara culture. "Here's an example," he says, waving a can of Tecate in the air. "The Tarahumara have a beer-based economy, yet somehow it works." Instead of cash, they like to trade in home-brewed corn beer, called *tesguino*, which inevitably leads to a good amount of inebriation in the name of commerce. "But they're also extremely hard workers," Noveck says.

The Tarahumara, it seems, just farm and party and run for fun, all the while staying in remarkable condition. In 1971, physiologist Dale Groom ran cardiovascular tests on Tarahumara adults and children, and concluded (as he'd write in the *American Heart Journal*), "Probably not since the days of the ancient Spartans has a people achieved such a high state of physical conditioning." Groom checked the pulse and blood pressure of Tarahumara runners during a five-hour race, and found their blood pressure went down while running, and their average heart rate—in the midst of banging out eight-minute miles—was only 130 beats per minute. But what most impressed Groom was something that didn't register on his instruments: after running 50 miles, the Tarahumara didn't even look beat. They stood around and chatted while Groom pumped the diastolic cuff.

During his years at Adams State College in Alamosa, Colorado, Joe Vigil coached 19 national championship teams. He also earned three advanced degrees. But nothing he'd seen on the track or in his physiology books left him prepared for what he witnessed at Leadville in 1993. The harder the Tarahumara fought their way through the Rockies, Vigil marveled, the more rapturous they became. Glee and determination are usually antithetical emotions, yet the Tarahumara were brimming with both at once; it was as if running to the death made them feel more alive." It was quite remarkable," Vigil now says.

Heart disease, high blood pressure, and lethal cholesterol are virtually unknown among the Tarahumara, Vigil would later learn. So are crime, child abuse, and domestic violence. Seekers used to climb the Himalayas to discover the secret of a serene, hyper-healthy life; Vigil now realized it lay just south of the

U.S. border. So after retiring in 2000, Vigil and his wife sold their home in Colorado, intending to spend the next few years studying the Tarahumara. But just before they were to leave, Vigil got a phone call. Actually several of them. A bunch of U.S. elite runners, among them, Deena Kastor, were begging Vigil to stick around and train them for the 2004 Olympic Games. How could he say no?

In 1994, Micah True had his own encounter with the Tarahumara at Leadville. He'd heard about their incredible performance the year before and wanted to see them in action for himself. But instead of competing against them (True already had run a few Leadvilles), he offered himself as a guide. He teamed up with a Tarahumara runner over the back half of the course, he says, and "we spent the next 10 hours together, and even though we didn't have much language between us, somehow we could joke and communicate." After the race, he was as obsessed as Vigil with learning the Tarahumara secrets, but unlike the coach, nothing anchored True to Colorado but a '69 Chevy pickup and a one-man landscaping business.

"I have no wife, no kids, no expenses," Caballo says, as he mops up the last of his frijoles with a scrap of tortilla. But the tricky part, he learned, would be gaining access. The Tarahumara, for very good reason, refer to most outsiders as "white devils." They may let researchers monitor their hearts, but not look into them.

"I did have one thing working for me," True says. "When you act out of love, good things happen. It's a law." He'll finish the story tomorrow, he says, when we meet for a run. But he leaves me with this thought: For centuries, whenever outsiders have tried to get close to the Tarahumara, they've responded by running. Away.

SO WHERE THE HELL are they? A few days before meeting Caballo Blanco, we were out here in ... in ... actually, I really didn't know where we were anymore. Salvador Holquín, a 33-year-old, semipro mariachi singer doubling as my driver, had been grinding and rocking his Dodge Ram truck in low, low gear since dawn, wheezing like a tramp steamer on stormy seas, trying to squeeze through logging trails so narrow that the passenger-side wheels were closer to the cliff's edge than I cared to look. I tried keeping track of our location with a compass and forest map, but my head was throbbing from smacking the roll bar every time we jounced to the axles on a rut, not to mention Holquín 's relentlessly ay-yay-yay-ing mariachi tapes.

Somewhere out here are the hidden canyon homes of the Tarahumara, though the Tarahumara might quibble with one detail. They call themselves

Rarámuri—the lightning-footed people. "Tarahumara" is the garbled name they were given by 17th-century explorers who didn't understand the tribal tongue. The name stuck, ironically, because the Rarámuri remained true to it by running away instead of hanging around to argue the point.

That has always been their way. Ever since Cortez's armored conquistadors came jangling into their homeland, and lasting through subsequent invasions by Mexican homesteaders, Pancho Villa's roughriders, and U.S.-backed timber barons, the Tarahumara have responded to centuries of blunderbusses, bull-dozers, and Kalashnikovs by simply avoiding them, retreating deeper and deeper into the labyrinthine Copper Canyons.

It's left them, today, one of the most remote people on the planet. Fewer than 40,000 Tarahumara remain, from a population of two million a century ago. No wheeled vehicles can make it to the bottom of the Copper Canyons, and few choppers would try; the gorges are a twisting maze of swirling drafts and sheer rock walls, many plunging deeper than the Grand Canyon. Only hooves and seriously determined legs can make it much farther than where we'd come to: the far end of a pathless forest, above Tarahumara huts and cave dwellings some 8,000 feet below.

We'd set out at noon yesterday from Chihuahua, driving southwest across the desert. Holquín had a general idea of the area, since he also helps recruit Tarahumara runners for the Ultramaratón de los Cañones, a 100-kilometer trail run through the Sinforosa Canyons each July. The Canyon Ultra, as it's known, is something of a cult attraction for the cognoscenti who idolize the Tarahumara, since it's one of the very few organized races they still run.

The defending champ is Arnulfo Quimare, a 24-year-old Tarahumara who may be the greatest runner you've never heard of. For the past three years, Quimare has defeated all comers. What's more, he took the title from his brother and has been defending it against his brother-in-law, which means that somewhere in the Copper Canyons, invisible to the outside world, a distance-running dynasty is forming.

"We nearly there?" I asked Holquín, once the road had narrowed nearly to the point of disappearing.

By way of answer, Holquín backed up, cut a hard right off the road, and started winding between the trees. We wandered like this for an hour, and then, as the sun set, we emerged from the woods to see three men silhouetted against the edge of a gigantic canyon. We pulled up next to them, stopped, and got out.

I'd rarely been in such an eerily silent spot in my life; there wasn't even a rustling branch to break the silence, yet I could still barely hear the one

Tarahumara who responded when Holquín pulled up and said, "Cuida va"—
Tarahumara for "How's it going?"

"CUIDA," THE TARAHUMARA BREATHED, soft as a sigh.

The other two didn't say a word. All three were dressed in homemade huaraches and one-piece tunics that hung short in the front and in a long, triangular
tail behind. The greetings over, we all stood in silence for a while, gazing at the
spectacular molten sunset receding from the far canyon wall.

Soon, a battered Jeep appeared, and another Tarahumara slid from the driver's seat. "Silvino," he introduced himself, shaking hands shyly with just his
fingertips. Unlike the others, he was dressed in work pants and Reebok sneakers. Last year, Silvino said, the Christian brother who runs the Tarahumara
school drove him to Mexicali, where he says a marathon offered a $10,000 first
prize. Silvino won, and split the pot: half the money went to the school, the
other paid for Silvino's new ride and duds.

"What was your winning time?" I asked.

Silvino spat into the dust. "No me acuerdo" (I don't remember).

"Will you race it again this year?"

He loogied again. "Maybe. If the brother wants to go, perhaps . . ."

However, Silvino perked up when he heard we were interested in meeting
Arnulfo Quimare. Every year, Silvino races the Canyon Ultra, and every year, he
finishes behind a member of the Quimare clan. He says he wants a rematch, but
not in some dull trail race, which Silvino somehow finds simultaneously too
short and too boring. He prefers an all-out *rarajipari*, the traditional Tarahumara
ball race. One village will send word that it's ready for a challenge; when a rival
village responds, they'll set a time, place, and distance. Three or four runners
usually compete from each village, but Silvino knows of rarajiparis that fielded
10 per side.

The night before a race, the two villages get together to drink and bet. Early
the following morning, the teams line up on a stretch of trail about five miles
long, unless the runners got too drunk the previous night and decided to call off
the race, as occasionally happens. The Tarahumara's taste for corn beer, by the
way, is not some form of aboriginal alcoholism, as anthropologist John Kennedy
explains in *Tarahumara of the Sierra Madre: Beer, Ecology and Social Organization.*
It's actually a clever cultural defense mechanism for a tribe that has powerful
emotions and no refrigeration. Because the Tarahumara are often too bashful to
act on passion, and too nonviolent to belt some annoying neighbor in the mouth,

they use regular beer parties, called *tesguinadas*, to simultaneously vent any built-up lust or anger, and make use of excess corn by fermenting it into beer.

So assuming the race-night tesguinada didn't get too nuts, each team will produce a small ball, carved with a machete from the hard wood of a guacimo tree. Then they're off . . . and for the next 24, or 36, or 40 straight hours, they'll do continuous laps back and forth over the course, kicking the ball along until they reach the prearranged distance, which can be anything from 100 to 200 miles. During the night, the nonracing villagers will light the course with okote-burning pine torches—and feed the runners water and piñole.

The year before, the other two members of Silvino's team dropped out in the middle of their rarajipari. For the rest of the night and into the next day, he raced on by himself, constantly surging and easing back to keep pace with the ricocheting ball, hunting it down when it caromed off the rocks. He was doubly lucky, Silvino says: he not only finished the 120 miles and won, but he also didn't piss blood for the next few days, as he has in the past.

This kind of action gets Silvino fired up. It's much more uncertain; consequently, more dramatic. No one knows in advance when the race will be, or who will show up, or how deep a crevice a ricocheting ball may need to be retrieved from in midrace, or who will take a midnight tumble and gash his head. But that's what real running is all about, Silvino tells me; any able-bodied Tarahumara can finish an ultramarathon, but there's no telling how anyone will fare during the long, lonely night of a rarajipari. For Silvino, it's the difference between a guy who runs races and a guy who runs.

At dawn the next morning, one of the Tarahumara agreed to guide us to Arnulfo Quimare's house. After a five-hour hike down a steep, faint footpath carved into the canyon by centuries of Tarahumara feet, we came to a river at the canyon bottom and picked our way upstream over the rocks. Finally, we arrived at a mud hut wedged almost invisibly against the canyon wall.

Quimare appeared in the door and blew his nose. Everyone in the family had the flu, he explained. His brother, Pedro, couldn't even get up from the mat he was resting on. Holquín pulled me aside. Because Tarahumara families share blankets at night in one-room huts and eat from communal pots of piñole, he whispered, the flu can last for months and incubate into a serious debilitator, and often a killer. "There's no way they're going to be able to run with you," he said. "He's making a real effort just to talk."

Quimare offered a basket of small, sweet limes and waved for us to sit. He's tall for a Tarahumara at nearly six feet, with a Prince Valiant bob, muscle-knotted thighs, and a quiet smile. We chomped limes and spat seeds for a while, and when I started to ask about his ultra victories, that's pretty much the response I got: chomping and spitting.

"How do you and Pedro train?" I began.

(Chomp, chomp, followed by long pause.) "We don't."

"Don't what—train together?"

"No," (chomp, chomp, pause), "... we don't train."

"Did you have a time you were going for?"

"No... I was just trying to pass whoever was in front of me."

Quimare was hospitable and considered his answers carefully, if only to come up with a good one so I'd stop asking and clear out so he could rest, but as Caballo Blanco had learned years before, the Tarahumara allow white devils to penetrate only so far. Beyond that... silence.

Eventually, we gave up and left the Quimares to their sickbeds. But just when I thought I wouldn't get a chance to see Tarahumara champs in action, I got an unexpected break. We'd wandered down to a little school by the river, where dozens of kids came pouring out for recess. They were dressed like their parents—the girls in long skirts, the boys in huaraches and hanging tunics—and they quickly formed two lines.

The head of the school, an uncharacteristically portly Tarahumara named Angel, appeared with two guacimo-wood balls. He quickly matched the boys up by height, then did the same with the girls. He tossed a ball to each team, then shouted, "Vayan!" Two kids dropped the balls and, using the tips of their toes and a deft flip-kick motion, sent them bouncing down the trail to the river. A stampede of boys broke out, while the girls hung back; they'd join after the boys had gone about a mile. The teams seemed evenly matched, but my pesos were on Marcelino, the tall, rangy kid in the red smock who'd ripped to the front.

But shortly after Marcelino had taken control of his team's ball and was steadily opening a lead, the genius of the rarajipari became apparent: it's endlessly and instantly self-handicapping. Because the trail was so rocky and twisty, the ball ricocheted madly, allowing the slower kids on Marcelino's team to catch up when he checked his stride to dig it out of a crevice. Even the smallest kids got a chance to shine: once Marcelino reached the river, he wheeled around and flipped the ball back up the trail, right to a pudgy little six-year-old who'd lost a sandal and his belt, forcing him to hop along and hold his tunic shut with one hand. Until Marcelino could catch up, Little One-Shoe was leading his team's fast break, and loving it.

It's like no kid's game I've seen before, and every kid's game. Everyone is trying to win, but no one really seems to care who does; the rules are simple and adjusted on the fly, and no adults are offering advice or gumming up the fun—no hockey dads at rarajipari races. The kids accelerate when they feel like it, downshift when they don't, and catch an occasional breather under a tree before jumping back into the fray. When the girls blend in a few minutes later, running as hard and gleefully as the boys, I'm reminded that the best speed workouts of my life were logged before I ever saw a stop watch, in kick-the-can battles involving two dozen kids and connecting backyards in the summers of 1970 and '71.

It's been too long since I last ran like a maniac through my neighbors' azaleas, and I've been paying for it in breakdowns, boredom, and fast-twitch muscle loss: Now that I see how the Tarahumara take the spontaneity and semi-shapelessness of kids' play and turn it into a lifelong running tradition, their ability to stay fast into their 50s and keep their legs immune from injury makes sense. There's a logic to the way kids play instinctively, and the Tarahumara never abandoned it.

That night, as we camped by the school, Angel told us his version of a horror story. "There's a Tarahumara village called Mesa de Hierba Buena," Angel begins. "Many of the best runners were from Hierba Buena. They had a very good trail that would let them cover a lot of distance in a day, much farther than you could get to from here." The trail was so fine, in fact, that the Mexican government decided to slick it with asphalt and turn it into a road. Now that it could be supplied by truck, Hierba Buena soon had grocery stores, and in them, soda, chocolate, sugar, butter—foods the Tarahumara had rarely eaten. They developed a taste for junk food, but needed cash to buy it, so instead of working their fields, they hitched to Guachochi to work as dishwashers and day laborers.

"That was 20 years ago. Now, there are no runners in Hierba Buena. We'll lose the Rarámuri ways," Angel laments. "The men will stop running. The kids won't eat the old way, just a cup of piñole at a time. It's terrible! There are Rarámuri who don't respect our traditions as much as el Caballo Blanco does."

"HU—!...HU—!" I'M TRYING TO shout "Horse!" but it keeps turning into a pant. I finally get it out, catching Caballo's ear just before he darts around an uphill bend and vanishes. My God, I'm not that out of shape, but the way Caballo is rock-hopping, he makes me look as sick as Arnulfo Quimare.

We'd set out that morning for a run in the hills behind Creel, and within minutes we're on a rocky, pine-needled trail climbing through the woods. It's not that Caballo is so fast; it's just that he seems so light, flowing as smoothly over a seriously gnarly trail as an expert mountain biker on a perfectly chosen line. "My whole approach to running has changed since I've been here," he says, once I catch up. "I used to have trouble with injuries, especially with my ankle tendons. Now I'm 50-ish, and they've gone away."

Caballo first came to Copper Canyons in the winter after meeting the Tarahumara runner at Leadville. Before leaving, he got on a Boulder, Colorado, radio station and asked for listeners to donate old winter coats. Once he had a pickup-load, he pointed his Chevy south. He handed out his coats, but didn't want to leave the canyons: Tarahumara women were feeding him piñole and hand-patted tortillas, and he was running each day on the most spectacular trails he'd ever seen.

But he wasn't included in the rarajiparis, or invited when anyone ran to the canyon top. He needed a way to break through, and the lesson of Leadville came back to him—be humble, and be funny. He started joking with the Tarahumara kids, neighing and stamping his feet. For the adults, he spun wild, bawdy tales, in his barely intelligible Spanish, of Ramón Chingón, his make-believe Apache friend. He didn't come in as the Great White Father; he was more like a goofy, sunburned cousin. He made himself fun to run with, so some of the Tarahumara began taking him along.

He stumbled badly at first, as he tried to follow the Tarahumara over rocks and scree. But he soon learned to stop relying on his long legs to keep up and, instead, mimic their short, quick steps. He chopped his long stride into thirds, pattering out three quick steps between rocks rather than one lunge. When he tripped, he didn't flail; he'd trust his body and find himself 30 yards up the trail, still on his feet.

One thing that struck Caballo about Tarahumara men is that they still run the way they did as kids; the rarajipari, after all, is the same game they played as five-year-olds. Caballo, consequently, avoids planned routes when possible. "I'm always getting lost and having to vertical climb, water bottle between my teeth, buzzards circling overhead," he says. Most of all, he began to acquire the confidence the Tarahumara possess beginning in childhood, their conviction that they can run until their minds decide to stop, and not their bodies. Before Silvino ran his first 150-mile rarajipari at age 16, he never had raced more than 10 miles. How did he train for a 15-fold increase? He didn't. "I just knew I could do it," Silvino had told me. Or then there is the 95-year-old man Caballo saw walking for five hours up the canyons. "No one told him he shouldn't," Caballo says, "and he never doubted he could."

Caballo soon saw the improvement in his running. Quick-stepping over such nasty footing, he found, made him not only more nimble, but also faster;

Caballo Blanco has more foot speed and resilience than Micah True ever had during his speedwork days in the U.S. "I do all my running on trails, and that's the difference," he explains. "I'm not battering myself by pounding and pounding over asphalt. I've learned to run Tarahumara-style—smooth, high-stepping, with no urgency."

Today, Caballo may be the only American training Tarahumara-style. After their brief rocket to stardom in the mid-'90s, the Tarahumara stopped coming to U.S. ultras. An American who had sponsored them got into one feud too many with race organizers and vowed not to bring them back. The Tarahumara didn't really care: the ultras offered little prize money and no special prestige back home.

So now, each March and December, Caballo organizes his own race. It's just him, a half-dozen or so Tarahumara buddies, and the rare gringo who signs on. "It's a blast!" he raves. The whole troop hikes across the canyon, camps out, then runs 20-some miles back the next day. Those who finish are crowned with T-shirts as new members of "Club Más Loco."

As he's telling war stories of past canyon races, the trail has suddenly opened on a limitless mesa, with giant standing stones all around and snow-capped mountains in the background. "Wow!" I exclaim.

"I told you," Caballo says. The mountain air is crisp and pine scented, and it's then, as I give in to the euphoric feeling of this perfect mountain morning and cruise along faster than I should, that I understand how he made the transformation from Micah True, oft-injured ultrarunner, to Caballo Blanco, long-ranging roamer of the Sierra Madre mountains.

We've hit our four-mile turnaround point, but even though I know it would be foolish for me to try more than eight on my first run at a 7,500-foot altitude, it's so beautiful out here and so fun to lope and bounce along over these trails that I'm reluctant to head back.

Caballo Blanco knows what I mean. "I've felt that way for the last 10 years," he says.

LE GRIZZ

BY DON KARDONG

> *The race begins at birth,*
> *and ends somewhere over*
> *the finish line.*

LIKE MOST STORIES, this one could begin almost anywhere. At conception. At birth. On the day I first began running. At the moment I discovered that, more than almost anything, I loved running through the woods, feeling like an integral, primitive, living part of the planet.

Perhaps the best point to begin, though, is at the moment I paid my $30 entry fee. Thirty dollars, after all, is not just three sawbucks. It signifies, rather, a commitment—in this case, a commitment to run 50 miles. And so I hovered, a detached observer far above my checkbook, watching myself sign on the dotted line. Apparently, I was actually going to do this thing.

For five years, I had heard of Le Grizz, a 50-mile race in Montana. For love of this event, friends from Spokane, Washington, had driven long distances, camped in freezing weather, eluded ravenous bears, and run, walked, and ultimately dragged themselves to a distant finish line. Then, the trek completed, they had soaked in hot tubs and consumed beer and pizza until their pains subsided, leaving only the memories of an extraordinary adventure to relate to the folks back home. Most, it seemed, remained delirious for days, professing to have enjoyed themselves.

I found this interesting. I had always been fascinated with ultramarathons (or "ultras"), had once even considered running 70 miles from the English town where I lived to the ancient monument of Stonehenge. The point? Some sort of neo-Druidic experience, I suppose, an athletic-religious-cosmic adventure. My friends thought I was nuts and talked me out of it.

Later I ran my first marathon, learning that it is not easy to run mile after mile after mile after mile. If strange things can happen in a race of only 26 miles, what might lay in the void beyond?

"Fifty miles is a whole new world compared to the marathon," noted the Le Grizz entry form. "It is a world of new knowledge of oneself, of self-actualization and of brotherhood."

Obviously, someone penned this line in the delirium of postrace hot-tubbing. Still, the lure remained considerable. I can't explain why we choose to challenge the extremes of human endurance—climbing Mount Everest, swimming the English Channel, or pursuing our own personal fantasy. But here's what I think: to explore boundaries is the reason for living.

For years, 50 miles sat on a backburner in my mind, simmering. Eventually, I succumbed.

THE NIGHT BEFORE

THERE ARE MOONS, and then, I swear, there are moons. On the evening before my first 50-miler, the moon that rose over the mountains behind the Spotted Bear Ranger Station was a real moon. Not a fat, lazy, mellow-yellow harvest moon or one of those fuzzy, sociable kind of orbs that smiles over urban landscapes. Rather, this was a piercing, ice-cold, nasty, I'm-the-eye-of-the-universe sort of moon that scattered the stars, scared wildlife, quieted the rocks, and glared at our assembled group in the campground below. We were, this moon let us know, unlikely to get much sympathy from Mother Nature for what we were about to do.

The temperature was falling like a stone through ice water. Before dawn, it would drop to 15 degrees. October in the Rockies is a gamble with loaded dice.

"There is always the outside chance, this being Montana," noted the Le Grizz entry form, "of foul, horrible weather."

Actually, we were lucky. We didn't encounter any of the snow, sleet, wind, or rain that have visited the running of the Le Grizz in prior years. "Runners alternated between feelings of depression and stupidity as the start time approached," noted the report of one such event.

This year it was simply cold. Naked cold. Dazzling-moon cold. You could see clearly a half-mile to the other side of the river. It was cold there, too.

Those who run ultras thrive on extremes. It is not enough, you see, to simply run 50 or 100 miles from point A to point B. We seek the added status that comes from tolerating extremes of temperature, navigating narrow trails, and scoring thousands of feet of elevation change in regions where the air is impossibly thin.

To enter Le Grizz, I had been asked to sign the following: "I understand that participating in the Le Grizz 50-Mile Ultramarathon may subject me to injuries and illnesses, including but not limited to hypothermia, frostbite, heat stroke, heat exhaustion, physical exhaustion, animal attack, falling trees, road failure and vehicle accident."

Yes, I understood. And I paid my 30 bucks.

I wasn't alone. More than 40 similarly disposed adults had signed up for Le Grizz, up from 25 the year before. Most gathered, along with family and friends, within a 5-foot radius of the campfire at the Spotted Bear Campground, trying to carbo-load before the pasta froze.

The group included Rick Spady and Jim Pomroy, two Montana runners who between them had won all five previous Le Grizz runs. Spady, the faster of the two, held the Le Grizz record of 5:50:56. He also presided over the firewood, a job that seemed more a reflection of his nature than a specific obligation of the course-record holder.

I have stood around a fair number of campfires in my life, and they all seem blessed with the same purpose: to evoke memories, inspire philosophical ramblings, and shake loose a few tall tales. Staring across the fire, one sees friends and strangers lost in thought. Their eyes, reflecting the glow of sparks from the fire, suggest the kindling of the mind. It is the look of human beings at peace, and also the look that flashes in the eyes of ax murderers just before the massacre. It is a look of ambiguous calm, and it appeared on the faces of the ultrarunners that evening.

As the night chill clamped down, most folks headed for the relative warmth of campers, tents, and sleeping bags, leaving only a few seasoned ultrarunners around the fire to tell tales of Leadville, Western States, and past Le Grizz struggles. They looked like woodsmen or hunters, or perhaps creatures that came sneaking out of the woods in the middle of the night, eyes gleaming.

But they were simply runners of long races, about to begin another. Above them, the eye of the moon blasted its icy light across the wilderness, promising nothing but the indifference of Nature to human dreams.

THE START

WE SPENT A ROUGH NIGHT in the forest. In theory, I had the best accommodations within 50 miles of the starting line. The camper I had rented came complete with kitchen, toilet, and sleeping areas for myself, my wife, Bridgid, and my two daughters, Kaitlin (age 4) and Catherine (age 2). More importantly, it had a heater.

In spite of all this luxury, I thrashed around inside the thing all night, trying to find a spot where I could stretch out and sleep. Sleep deprivation became one more hardship to suffer in the spirit of ultrarunning.

Awakening on the morning of the run, I thought first of food. I ate cereal, cookies, and whatever else seemed to speak the language of carbohydrates. Though not full, my stomach was engaged, which would hopefully give my body a chance at surviving the hours and miles ahead.

Outside the camper, runners and friends scurried back and forth, puffing clouds of warm breath in the air while searching for food of their own. Many were dressed in custom-made yellow and black tights, the uniform of the day for those of us from Spokane. In the midst of my apprehension, the gaudy tights helped lighten the load. After pulling on a pair, I left the warmth of the camper and went hunting for the race director, Pat Caffrey. He was busy handing out race numbers at one end of the parking area.

Caffrey—the force behind Le Grizz—is the race director, the starter, and the man in charge of almost everything. Most importantly, he writes the funny things about Le Grizz on the entry form and other race materials, helping the reader forget what a gruesome thing a 50-mile run can be.

"Contrary to Yuppie Myth," wrote Caffrey about the atrocious weather that plagued Le Grizz runners in 1985, "people become wild animals, not environmentalists, when confronted with such a wilderness experience."

I understood that sentiment. After picking up my number and hustling to the line a few minutes before the eight o'clock starting time, as ready as I was going to be for this thing, I shivered relentlessly as Caffrey began a round of instructions, jokes, and (at 15 degrees!) information on how to buy leftover Le Grizz T-shirts.

"Brrrr. Grrrrr." I muttered. Others around me agreed.

"Today's temperature marks a Le Grizz record," Caffrey noted, grinning. Our frozen lips couldn't manage a comment. Finally, raising the starting weapon, a 12-gauge shotgun wound with electrical tape, the man behind Le Grizz fired a single blast that echoed in the depths of the wilderness.

Numb, we were off.

Zero to 10 Miles

THE START OF MOST ROAD RACES is a flurry of arms, legs, elbows, and adrenaline. The start of Le Grizz seemed more like the opening of Macy's doors on the day after Thanksgiving. People hurried, but within recognized bounds of propriety. We had time, plenty of time, to complete the task.

It had been so complicated just getting going that morning—finding food, going to the bathroom, making sure cars would start (several needed considerable coaxing), deciding on the right combination of clothing, etc.—that I began to relate to Le Grizz as it should be. Not as a race, but as survival.

I *will* overcome all this. I *will* get to the finish.

Other than finishing, I couldn't decide on an actual race goal. To win? To break six hours? I had nothing to base my expectations on, so I had settled on simply running the distance at a comfortable pace and scaling whatever obstacles lay in the road ahead.

After a mile or so, as the numbness in my quads, hands, and face began to subside, I found myself running with Spady. We discussed ultramarathon training. Spady argued the value of the weekly long run instead of extremely high overall mileage. That system had kept him generally healthy and made him a top contender in races of 50 and 100 miles.

"People shouldn't worry so much about total mileage," said the course-record holder. "They'd do a lot better if they'd get out there and just keep going for six hours."

Long training runs, the kind that help ultrarunners, require a different perspective on the sport. Years ago I had tried adding 30-mile runs to my marathon training. One evening in 1971, I left home in the dark on an out-and-back course, 15 miles each way. After half an hour, I was running down a major highway; blinded by headlights and contemplating death. Thirty minutes later, I turned onto a country road, and things grew quiet. Only the breeze in the trees and my padding footsteps broke the silence. It was more like a dream than any training I was accustomed to. Suddenly an owl called *whoooooooo*... from a telephone pole.

I'm sorry, but this couldn't be called training. This was weirdness. It was also my last 30-mile training run for a decade.

That's why I was so worried about Le Grizz. "Things get really weird after 35 miles," noted Von Klohe, a Spokane friend and ultrarunner who advised me on my Le Grizz training. Ultrarunners always say things like that. Then they chuckle.

As Spady and I ran along discussing ultramarathon training and racing, he reported the splits from his past Le Grizz runs. They made me nervous. The man was talking 6:10 and 6:20 mile pace—much faster than the times I planned. Hearing these splits, I grew anxious for a reason to let him go. That opportunity came at about 7 miles in the form of my support crew, my family. As we headed up a slight incline, I spotted them ahead.

The Le Grizz weekend represented a watershed for the Kardongs. It was our first night of camping together, at least if an evening in a heated home on wheels can be called camping. Things had gone well so far, but Bridgid and I both remained apprehensive about how well our two girls would tolerate six hours of riding in a camper while Dad slowly whittled himself to a nub. To get them in the spirit of things, I had put Kaitlin in charge of Dad's cookies.

Seeing my crew alongside the road at 7 miles, I drifted off Spady's pace, slowed, and stopped for aid. Kaitlin handed me a bag of unopened cookies. Bridgid was in the camper, changing Catherine's diaper.

A well-trained support crew is essential to success in ultramarathons. They provide quick access to fluids, food, and emotional support. As I ripped open the package of cookies, wasting precious time and energy, I realized I had forgotten to give my crew any information about what it was they were supposed to do.

Up ahead, Spady was disappearing around a corner.

10 MILES—1:06:48

I'M NOT SURE EXACTLY HOW FAST I expected to go through the various 10-mile check points, but 1:06:48, including one aid stop and a pee break, seemed about right. I was running steadily, comfortably; Spady was nowhere in sight.

The main problem I had faced so far, other than an undertrained support crew, was clouds of dust from support-crew vehicles. It had been a dry summer and fall in the Rockies. As vehicles leapfrogged from aid station to aid station, they kicked up billowing clouds of dust, which threatened to smother those of us on foot.

Spady had speculated earlier that the dusty conditions would last until about 15 miles, when the bulk of the traffic would be behind us and the air would clear. He proved to be only slightly off the mark. After 10 miles, dust and traffic began to fade, replaced by the full beauty of the countryside through which Le Grizz travels.

Hungry Horse Reservoir sits on the western side of the continental divide in northwestern Montana, just south of Glacier Park. Waters from here flow in convoluted fashion through Montana, Idaho, Canada, and Washington, eventually joining the Columbia River. The Le Grizz course follows a road along the south-west side of Hungry Horse Reservoir, affording participants still in control of their faculties an exquisite view across to the Great Bear Wilderness area.

The sight itself is worth the drive (though perhaps not a 50-mile run), especially in the fall. In this part of the country, most of the conifers just hunch their shoulders and settle in for the winter with no major transformation. The tamaracks, though, change from green to gold, then drop their needles like any deciduous tree. At the same time, aspens, birches, cottonwoods, and alders are busy turning color among the evergreens, splashing their hues across the hills. The aspens in particular stand out among the forest giants, brilliant gold, shimmering with the slightest breeze as if charged with electricity.

On this day, too, the moon had joined the scenery, preceding us most of the way. Hanging just above the trees, it had grown less and less harsh, deferring to the ascending sun and the blue sky. The moon had, I imagined, given up glaring at us, grumbled, and simply accepted the lunacy of human beings.

Now that the dust had settled, running through this scenery became distinctly pleasurable. Fifty miles began to seem possible, reasonable, even easy. The view was gorgeous, my legs felt strong, and the temperature had warmed to a comfortable level. I was really enjoying myself.

The attraction of Le Grizz—the combination of scenery and challenge—grew clearer. It was the ability to run without effort through natural splendor. It was the calm of the forest and the joy of self-propulsion. It was the combination of two loves, running and wilderness, that induced euphoria. I smiled. This was wonderful. And then I hit the first big uphill.

I wouldn't call it a monster—just a steady, continuous upgrade of perhaps a half-mile. When it had passed, my euphoria had dimmed. I was no longer convinced of my ability to travel another 40 miles. My quads had complained on the way up, the first signal of problems lying ahead.

With five hours of running left, the joy of the forest began to give way to the reality of the long road through it.

Misery would come later. For now, miles 10 to 20 became a task, a goal within a goal: I must *get* to the 20-mile mark.

Mentally, the secret to running 50 miles lies with the process of putting miles behind you. Ten miles represents one chunk, 20 miles another. It's a little like filling a garbage bag with aluminum cans. Crush the can; throw it in the bag. Crush another; throw it in the bag. Crush it, bag it, crush it, bag it, crush it, bag it. This is not an elegant process, and at times it seems both endless and meaningless. Eventually, though, the bag is full.

At 13 miles, my support crew appeared again, better prepared this time. I took a swig of defizzed Pepsi, asked them to meet me in another 3 miles or so, and trotted off. They showed up again at 17 miles, where Kaitlin handed me a half-glass of Pepsi and Bridgid announced that I was ahead of Spady.

"I don't think so," I answered. "He went ahead at the first stop, and I haven't passed him."

"The only guy I've seen is that other runner," she said, referring to someone who was running as part of a relay team. "I'm sure you're ahead of everyone else."

"I don't think so."

I downed the pop and headed off again. Whether I led or not seemed irrelevant. I needed to relax, conserve energy, try to go with the flow. I hadn't even reached halfway yet, but already the tightness was growing, from my stomach to my knees.

20 MILES—2:12:58

TWENTY MILES. A long Sunday morning training run, the kind that drains my legs for at least a couple of days. This time, though, 20 miles marked only the beginning. Thirty more lay ahead.

The split time was encouraging. My pace had held up nicely for the second 10, but was I making a big mistake? Just prior to 20 miles, I had passed the relay runner. Now I began to suspect that Bridgid was right: I was in first place. I couldn't figure out what had happened to Spady. I began to suspect that he and his crew had played some kind of trick. Perhaps they were leaving me to my own devices, the neophyte ultrarunner, to dig my own grave. Was I running too fast?

Whatever the answers, I consciously slowed myself down and concentrated on getting to 30 miles. Seeing my support crew a short while later, I stopped for more fluid and a molasses cookie, hoping to delay the complete depletion of my dwindling energy reserves.

Every marathoner knows that at a point near 20 miles, the body sends out notices saying, "Enough already." Running becomes geometrically more difficult, fatigue seems to encompass the body, collapse is imminent, and depression sets in. All this happens between one toe-off and the next heel-strike, don't ask me how. Marathoners call it hitting the wall.

In an effort to avoid the wall, ultramarathoners eat on the run; I hoped that the occasional sugary pop and cookie that I consumed would do the trick. However, any attempt to keep the body adequately supplied with energy during a

50-miler can meet with only partial success, and I knew I would soon be running on empty. As early as 20 miles, I had begun to feel slightly dizzy, moderately disoriented.

An ultramarathon teaches you that, as the Zen masters have always insisted, body and mind are inseparable. The mind does not sit in the skull, happily piloting the body from checkpoint to checkpoint, detached from the organism's needs. As the body staggers, so does the mind. They are, my friends, connected. If you don't believe me, try a 50-miler.

Earlier my smoothly running body had made me feel euphoric. Now it was doing a bang-up job of foisting paranoia on the mind. Hungry grizzlies, I grew convinced, were watching me run.

The Le Grizz entry form (aka Pat Caffrey) says the following about midrace wildlife: "The road is lightly traveled in October and goes through wild, mountainous country where grizzly bears still roam. Other mammals, such as deer, elk, moose, black bear, mountain lion, bobcat and coyote, are common."

In this year's final instructions, Caffrey had added the following: "The Montana Department of Fish, Wildlife and Parks has been trapping our grizzly bears from the west side of the reservoir. Six have been removed recently. If this continues, you may be running 'Le Traps'!"

Ultrarunners may be able to laugh at adversity, but when you get right down to it, grizzly bears are not funny. Like sharks, they eat people, and generally without benefit of music.

"Don't worry," a ranger at Glacier Park once told me. "Grizzlies will only attack if you surprise them, invade their territory, or come between them and their cubs." Those were three things, I explained to him, that a runner could do without realizing it.

A grizzly bear can run up to 30 miles an hour, meaning it could give Ben Johnson a head start and still feast on his carcass at 80 meters. Grizzlies are both unpredictable and quick on their feet.

So there I was, running out in front of the ultraparade, a mostly solitary figure traveling through the wilderness and enjoying the scenery, when it suddenly dawned on me that I heard crackling noises in the bushes.

I've spent enough time in the woods to know that even a tiny animal, a chipmunk, for example, can make a lot of noise. A bear, then, ought to sound like a rock slide as it snaps branches, crushes dry leaves, and generally bullies its way through the forest. So argued my rational mind, insisting on its ability to make an objective judgment about the crackling of twigs. But, I tell you again, the mind is connected to the body—in this case a body with a tank approaching zero.

"The grizzly could be standing very still, waiting to run me down," the mind mused. "He's probably watching me right now. My black-spotted tights, which accent the giraffeness of my legs, are probably invoking some sort of predatory response in the bear *at this very moment.*"

In a past Le Grizz, one of the Spokane runners had spotted a pile of fresh bear dung in the road. ("Right about this point in the race," my weakening mind noted.) Another Spokane runner had responded to the crackling and crashing in the underbrush by stopping to throw rocks, a sure sign of glycogen depletion.

I told myself that, should I suddenly encounter a big Yogi, I would respond more appropriately, which meant . . . well, anyway, I would *not* throw rocks. Meanwhile, as I continued toward the halfway mark, I tried to relax and imagine that the sounds I was hearing were made by chipmunks, birds, and other creatures that used to delight Snow White and not by the sort of animal that can remove a runner's head with a single swipe of its paw.

MARATHON—2:56:14

IN THE 1976 OLYMPICS, I ran the marathon in 2:11:16. Thus, a time 45 minutes slower than that should not have pleased me, but it did. Passing the marathon mark in 2:56:14 went much more smoothly than I might have expected.

There is no such thing as an "easy" marathon. Twenty-six miles of easy running still produces sore, tight, fatigued muscles and a mind that is tired, scattered, and testy. Body and mind have had it. This, the duo agrees, would be a good time to stop.

In the very first Le Grizz Ultramarathon, in 1982, runners crossed this point, indicated by 26.2 MILES written in red paint on the road, and immediately observed an arrow pointing down the road with the inscription THE UNKNOWN. I imagine Pat Caffrey on the evening before the run grinning devilishly as he wrote this.

Passing the marathon point this time, I had several thoughts. One, I was *more* than halfway. I had fewer miles to go now than I had already covered. The feeling was similar to what I've experienced during a track workout after completing six out of ten 440-yard repeats. An odd sort of relief blossomed. The garbage bag was more than half full.

Two, I needed to get to 30. In an ultra, the satisfaction of reaching a mile point is short-lived. I wanted to reach the next major milestone immediately.

Three, I needed a potty stop. My stomach had been bothering me for the past 10 miles, and I thought a trip to the bathroom would help. Seeing my support crew ahead, I pulled over and headed into the van for relief.

There's a Disney cartoon in which Goofy puts on a pair of stretch pants without taking off his snow skis. That's how I felt trying to do my business in the tiny camper toilet. I figured afterward that it had taken at least 3 minutes, most of which involved logistics rather then function. I spent thirty seconds or so convincing Kaitlin and Catherine that they didn't need to visit me during this activity.

Back on the road I felt much better. Part of me worried that Spady might have caught and passed me during my prolonged pit stop, but mostly I was concerned about monitoring vital signs rather than staying ahead of anyone.

30 MILES—3:25:20

I DIDN'T TAKE MUCH SOLACE from reaching the 30-mile checkpoint. I could only think: 20 miles left—the length of my Sunday morning long run. Too many miles.

Even the time, 3:25:20, evoked no particular response. More importantly, I had forgotten to share some important information with Bridgid. I had meant to warn her about the drastic personality deterioration I expected would soon strike me. When blood sugar drops, the "personality," a supposedly fixed set of human traits and attributes, proves to be about as permanent as Mount St. Helens: ordinarily reasonable and pleasant folks become nasty, whining, hopeless idiots.

This once happened to a friend of mine who, preparing for a marathon, decided to follow the carbohydrate-depletion routine while living in the vicinity of his wife, which proved a big mistake. When she served a meal that didn't meet his standards, he complained loudly and stomped off to the nearest supermarket. An hour later he returned, looking sheepish.

"I went to the store, but I didn't eat anything," he confessed. "I just walked around."

"For 45 minutes?" his wife asked incredulously. It was true. This is fairly typical behavior for a runner whose leg muscles have cannibalized all the body's fuel. It's best to steer clear of such folks.

My support crew, though, had agreed to stay with me. Even if I became so rude and disagreeable that they would rather hand me over to the grizzlies. We were clearly entering a danger zone of intrafamily relationships. When the camper appeared again, I vowed to issue a warning.

"Do you need anything?" Bridgid asked sweetly.

"No, but I'm going to start getting nasty pretty soon," I answered obliquely. Bridgid has watched me slowly deplete before. She knew exactly what I meant.

For the next few miles, the road seemed to climb steadily, rising fairly high above the reservoir. The going got tough, and I labored hard at it. At 33 miles I stopped for fluids, nearly threw up from the ensuing nausea, and began walking to regain my equilibrium. Just then Bridgid pulled up beside me in the camper.

"I think you slowed down a bit," she said innocently, forgetting about my increasing depletion. I stared ahead morosely and kept walking. Fortunately, I wasn't carrying a weapon.

Suddenly, some kind of large bird, a pheasant, perhaps, took flight from the bushes. It may have been frightened, but I was terrified. My heartbeat soared.

I began to feel the way I had when I reached the final miles at the Ultimate Runner, a pentathlon of running events I had entered a year earlier. I would travel 1 mile at a time, rewarding myself with a short walking break and a drink at each mile marker. I thought a similar system might help me get through Le Grizz, so I asked my support crew to meet me at every mile marker.

40 MILES—4:38:17

I AM ENTERING A WORLD not of sight or sound, but of mind. And the sign-post up ahead says: LE GRIZZ—40 MILES.

"Ultramarathons are for the patient and calculating runner," says the Le Grizz entry form. "You are in charge of your body, your mind, your run." Well, maybe. At 40 miles, though, it sure as hell didn't feel like it. The next 5 miles would prove the hardest of the day. Along with the general beating my legs had taken, my stomach continued to rebel, and my mind drifted from thought to thought like an explorer without a compass. At one moment I'd feel certain that I could win my first 50-miler in less than 6 hours. The next moment I would be struggling against the urge to walk the rest of the way.

For some bizarre reason, a good part of my concern during these miles focused on having Bridgid stop the camper exactly at each mile mark, not 50 or 100 meters down the road. For Bridgid, though, driving along searching for the white mile marks in the road proved to be incompatible with supervising two camperbound preschoolers. Mile after mile, she missed them. And mile after mile I repeated my whining request that she drive to the exact mile-marker locations.

"I don't know why it's so important to me," I told her at 43 miles, "but please stop right on the next mark."

Later on, a Snickers bar in one hand and a beer in the other, this kind of behavior seems so foolish. Unfortunately, after 40-plus miles of an ultramarathon, it seemed divinely ordained. It was crucial that Bridgid stop where I directed.

Closing in on the 44-mile mark, I grew incensed. Bridgid was not there! After all my begging, she still wasn't on the mark! I cursed. I may have even picked up the pace a bit, anticipating that I'd see the camper around the next turn. She wasn't there either. One more turn. Still not there. Suddenly I realized the awful truth: Bridgid had missed stopping at 44 miles altogether. I would have to run all the way to 45 miles!

God, what a cruel, cruel world, in which a man has to run *2 miles* without a support crew. I screamed something into the forest. Something about Bridgid. To this day, only the trees and wildlife know what I howled.

I wanted to cry, to stop, to lie down and never get up again. Somehow, though, I kept going, step after painful step. Finally, an eon or so later, I reached 45 miles.

"I can't believe you missed the last mile-point," I whimpered.

"I'm sorry," Bridgid replied. She seemed sincere.

My time at 45 miles was 5:18:40. I drank another half-glass of defizzed Pepsi and walked down the road. Ten seconds later, I threw up.

"It never always gets worse," Dan Brannen, a longtime ultrarunning aficionado, had explained prior to Le Grizz. He suggested I should remember those words when the downward spiral of bad to worse to even-worse-than-that seemed unbroken, infinite.

"Eventually," said Brannen, "something will get better."

And it was that advice, that odd nugget of wisdom, that ran truer than anything else at 45 miles. It never always gets worse. We're talking about life now, not just ultramarathons. Or at least life in the downward spiral. "Survive," we tell ourselves and others in the throes of despair. "Endure. It will get better."

Perhaps the attraction of ultrarunning lies in the simple distillation of this: the ability to envision a distant goal—another time and place when things will be better—and to survive the worst until then. This vision embraces both the survival instinct that unites us to other creatures and the imagination and willpower that catapults us above them. "I *will* make it," says the determined mind, and the body grows convinced.

Suddenly, as if on cue, I felt better. I rallied. Only 5 miles to go.

I sensed again that I might win this thing, might even break 6 hours. Those particular aspirations had been buried beneath a stack of miles for the past 3 hours. Even now, the truly relevant goal was to keep going at any pace without walking.

The final miles were more or less a blur of hills, sore quads, elevated spirits, low blood sugar, and human conviction. The last two seemed especially tough, as I skipped the final aid station in the hope of breaking 6 hours.

"Dad looks pretty good again, doesn't he?" Bridgid said to Catherine, who was now riding happily in the front seat with Kaitlin.

"Yeah," she answered cheerfully in 2-year-old-ese, "he no throw up now."

"In a 50-miler," says the Le Grizz entry form, "one competes against one's own limits, not someone else's limits. To finish is to win."

After 5 hours, 58 minutes, and 37 seconds of running, walking, pit stops, vomiting, despair, and determination, it was over. I had won. I finished.

Epilogue

EXACTLY TWO STEPS AFTER crossing the Le Grizz finish line, I stopped. Bridgid escorted me to the camper, where I found I couldn't climb high enough to get inside. My quads simply, absolutely, refused to lift me. Eventually Bridgid managed to push me inside, where I pulled on warmups and commenced to eating.

Soon Spady dropped by, looking much, much better than I felt. He had struggled with stomach problems all day, but still finished second in 6:19:57.

In chatting with other finishers, I discovered that one had actually seen a grizzly at the 18-mile mark. So was it depletion-induced paranoia or a sixth sense that told me something was drooling in the bushes as my tights flashed by?

All the runners who completed Le Grizz were eager to share their adventures, but I noticed they were even more eager to begin eating unhealthy things—candy, pop, Ho Hos, fried chicken. Someone who has just run 50 miles is in no mood for alfalfa sprouts. We paid our dues, expended tens of thousands of calories. It was time to chow down.

After we had consumed beer, chicken, and assorted junk food and watched a moose graze across a lake near the finish area, the sun was dipping toward the horizon. Caffrey finally called us to huddle together for the awards ceremony.

In an event as personally challenging as a 50-miler, organizers seems to feel that, since they told you "to finish is to win," the least they can do is prove they mean it. Everyone gets a trophy.

I accepted my award with pride—it's the only trophy I've chosen to display in public. It has a shellacked wooden base and a figure of a grizzly bear standing on its hind legs, looking fearsome. That bear has, I imagine, just spotted a skinny human being in yellow-and-black tights running through its domain.

For a week after Le Grizz, I hobbled down the hallways of the building in downtown Spokane where I work, hoping someone would question the reason behind my limp. ("Oh, that? Nothing serious, really. Just tired legs from a 50-mile run. That's right, 50.") Gradually, my muscles began to rebuild. In a strange way, though, I relished the residual pain—evidence of my journey through the world beyond the marathon.

And after that?

The Le Grizz entry form says this about the postrace period. "You might feel burned out for four days as a result of energy depletion. Then comes some euphoria."

Spady had put it differently when we chatted right after the run. "I've got some real bad news for you," he said, grinning somewhere beneath his Fu Manchu. "In about three days you're going to think you had fun out there today."

He was wrong. It took almost a week.

FOLLOWING
TERRY FOX

BY JOHN BRANT

After losing his leg to cancer, Terry Fox set
out to do the impossible: run 5,300 miles across his native
Canada, one five-hour marathon at a time.
He died before he could reach his goal, but retracing his route
26 years later shows his legend to be very much alive.

JANUARY 2007

YOU MIGHT NOT BE able to find many people who saw him," Darrell Fox warns me as he drops me off at my Toronto hotel. "Twenty-six years is a long time. People die; people move away." Darrell has reason to be a bit skeptical. Where do you start to write a story about Terry Fox, to many the most influential distance runner of the last half century or, as 32 million Canadians politely but passionately maintain, of any era? How do you compete with the biographies, the feature films, the TV documentaries, the narratives in school textbooks? Highways and stadiums have been named after Terry Fox; in a 2004 poll among Canadians, he was voted the second greatest Canadian of all time in any field.

During the spring and summer of 1980, on one good leg and one prosthetic leg, Terry Fox ran more than halfway across Canada, a total of 3,339 miles, logging nearly a marathon a day over 143 days, and through his Marathon of Hope raised more than $23 million for cancer research. On the 143rd day, he was forced to stop; the cancer that took his leg had spread to his lungs and would kill him in the summer of 1981. He was 22. Each year since, on a Sunday in September, Terry Fox runs have been held, growing to more than 4,000 venues in 56 nations. These noncompetitive 5-Ks and 10-Ks, along with other efforts by the Terry Fox Foundation, have raised close to $370 million.

Thus far the Canadians I've talked to about Terry, like his younger brother

Darrell, have supported my project, but with a sardonic undertone. *Don't come waltzing up from the States, mister, and try to tell us something new about Terry.*

My plan is to drive a portion of the Marathon of Hope route west from Toronto, call the directors of the Terry Fox runs in the towns along the way, and see what sorts of memories, influences, ripples, and reverberations turn up. I already know that, regardless of age, almost everyone in Canada has a Terry story to tell, and, a quarter century after his death, he is almost always referred to in the present tense. During this week in mid-August, I will go all the way to the end of the line, to the statue of Terry by the Trans-Canada Highway in Thunder Bay, the city where he ran his last mile.

That's a round-trip distance of more than 1,700 miles. On the night before departing, over a cold Molson in my hotel near the Toronto airport, I study a map of Ontario, a province so wide that it encompasses two time zones. And I first voice the question I will repeat a hundred times over the next several days.

How in God's name did he run this far?

I recite the names of the towns I will encounter—Parry Sound, Sudbury, Blind River, Sault Ste. Marie (known in Canada as the Soo), Marathon (Marathon!), and my favorite, the one I keep whispering because of its homely but soulful sound and its remote location on a distant corner of Lake Superior: Wawa.

AN UNNATURAL STILLNESS SEEMED to have come over the town on that August day in 1980. As 16-year-old Shelly Skryba walked across Wawa, Ontario, she wondered where everyone could be. Men should be punching out from the day shift at the Algoma Ore mill, women should be out weeding their gardens, and kids should be out riding their bikes. At this point in the summer, on the far northeast corner of the cold lake, you seldom wasted a sunny day.

About 3,700 people lived in Wawa, which was known for its 28-foot-high metal goose welcoming motorists off the Trans-Canada Highway; the word *wawa* means "wild goose" in the Ojibwa language. Embarrassed by its rather silly sound in English, civic leaders had changed the name to the more dignified "Jamestown" in the 1950s. The new name failed to catch on, however, and it soon reverted back to the original.

Typically, from October through April, and some years well into May, winter seized the town. Snow often closed the highway, isolating Wawa on a bleak edge between ice-locked Lake Superior and Canada's vast, granite-studded Precambrian Shield. In the summer, dense morning fog drifted off the lake, forcing truckers to inch up and down the steep grade at Montreal River east of town.

The town, the lake, the highway, summer's dwindling days: As she neared her boyfriend Earl Dereski's house, the dime dropped for Shelly. She suddenly remembered why the streets were empty today. Terry Fox had run into Wawa.

Shelly had not been granted a carefree childhood. Her father had worked at Algoma Ore. When her mother was stricken by multiple sclerosis, Shelly and the rest of the family moved to Sault Ste. Marie, the nearest urban center, for medical care. There, unfortunately, the couple's marriage foundered. Following the divorce, Shelly moved back to Wawa, where she lived with her grandmother.

Shelly daydreamed often during that summer of 1980, thinking about the house that she and Earl, also a mill worker, would live in one day after they got married. She imagined having a daughter who would graduate from college and accomplish great things. But all that dreaming almost kept her from seeing the fantasy running in her direction.

She had been late jumping onto the Terry Fox bandwagon. One day a few months earlier, Shelly got home from her summer job at the local tourist agency, eager to change clothes and go meet Earl. "Hello," she called as she walked into her house.

"In the kitchen," her grandmother, Elma, responded. Shelly headed that way. Her grandmother was listening to a news report on the radio. "He's made it to Toronto," she announced. Elma pointed to a map of Canada spread out on the table, running her finger from St. John's, Newfoundland, where Terry had started to run in April by dipping his prosthesis in the Atlantic Ocean, over to Ontario, and then all the way to Vancouver, near his hometown of Port Coquitlam, British Columbia, where he was due to arrive in September. When finished, he would have run a total of more than 5,300 miles. "Just look at what this young man is doing!"

Terry had trained years for the run, preparing his legs—both the good one and prosthetic one—for what was in store. The prosthetic was a standard model, outfitted with a few primitive modifications for running; a metal valve, for instance, had been replaced with one of stainless steel so it wouldn't rust from sweat. During the Marathon of Hope, he would start running most mornings at 5, moving with a stride that consisted of two hops of his whole leg and one of his prosthesis, moving at roughly an 11-minute-per-mile pace. Terry would turn testy sometimes when challenged on his athletic integrity.

"Some people can't figure out what I'm doing," he had said in June. "It's not a walk-hop, it's not a trot. It's running, or as close as I can get to running, and it's harder than doing it on two legs. It makes me mad when people call this a walk. If I was walking, it wouldn't be anything."

He would run two miles, take a brief water break at the van that his best friend, Doug Alward, drove beside him, run another two miles, and then take another break. Terry continued this routine until he covered 14 to 16 miles, usually finishing his morning stint by 8. He would rest for three hours, then run another 10 to 12 miles, regardless of heat, cold, crowds, or headwinds.

In the afternoons and evenings, he gave interviews and addressed audiences in community halls and school gyms. As he spoke, a representative of the Canadian Cancer Society would move among the crowd, collecting bills and change in plastic trash bags and wrinkled grocery sacks. Every cent went directly to fighting cancer; all expenses for the Marathon of Hope were separately donated. He declined all sponsorship offers and displayed no advertising logos, not even a T-shirt with the name of a college or hockey team. The only hint of a corporation's presence were the three parallel stripes on Terry's dark-blue Adidas Orions.

He and Doug would spend the night in the van or, as they moved through Ontario and Terry's fame grew, in donated motel rooms. At 5 the next morning, they would return to the spot where he had stopped running the day before, which Doug had marked with a small stack of rocks piled by the highway. Making sure to set out from behind the rocks, Terry began the ordeal over again. He was determined to run every inch of the distance across Canada.

As he came closer to Wawa, millions of Terry Fox fans assumed that he was only halfway through his journey. No one could imagine that he actually approached the end: both of his epic road trip and of his brief life. But in terms of impact and influence, of inspiring hope and courage, of achieving fundamental progress in the fight against cancer, Terry was just getting started. "The way I think about Terry," says Alward, speaking not altogether metaphorically, "is that he's not really dead."

IN 1976, DICK TRAUM became the first person to finish the New York City Marathon on a prosthetic leg. A few months later, in early 1977, in Port Coquitlam, British Columbia, 18-year-old Terry Fox developed osteogenic sarcoma, a rare type of bone cancer, which required his right leg to be amputated six inches above the knee. The day before the amputation, Terry's former high school basketball coach happened across a copy of *Runner's World* with a story about Traum running New York. The coach brought the magazine to Terry that night, thinking the story might encourage him. The kid looked at the story but didn't say anything. The coach worried that he'd committed a terrible gaffe. But Terry kept studying Traum's photo. Finally, he said, "Thanks, Coach," and put the magazine aside.

Terry had a dream that night. He dreamed that if some old walrus like Traum could run the New York City Marathon, well...

Four years passed. Terry became world famous; then he died. He was honored with a memorial distance run, and because he had inspired the kid, Dick

Traum was invited to Toronto to participate. At most American road races, Traum was the only disabled runner; he was astonished by the number of disabled athletes running the Canadian event.

He went home and reported the experience to Fred Lebow, the New York City Marathon race director. Lebow encouraged Traum to recruit disabled runners for the marathon, and thus was born the Achilles Track Club, which has grown into the largest and most influential organization of its kind in the world. "It didn't really come from me or that magazine story," says Traum, who remains president of the Achilles club. "It all came from Terry's dream."

LEAVING TORONTO AND HEADING WEST, I get held up in morning traffic. It takes me more than an hour to cover 10 miles—not a great deal faster than Terry's pace. Two hours north of the city, I approach Parry Sound, the hometown of hockey legend Bobby Orr. When they met during the run, Terry showed Orr his prosthesis, and Orr showed Terry the scars from his knee surgeries.

The expressway narrows to a two-lane highway and the traffic calms. I catch glimpses of Georgian Bay—shards of a blue dream—and listen to a CBC call-in show about minor-league hockey goons. Most days during the Marathon of Hope, despite his excruciating effort (at times, for instance, the chafing of his prosthesis rubbed his stump so raw that blood dripped into his shoe), Terry also had a blast.

"I loved it," he told a reporter after the run. "I enjoyed myself so much, and that was what people couldn't realize. They thought I was going through a nightmare, running all day long.... Maybe I was, partly, but still I was doing what I wanted.... Even though it was so difficult, there was not another thing in the world I would rather have been doing."

AS THE SUMMER WORE ON, as Terry's story percolated across the nation, Shelly grew more interested in Terry and his run. She wasn't nearly as consumed by the Marathon of Hope as Dory, Earl's sister, was. Dory had filled scrapbooks with pictures and stories of Terry, as if he were a rock star. Still, Shelly sensed that he wasn't just a media darling. He wasn't doing this to stoke his ego or strike it rich. Terry reminded Shelly of the Ontario pioneers she had studied in school, who had paddled across Superior to deliver medicine to sick children. They weren't trying to be heroes; they were just doing what was necessary. Terry seemed to have the same attitude. He was just a plodding Canadian kid—average in school, average as an athlete—who had somehow been chosen for a wonderful, terrible mission. Before Terry, people died from cancer, but they were ashamed to talk about it. This boy from Port Coquitlam wasn't ashamed. Every day, Terry showed his cancer to the world, and the world would never be the same.

Millions of Canadians were drawing similar conclusions. Once Terry had moved through Quebec, there were no more pudgy lifestyle-section reporters puffing alongside him so they could write what running with Terry felt like. The flavor of the news reports changed. The stories took on a respectful, almost reverent tone. The TV showed thousands of people massed in Nathan Phillips Square welcoming him to downtown Toronto. Women in hair curlers hustled out from beauty parlors to watch him run past. Little kids shoved pennies into his hand. NHL superstar Darryl Sittler, Terry's own hero, looked starstruck as he stood beside Terry.

Shelly watched the TV news reports with growing fascination as the Marathon of Hope parade—an Ontario Provincial Police cruiser, Doug Alward and other crew members in their smelly van, an RV carrying a staffer from the Canadian Cancer Society, and, on foot, a one-legged man wearing ragged gray shorts—lurched west toward Wawa.

LYNDON FOURNIER IS A 47-year-old executive for the financial firm ScotiaMcLeod in Mississauga, Ontario. His corner office is filled with Terry Fox memorabilia: photos, newspaper clippings, and certificates of appreciation from the Terry Fox Foundation. Each year Fournier leads the office fund drive for the Terry Fox Run. One of his most prized possessions is a pair of Adidas Orion TFs. In 2005, to help commemorate the 25th anniversary of the Marathon of Hope, Adidas came out with the TFs, a retro model of the original Orions Terry wore on his run. One of his used shoes—a right-footed one, which he wore over the foot of his prosthesis—sits under glass at an exhibit at the Terry Fox Public Library in Port Coquitlam. Battered, stained, torn, worn down to the midsole, the shoe seems like a relic of a medieval saint. The foot bed of the commemorative TF was embossed with a color map of Terry's marathon route and sold for $100. Adidas donated all proceeds to the Terry Fox Foundation. It wasn't easy to find a pair. Nationwide, 40 percent of retail locations sold out on the first day, and 75 percent in the first week. Fournier had to pull a few strings to get his pair. He looks at the shoes every so often, for inspiration. They have never touched the ground, of course, and Fournier wouldn't dream of running in them.

IN SUDBURY, I HAVE LUNCH with a man named Lou Fine, who, in 1980, as district supervisor for the Canadian Cancer Society, accompanied the Marathon of Hope over its final six weeks. "I told one lie to Terry," Fine confesses to me. "When we got to the town of Marathon, halfway between Wawa and Thunder

Bay, he got tendinitis so bad in his good leg that he couldn't go another step. One of Terry's supporters got us a small plane, and we flew to the Soo to see a doctor. The doc looks at his leg and says, 'You gotta take a day or two off, son, or at least cut down to 13 miles a day.' Terry, of course, says the hell with that.

"We were all set to fly back to Marathon, and that's when I told Terry my lie. I made up a story that fog had closed the airport in Marathon. We would have to catch a bus, and wouldn't you know it, there wasn't another bus coming through town until the next day."

Lou gives a dry laugh. "To my amazement, Terry bought my BS. He let himself rest for two days—two of the three days he took off out of the 143 days on the road."

ON HIS WAY TO WAWA, Terry had followed a convoluted course through heavily populated southern Ontario, adding hundreds of draining miles to his route in order to collect as much money as possible for cancer research. Finally, in mid-July, he worked clear of the Toronto megalopolis and began running up Highway 69 along the eastern shore of Lake Huron, onto the edge of the rocky Precambrian Shield and the great boreal forest carrying north to the Arctic.

At Sudbury, Terry picked up Highway 17, the southern arm of the Trans-Canada Highway, which carried him due west, into the morning fog and mus-keg, along the blue deeps of Huron and Superior, through Blind River and the Soo and finally, in mid-August, to Wawa. Now, late on that Monday afternoon, he was about to speak at the community center. Shelly raced across town and squeezed into the arena as Terry took the stage.

In front of 700 citizens, Terry looked exhausted. On this day, number 129 of his run, he had completed one of the hilliest portions of his cross-country expedition, and yet was only 30 minutes off his scheduled 3 p.m. arrival. "I guess I was spurred on by the challenge of it. Everybody kept talking about the hills—Montreal River, Old Woman Bay—especially Montreal River," Terry told the crowd. Shelly listened intently. "But when I got to the top of it, I said, 'Is that it?'" Shelly broke into a smile.

Watching him, her first thought was that this must be what it was like seeing the Beatles. He had curly hair, a deep tan, and a white smile. He was pure muscle from all the running. At the same time, the angular machinery of his prosthetic leg made him seem like a vulnerable little boy. Shelly and her girlfriends were practi-cally passing out looking at him. And besides being gorgeous, he was modest.

"I'm not the one who is important here," Terry told the crowd. "This whole thing isn't about me at all."

The people in and around Wawa raised more than $15,000. Donations included $500 from a Wawa motel, $88 from the sale of homemade blueberry pies, and a gold-plated goose. Another $1,000 or so came from motorists who donated directly to the caravan. Terry told the people of Wawa, before leaving the center, why every dollar was important. "I've been on the road four months and I'm sore. It's hard for people to comprehend what it's like getting up and running every single day. All we're trying to do is help this cause."

IN EARLY 1993, 14-YEAR-OLD Nikki Parkinson developed a sharp pain in her shoulder. She assumed it was due to tendinitis caused by the stress of being a competitive swimmer. The pain persisted, however, and specialists in her home-town of Toronto discovered that a malignant tumor had invaded her shoulder joint. Parkinson had been stricken by osteogenic sarcoma, the same type of can-cer that afflicted Terry Fox. If, as in Terry's case, Parkinson's tumor metastasized, it would spread to vital organs and kill her. But that was where the similarities between Terry's cancer and Parkinson's ended. "When I came out of the biopsy and got the diagnosis, I asked my mother if I was going to die," Parkinson says. "She looked me in the eye and told me no."

Instead of a 50 percent chance of survival, which was what Terry faced, Parkinson's chances stood at 85 percent. Instead of amputating her arm, sur-geons at a Toronto hospital performed reconstructive surgery in which Parkin-son's malignant shoulder joint was replaced by one from a cadaver and reinforced with steel rods. It was an innovative surgical technique unheard of in Terry's time, developed in large part due to funding from the Terry Fox Foundation.

After surgery, she underwent a chemotherapy regimen, at the end of which she was diagnosed cancer-free. She went on to graduate from high school and college and earn an advanced degree in human genetics. One day, Parkinson says, she hopes to work with cancer patients at the same hospital in which she was cured. "Terry is the reason that I'm alive," she says. "In more ways than I can count, he is my hero."

I STOP ONE NIGHT in Blind River, about 250 miles southeast of Wawa, on the northern lip of Lake Huron, and stay at a motel on Highway 17, the same one Terry stayed in when he came through the town. The owner tells me that guests often ask about him. The waiter at the Chinese restaurant across the highway remembers the day Terry ran through Blind River, and so does Wayne Rivers, the local taxi dispatcher.

"He makes me proud to be a Canadian," Wayne told me, as if Terry were due in Blind River tonight.

I plan to get up just before 5 tomorrow morning and run a few miles in Terry's footsteps. I watch the sun set over the lake, go to bed early, but sleep poorly. On some nights during his run, despite his exhaustion, Terry also had trouble sleeping. By the time he reached Blind River, in what turned out to be the marathon's final few hundred miles, the signs of decline must have been undeniable—the dry cough and double vision that Doug and Darrell assumed were symptoms of the flu.

The next day I rise as planned. The same hour that Terry rose. He would have gotten out of bed and likely said a quick prayer. (Although he never made a show of his faith, he had read through the entire New Testament during his final months of training for the run.) He would have stepped into his prosthesis the way another man steps into his jeans. He would have washed and dressed and stuffed his gear into his pack and then headed out to the parking lot where Doug and Darrell, Lou Fine, and the Ontario Provincial Police trooper waited by their respective vehicles.

"If Terry said, 'Good morning, Lou, are you still fine?' then I knew he had slept well and we were in for a smooth ride," Lou had told me in Sudbury. "But if he just walked right past without a word, I knew that our morning was going to be interesting."

I turn left outside the motel and run past the 24-hour coffee shop, the dark Chinese restaurant, and the park by the mouth of Blind River. Terry's sea-to-shining-sea marathon appears possible at this hour. When he ran this stretch of road 26 years ago, it must have seemed a sure thing. He was 22 years old; the cough and double vision had to be symptoms of the flu. He was more than half-way across Canada now, more than halfway home.

I had learned, however, that Terry rarely thought in such abstract terms. When he reached the streetlight, he thought about making it to the gas station. When he reached the station, he thought about running to the water tower on the edge of town.

But no matter how iron your discipline, sometimes your mind drifts. On this morning there are no dogs howling or monster semis batting past with a back draft that knocks you halfway across the highway. The fog lies softly over the muskeg in the last of the moonlight. The breeze is cool off Lake Huron, and the dawn light lacks the day's punishing glare.

Sometimes a farm family would be out at dawn to greet Terry and offer a doughnut or a cup of tea. But not today. It's just the police cruiser up front and Doug and Darrell in the van beside him and Lou in the RV, riding sweep. No sweaty crowds, no reporters asking why. The springs on his prosthesis make a steady mechanical squeak. Now the light is rising. A half mile up the highway, a granite outcropping takes shape out of the fog. Terry sets aim at the rock, emptying his mind, keeping his pace, moving west.

SHELLY SKRYBA CRIED ON the day Terry Fox died, June 10, 1981. It had been nearly 10 months since he had come through Wawa. She saw him leave town that evening, and then two weeks and 293 miles later—after running through cities like Thessalon and Marathon—he came to a spot on the highway a few miles east of Thunder Bay and stopped, brought to a halt by crushing chest pains. Three years earlier, when the surgeons had sawed off his leg at the hospital in British Columbia, Terry had convinced himself they had also cut out his cancer; he had willed himself inside that charmed circle of osteogenic sarcoma survivors, the 50 percent who were cured.

But it was now plain that, to his and the world's grief, he'd been running outside that circle all along. Before the amputation, seeds of carcinogenic cells had migrated to Terry's lungs and had now bloomed into an inoperable secondary cancer. The Marathon of Hope was suspended in midstride. Terry was flown to a hospital not far from his home, where, after a 10-month decline, he died.

Since his death, the Terry Fox Foundation has continued to raise money for treatment-based cancer research chiefly through donations gathered at the Terry Fox Runs. Over the years, the foundation, led by Darrell Fox, has maintained tight control over Terry's name and brand and has shown the same kind of disciplined focus for fund-raising that Terry displayed. For instance, in 2000, Darrell turned down a request by the Canadian mint to sell a Terry Fox commemorative coin set marking the 20th anniversary of the Marathon of Hope; portions of the profits would have gone to the foundation. Only after the mint came forward with a new proposal in 2005—it would produce a general-circulation silver dollar embossed with Terry's image—did Darrell say yes. "Terry's original goal was to raise a dollar from every Canadian," Darrell had told me before I set out on my trip, "so the symbolism was perfect."

Like Shelly, much of Canada was in tears the day Terry was buried. The CBC televised the funeral live from Port Coquitlam. By that time, Terry was already half legend. There had been a telethon with Gordon Lightfoot and other stars. Prime Minister Pierre Trudeau made a speech. Millions of dollars had poured in from every province in Canada and around the world. Plans formed for the first Terry Fox Run that September.

After his funeral, the media stories about Terry worked down to a trickle. Life returned to normal in Wawa. The men punched in for their shifts at Algoma Ore, the big trucks boomed by on the Trans-Canada Highway. In the summer the fog drifted off the lake, and in the winter the iron cold clamped down. In September, just after the start of the school year, the kids ran around the playground in memory of Terry Fox.

JASON BIELAS ANSWERS the phone guardedly. Why would a sportswriter be calling? But when Bielas, a 31-year-old postdoctoral fellow in the department of pathology at the University of Washington Medical School in Seattle, hears the name Terry Fox, he relaxes. Somehow, whenever Terry is involved, no connection is too far-fetched. There always seems to be a thread to follow.

So Bielas discusses his recent work. He is helping develop a reliable laboratory test for measuring the level of cancer-associated mutations in DNA. With an accurate mutation-level test, Bielas explains, thousands of unnecessary surgeries could be avoided each year. But Bielas also talks about his challenges: Federal funding to the lab has just about dried up. Only 10 percent or so of the NIH grants his department applied for this year in the United States have been approved. Which leads the conversation back to Terry. Because Bielas is the recipient of a $40,000 Terry Fox Foundation research grant, Bielas doesn't share his colleagues' anxieties. He can continue his work in the way he sees fit. This makes Bielas feel lucky, and somewhat guilty, and also, especially at this time of year, a little homesick for Canada. Each September, when he was growing up in Toronto, Bielas would do the Terry Fox Run at school. Of the 4,000 Terry Fox runs, only a few are held in the United States. When Bielas mentions Terry Fox to his American friends, he rarely gets more than a blank look in return.

IN 1981, AT THE AGE OF 17, Shelly married Earl Dereski, and they soon had two daughters. Shelly worked on being a mother for 10 years, then went to college and earned a nursing degree.

Life was fine except for one thing: Taylor, the couple's second child, was always sick. She was constantly missing school; she didn't have the same energy as other kids. Shelly took her to the doctor and they ran tests, but they couldn't find anything wrong. The pattern continued through the summer of 1998. Taylor was sick when she started high school in September, and by Halloween she was too weak to get out of bed. Shelly took her to the hospital in Wawa, but the doctors still couldn't find anything wrong. Taylor went home and collapsed into bed. In the middle of the night she was burning up with fever and her pulse was racing. Her mother put her in a cold tub. They got through the night, and at first light Shelly drove Taylor down to the emergency room. X-rays revealed a foggy mass in Taylor's left lung. The doctors diagnosed pneumonia and put her on antibiotics. But Taylor's condition worsened.

Over the next week, Taylor grew increasingly delirious. One night, Taylor lay quietly in bed, when she said to her mother, "I know why I'm sick."

Shelly didn't like this. "Why?"

"Grandma Myrna wants me to come visit."

Shelly went cold. Her mother, Myrna, who had suffered from MS, had died before Taylor was born. Shelly hardly ever talked about her.

At the end of the week it was decided that Taylor should be seen by specialists in the Soo. There, doctors detected a tumor sitting at the opening of her left lung. The next day a medevac helicopter flew Taylor and her mother down to the Hospital for Sick Children, in Toronto, one of the world's leading pediatric hospitals, which was popularly known by its nickname, Sick Kids. Specialists verified that the tumor was malignant and had gradually cut off the blood and oxygen supply to the organ. The lung had stagnated, collapsed, and filled with pus. The simmering infection was what had made Taylor sick all her life and was now threatening to kill her.

"At the time, I was too scared and worried to remember that secondary lung cancer was what killed Terry," Shelly would later tell me. "But at the same time, I couldn't help but think of him. Terry Fox was all over Sick Kids."

On a practical level, Terry's influence was tangible in the hospital's radiology and chemotherapy, its surgery and physical therapy: over the past decade, these and other healing arts had dramatically advanced due to support from the Terry Fox Foundation.

But Terry was also present in other ways. His picture, for instance, looked out from the T-shirts of the young patients on the oncology floor. These kids had grown up with Terry Fox. They had listened to their parents tell stories about him around the dinner table, had studied him in the classroom, and had run in his memory on the playground. Now, as they engaged cancer themselves, Terry was their guide and companion.

DRIVING HIGHWAY 17, I APPROACH Wawa seemingly by the inch. Bombing rain eclipses the Montreal River grade, and the CBC drifts out of range on the radio. The 18-wheelers throw up fiendish curtains of water. Over the past day or so behind the wheel, I've begun thinking out loud, but not exactly talking to myself. Terry, I complain, as, semi-blindly, I pass another truck on the rainswept highway, why did you have to run so damn far?

A hundred miles west of the Soo, I stop for gas, coffee, and to call ahead to Wawa on a pay phone; my cell phone doesn't work in Canada. I dial the race director of the annual Terry Fox Run in Wawa, but I'm doubtful she'll be home on a Saturday afternoon. I'm right; a young voice answers, her daughter's voice. Her mother and father are down in the Soo for the weekend, she says. She would normally be there, too, but on the spur of the moment she decided to drive up to Wawa for a fishing derby, which is currently suspended by rain. It was purely by chance that she had answered my call.

I stammer out my case anyway... magazine in the States, traveling through, thought I'd take a shot... the kid must think I'm a lunatic. But she hears me out calmly and says she'd be happy to talk with me. In fact, Taylor Dereski says, she has her own Terry story to tell.

ON NOVEMBER 23, 1998, surgeons removed most of Taylor's lung, leaving a long, hook-shaped scar across her back. She returned home to Wawa, where she missed the remainder of her freshman year in high school. Taylor quickly caught up, however, and in ensuing years, short of some type of vigorous exercise, savored all the pleasures that her disease previously had denied her. She developed a passion for fishing. She graduated from high school and immediately settled on a profession. "Because of the model of my mother, I hope to become a nurse," Taylor says, sitting in her parents' apartment. "Due to my own experience with cancer," she adds, "I'd like to one day work with kids with cancer."

Taylor pauses. At 22, she is the same age that Terry was when he ran through Wawa, and radiates the same sense of life that jumps out from his photos. "My mother talked about Terry a lot, and we learned all about him in school," she continues. "I don't mean to sound spooky or cornball, but having gone through the same thing as he did, and with him actually visiting Wawa, I feel like I know him."

IN SEPTEMBER 2002, Shelly Dereski noticed that something had changed about her hometown. For the first time since 1981, Wawa lacked a Terry Fox Run. There had been no deliberate slight; people hadn't forgotten Terry. The run organizer had simply moved away, and nobody picked up the ball. Shelly was horrified.

"How could there not be a Terry Fox Run in Wawa?" she says. "With my daughter being a cancer survivor, I had a direct connection to him. And Terry ran through Wawa. I saw him."

So Shelly volunteered to become the town's Terry Fox Run director. She didn't know anything about the job. She called the run director in Thunder Bay to get advice and sent away to the Terry Fox Foundation for an organizer's kit. Soon Terry's photo appeared on the same bulletin boards and store windows where the original Terry Fox posters had hung during that golden month of August 1980, when millions of people followed each mile of his magical run through northern Ontario, step by syncopated step. Shelly was young then, and she dreamed of having a beautiful daughter someday. Something profound had touched this cold little town, delivered by a one-legged man who paused here during his long run home.

Shelly had Earl lay out a 5-K course around the high school, while she organized a barbecue at the finish line, and a few hundred people came out, raising $2,600 for the foundation. For the next few years the turnout grew, and in 2005, during the Marathon of Hope's 25th anniversary, townspeople contributed more than $5,000. Taylor's diminished lung capacity did not allow her to run or walk at the event, but one year, as a cancer survivor, she cut the ribbon at the starting line.

Her mother was happy. Terry Fox had returned to Wawa.

ON THE THIRD SATURDAY in September, a month after my trip through Ontario, I drive north from my home in Portland, Oregon, through Washington State, under the Peace Arch border crossing, and into British Columbia. I spend the night at a motel in Port Coquitlam, just outside of Vancouver, watching the replay of a 2005 TV movie about Terry Fox and the Marathon of Hope. I'm impressed by the actor playing Doug Alward. The next morning I meet the real Doug Alward, a shy, intensely private man, and together we go to the Terry Fox Hometown Run in Port Coquitlam.

Near the starting line before the run, Alward shows me the various memories of Terry that have been gathered on a bulletin board. Noting Alward's interest, but having no idea who he is, a race volunteer asks him if he has any stories to share. Alward starts to speak, then catches himself, gives an awkward smile, and decides to walk away. I follow him.

At this same hour, in their respective time zones around the planet, Terry Fox runs are rolling in hundreds of towns and cities, including Toronto, where I picked up Terry's trail, and Wawa, where for reasons beyond my ken, the trail always seemed to lead me. There are still a few minutes before the start, and to pass the time I ask Alward about his memories of Wawa.

"Everything about that day was a blur," he recalls. "I vaguely remember the big white letters etched into a hillside on the highway."

Doug explains that their start that morning had been delayed because a film crew wanted to get a shot of Terry running up the nearby Montreal River grade. At his habitual 5 a.m. starting time, however, Terry would have been climbing the hill in darkness. So they waited an hour so the crew could shoot in daylight. "At the end of the day we had to pay the price," Doug tells me. "After leaving Wawa, Terry still had to run another 90 minutes to reach his quota for the day."

At that moment the ribbon is cut at the starting line. Alward, a 2:45 marathoner at age 48, takes off into the morning drizzle. I chug along in the middle of the pack, connecting Alward's story with my own memories of the town, the lake, the highway, and summer's dwindling days.

THE FAST
AND THE CURIOUS

BY ROBERT SULLIVAN

> In New York City's Fifth Avenue Mile,
> a middle-aged runner with big ideas wondered
> if he could hang with the elites.
> Then the gun went off.

JUNE 2006

IWAS AN ELITE runner for a day, or more precisely, a faux-elite runner for a day. And even though I suffered physically and emotionally and in ways that I may only understand many years from now, I loved every moment.

It was a perfect September afternoon in New York City, and the Continental Airlines Fifth Avenue Mile ran from 80th Street to 60th Street on Fifth Avenue, or 20 beautiful and usually cab- and Mercedes-filled blocks. The actual elite racers were all very tolerant, if not nice, to me, but one big difference between me and the elite athletes running that day was that they had been training for the race, running all year, scheduling the event on their calendars months before. I, on the other hand, pretty much just showed up.

I had gotten a call a couple of days earlier from a running insider seeing if I might want to, well, run the men's elite mile in the Fifth Avenue competition. Now, as it turns out, the same day that the elites are running, there are mile races for nearly every age group, from 20- to 29-year-olds to people 70-plus. You know, regular weekend-warrior types. But not thinking it through, I said, "Sure, put me in against the elite men," because although I have never actually trained as a miler, I have very actively imagined running a mile really, really fast. I would be running the Walter Mitty position in the Fifth Avenue Mile, except that unlike Walter Mitty, I would not be just daydreaming a race with the fastest runners in the world but actually experiencing it, with ESPN cameras, with crowds watching, where, if I passed out, I might be trampled by elite mile-running athletes or, depending on my time, the Fifth Avenue bus.

That day I was trying my best to look like a 20-something elite runner, not an easy act for an undersize, balding, 42-year-old father of two who hasn't run a timed mile since high school, much less trained for one. For the record, my credentials are as follows: Though I am not the worst runner in the world, I am way back from the best. I run five or six days a week, somewhere between five and seven miles, and if I really push it, I run around a seven- or eight-minute-per-mile pace, albeit for very limited distances. Like many nonprofessional runners in America today, my specialty is downhill. Not including the hair I have left, I weigh in at around 150 pounds, my weight and body and general health being the main reasons I run, as opposed to my competitive nature, which science has not yet developed tools sensitive enough to measure. As a runner, my goal is to stay alive while occasionally partaking in things like desserts and fermented hops.

I received my invitation on the Wednesday before the Saturday race and "trained" on Thursday, during my daughter's soccer practice, though training turned out to be me running in circles around a field of soccer-playing 9-year-olds as fast as I could, my daughter shaking her head when I pulled up out of breath. I also attended a press conference on Thursday, at which reporters interviewed some of the fastest milers in the world—such as Carrie Tollefson, Craig Mottram, and Alan Webb—and not me. At the conference, the CEO and president of the New York Road Runners, Mary Wittenberg, said things that made me nervous, such as, "These runners are gonna cruise!" I met Scott Raczko, the coach of Alan Webb, the 22-year-old favorite in the race, who's best known for breaking Jim Ryun's high school mile record in 2001. Pathetically, I beseeched Raczko for advice on how I might proceed vis-à-vis training, given that I would be racing the fastest runners in the world in about 48 hours. "Just keep doing what you're doing," he said. I even met Webb. He seemed very focused—even just shaking hands he was beating me—and though he greeted me kindly, his body language said, "You're kidding."

But I was not, or not really. I was really going to give my best shot, and so, as I often do, I rested on Friday. At four in the afternoon, I went to an elite runner logistical meeting that the New York Road Runners hosted in a hotel suite. Prior to becoming a faux-elite runner, I did not know about logistical meetings. At logistical meetings, we elite runners talk to each other about past races and our flights coming in and, in one case, about how, except for me, a New Yorker, we couldn't believe how many people are runners in Central Park, as opposed to, say, muggers. I talked to Webb's father about New Jersey, a noncompetitive subject, and to the woman in charge of drug testing everybody, and caught myself hoping I would go so fast as to be accused of using steroids. As we sipped free elite-athlete bottled water, Sarah Schwald and Jason Lunn let me in on their conversation about training in the Rocky Mountains, where they take advantage of lower oxygen levels to prepare their lungs for the stress of running a mile at high speeds. "Just relax," Sarah said. "You'll be fine." I think she might have noticed that I was hyperventilating, the thought of lung-stressing stressing me out.

David Monti is the Road Runners' professional athletic coordinator, the guy who answers your questions if you are an elite athlete and tells you about weather and road conditions (cool and dry, though there was a possibility of overnight rain), about how we would conduct our postrace interviews if we won, and about how we would get $10,000 if we broke a course record, something that would require not only illegal drugs on my part but also surgery. Monti handed out special elite-athlete T-shirts. "I don't want to see these on eBay tomorrow," he said. I think I saw Webb grab one for his dad, who looked pretty psyched.

That night, I rested more, alongside my wife, in the stands at a Yankees game. (I know, I should have been in bed, but we'd had the tickets for six months and had not been on a date since early in our marriage.) As far as hydration went, I drank only half a beer. Just to give you an insight into the kind of punishing self-sacrifices I was making, it was light beer. Between innings, I came up with a race plan with my newly appointed coaches—i.e., my wife and Bobby, the fireman from Queens who sat near us. If I could do about a 1:45 for each quarter mile, then I would finish in seven minutes, a time I figured would preserve my reputation as a 42-year-old balding old guy and not embarrass the New York Road Runners for letting me in the race. The major variable was nerves. Nerves had caused me to break out in hives for my SATs 24 years earlier. Would they allow me to even finish the race? Bobby the fireman, also hydrating during the game, didn't see a problem. "You'll be fine," he said.

Webb mentioned that he had run the course a couple of nights before the race. Thus, I made the point of driving to the Yankees game when I'd normally take the subway. That way, on the way home, I could also check out the course. By midnight, an hour or so after the game, Fifth Avenue was quiet, an express bus sprinting past the beautiful townhouses on the left and Central Park on the right, a few lost-looking tourists walking alongside the dark park. I drove slowly and counted off the blocks, the mile seeming long, the road looking rough. Getting to bed late, I felt as ready as I would ever feel, which is not very ready.

THE MORNING OF THE RACE, I showed up in the elite hotel suite with about five or six pounds more gear than the actual elite runners, who carried small backpacks containing only small water bottles and a couple of extra pairs of socks. I had packed street clothes, not realizing that I was not going to have the energy to change after the race. I was very happy to learn from several of the other runners that part of the elite-athlete regimen in the morning is espresso from the espresso machine that was in the elite suite. I threw back a few, as if I needed to be any more amped up. After what I now realize was probably too much espresso, I rode the elevator with Sinead Delahunty-Evans, an Irish runner who lives in Boston and in 1995 won the women's Fifth Avenue Mile in 4:25.2. It seemed that Delahunty-Evans was, frankly, going down a lot faster than I was.

We dropped off our things in the elite runners' tent, my gear taking up most of the table, and then walked up Fifth Avenue toward the starting line. In all the hours that I spent preparing for and then running the Fifth Avenue Mile, it was only at this moment that I thought any of these really fast guys had any interest in being anything like me. We were crossing 59th Street on our way north to the race start at 80th Street when Kevin Sullivan, a Canadian racer who, from his height (six feet) and build (sleek, athletic), bore no relation to me despite the last name, looked at me and lamented. "I wanted your number," he said. Unfortunately, with the mile start just minutes away, I was slowly losing the ability to communicate verbally in any way. Meanwhile, Sullivan, with a mile PR of 3:50 set in Oslo in 2000, was going on in a relaxed manner. "Ninety-nine," he said. "That's Wayne Gretzky's number, and I went to the same high school as him. I saw it and I thought it was mine and they told me it was yours."

I looked up at him and said, "What can I say?" Or at least that's what I think I said—I couldn't hear much over my pounding heartbeat.

When we got to the starting area, the nonprofessional racers had already begun their heats—and that was when it hit me precisely how unprepared I was: it was when I saw over-60-year-old, non-elite runners racing. I won't pretend that on Friday night at the baseball game there weren't moments when, half drunk on half a light beer, I imagined myself breaking from the pack—the old guy!—and finishing first and winning a Nike contract for old non-elite runners. Now, I wondered what the hell I was doing. On the sidewalk up near the starting line, in the glorious blue-skied Fifth Avenue morning, the elite athletes quietly stretched. I did the four or five stretches that I normally do and then realized that these guys were still stretching muscles I was only faintly aware of; they had their knees near their ears a lot of the time. Kind of faking a stretch (and getting more jittery now), I chatted up Kevin Sullivan, in an act of desperate bonding. "Just out of curiosity, would you ever have a beer the night before a race?" I asked. He shook his head and frowned. "No," he said.

At this point, with warmup directions I had printed out from the Internet in hand, I was ready to begin warmup sprints—six 50-yard dashes. That was when Ray Flynn spotted me. Aside from being a former champion junior miler (his 29-year-old Irish junior mile record of 4:02.6 was broken only in 2004), aside from having run the Fifth Avenue Mile as an actual elite runner, aside from currently representing as a sports agent a lot of elite athletes who have competed in the Olympics (such as Webb, who kept walking past me and was now looking so focused that I was avoiding looking at him the way you avoid pointing a laser at your eyes), Ray Flynn is a nice guy. As such, he seemed to take pity on me, a faux-elite runner, the way you would take pity on a dog about to run onto a freeway.

"I'm going to do six of these?" I said, pointing to the warmup directions.

"No, you're not," he said. He inspected the computer printout. "You're going to try two of these."

I did what Flynn said. In between strollers, Rollerbladers, and calm-looking pedestrians, I ran into Central Park and sprinted frantically back and forth between the park entrance and the park's main road, where I kept seeing a pack of elite female runners flying past, gliding like a herd of gazelles. I finished and returned to the starting area. "How do you feel?" Flynn asked.

Who knows how I responded? For it was time to race, and I was in a zone that only a faux-elite-runner-for-a-day can know, a zone that brings a woozy realization that this could go really badly and maybe be captured and repeated on evening TV sportscasts forever, as a blooper.

The next thing I knew I was on the starting line with nine other guys, guys like Craig Mottram, who, at 25, is a retired triathlete and the holder of the Australian record for the mile (3:48.98); Jason Lunn, fifth in the 1500 meters at the 2004 U.S. Olympic Trials; and John Itati, a Pennsylvania-based Kenyan who won the Fifth Avenue Mile (3:56) in 2003. The announcer began to call out the elite runners. People applauded and cheered. Then the elite runners strutted and milled, hands on hips, shaking arms, concentrating, me smiling awkwardly and not knowing what to do with the rest of my non-elite body. I said hello to Anthony Famiglietti, a New York–based runner whose best mile is 3:58.23, and then regretted it. "I can talk after the race," he said. Then the announcer, sounding pretty incredulous, announced me as a guy who "wanted to experience what it is like to run with elite runners," or something like that. People did not cheer; people didn't know what to do. And who can blame them? Never have I felt so out of place. It was like waiting outside the dressing room of a women's clothing store, naked.

There was no pushing and shoving. There was very little talking, if any. No one smelled, since I was really the only one perspiring profusely. I had worn regular running gear—shorts and a white T-shirt, and my only fashion error was not going with a tank top. I would have checked the elites' shoes, but I was getting dizzy when I looked down. They called us to get on the mark. The gun went off ... and I'm telling you, it was as if I had been shot—perhaps by the starter gun, perhaps by a Good Samaritan—because my body went into a running shock, a kind of shock that doubtless made me appear to the spectators as a running joke. Warm fluids and stars flushed through me and whirled around my sentient self in such a way as to suddenly whoosh my limbs forward without any input from me; I was on automatic faux-elite runner, a kind of hyperadrenaline rush that I have never felt before and, frankly, hope never to feel again. I figured I was running really slowly, given that the pack was racing ahead, but, like I say, I was not able to do much figuring. I do know that the actual elite runners all veered a little to the right and, in an effort to distinguish myself in some way, I headed toward the left. That's all I can really remember about the first quarter mile, other than being scared out of my mind.

Of the second quarter mile, I remember being in the middle of the street in New York City and hearing someone breathe in a manner that I would call bison-esque. I remember realizing it was me. My breathing sounded as if I had just finished a long race. I also remember hearing someone cheer me, some poor confused person. I could not sense my time, so nerve-fueled was I. I could only see the runners moving far, far ahead, just a pack of runners, so that I stopped caring about them. My plan to run a 1:45 for the first quarter was officially out the window because I just wanted to finish. Please, please let me finish.

I returned to semi-awareness somewhere in the vicinity of the halfway point, when I passed over the crest of a small hill and looked down Fifth Avenue and saw a pack of flashbulbs going off at what I assumed was the finish line, indicating to me that the actual elite athletes were finishing.

When I subsequently realized that I was the only "elite" still running, the course took on a different feel; the Fifth Avenue Mile felt so empty, highlighting the question that is often at the heart of running when you are pushing yourself: Why? At one point, I heard people laughing at me, which, given my condition, was like laughing at someone in a trauma ward. And yet it was this laughing that inspired me to take control of my breathing, or try to. Next, I was faced with a challenge that the elite runners rarely contend with: the police, thinking that the race was over, began to remove roadblocks, which would allow people and cars back onto Fifth Avenue. Thinking semi-clearly, I put my fingers to my mouth and gave my best taxi-calling whistle. (In a loud whistling competition I would be an actual elite athlete.) The cop was totally cool. "Ooh, sorry, buddy," he said. And then he cheered me on. "You're almost caught up to 'em."

As I passed the marker for the last quarter mile, two things were happening: (1) My brain functions were returning; (2) I was clearly feeling kind of sick. At this point I made my most elite-athlete-like move, the move I am proudest of, even if it probably wasn't measurable: I kicked it out, giving it all I had, which was not much, but there you have it.

I WOULD SAY THAT ARRIVING at the finish line in the wake of elite runners was like arriving a few hours late to a party that's already been over for a week and the people hosting it have moved away. I tried to avoid the cameras and post-trace interviews while I was looking around for garbage cans to offer my comments to. In a minute, I found my wife and daughter, who, they later told me, were thinking that maybe I had not run, after waiting and waiting and, yes, waiting for me to cross the line. "When we saw the professional women racers running so fast, we thought you'd be too embarrassed to run," my daughter said.

"Are you all right?" my wife asked.

I was told my time—6:16.95, which was fine by me—and then the thought of tossing my cookies passed. In a few seconds, I was breathing like someone with bronchitis who smokes four packs of cigarettes a day, which made it difficult to share my time with the elite runners, none of whom were even winded. Apparently, Craig Mottram, the Australian triathlete turned full-time runner, had beaten Alan Webb in the final stretch, coming in at 3:49.9. Back at the elite tent, the elite runners all made me feel like a champ, smiling and telling me how great I had done, a feat of championship performance in itself, in that, from what I can gather, I looked like crap. Then again, even if my lungs would ache for the next three days, I have to say I was feeling pretty good. Though I was beginning to be hunched over, I was on a postmile high. I was even thinking of trying again next year, in the non-elite competition. After all, on that afternoon, in that crowd of elite runners, in a pack of the best runners in the world, I had come in tenth, which was not bad at all.

WONDER BOY

BY BILL DONAHUE

*Take a trip to Bhubaneswar, India, and witness the circus act
surrounding Budhia Singh, the prodigy who ran 40 miles at age 4.
This alarming, astonishing feat brought lots of questions—
about his caretakers, his exploits, even the nature of celebrity.
But first: Is his story a fable, a miracle, or a nightmare?
Or all three?*

AUGUST 2008

IF YOU STAND LONG enough by the temple complex, you will see them—
the pilgrims—weaving on bare feet through the choked, filthy side streets,
past bone-thin wandering cows and past amputee beggars and street children and mangy dogs sprawled on their backs on the cobblestone.

Patiently, the pilgrims pick their way through the mayhem of Puri, India,
until they catch sight of the terraced white spires of Jagannath, a labyrinth of
some 120 temples. Then they drop to their knees and pray—and, watching, you
see how the gritty physical world and the shimmering spiritual realm are deeply
intertwined in India, sometimes in strange ways.

ON THE MORNING OF May 2, 2006, a little boy stepped into the streets of
Puri, in running shoes. Budhia Singh was 4 years, 3 months old. A slum kid from
a nearby city, Bhubaneswar, he wore bright red socks and a collared white tennis
shirt that drooped to midthigh. His task that morning, as prescribed by his
coach, Biranchi Das, a one-time all-India judo champ, was to run home: 43 miles
back to Bhubaneswar, the largest city in the state of Orissa, through the rising
heat of northeast India's most sweltering season.

If all this sounds stranger than a fairy tale, consider that Budhia is now a
celebrity in India. He's starred in a popular music video in which he runs, does

judo, and unleashes a hip-hop chant, "I am Budhia, son of Orissa." Indian newspapers regularly hail him as a "wonder boy" bound for the Olympics.

As he stood in Puri, Budhia was said to have run six half-marathons and train 120-plus miles a week. Sometimes he ran barefoot on asphalt. Almost always, he ran without hydrating. "If he drinks while running," reasoned Das, "he will go weak."

This run wasn't a race; it was a test with a spiritual resonance. Budhia was traveling a route that millions of pilgrims had ridden in buses: running north from Puri, with its 900-year-old holy shrine, and past the Sun Temple, a World Heritage site boasting exquisite stone carvings. Das had alerted the media and worked his connections with the Central Reserve police force. A squadron of officers and cadets in khaki shorts was ready to run with the boy. Budhia stood hip high among them. He looked little and fragile.

In time, Das would be pilloried by critics arguing that no 4-year-old should be forced to endure the ardors of long-distance running. Three days after Budhia's Puri run, Orissa's Minister for Women and Child Development would sweep in to arrest Das, who was also the boy's foster father, on charges of child cruelty. Later, newspapers would air lurid accusations. Budhia's mother, Sukanti Singh, alleged in 2007 that Das hung her son upside down from a ceiling fan, splashed him with hot water, and branded his skin with the name "Biranchi Sir." Budhia himself told reporters, "He locked me in a room for two days without food." His mother took him back from the coach.

All very damning, except that a medical report, conducted by a neutral forensics specialist, Sarbeswar Acharya, revealed that the scars on Budhia's body were three to six months old. They were not caused by scalding water, Acharya opined, and not corroborative of Sukanti's claims. And a newsbreak in the spring of 2008 only deepened the mystery.

On April 13, 2008, Biranchi Das, 41, was murdered—shot dead outside his judo hall. The prime suspect, a gangster named Raja Acharya, who faces some 30 unrelated counts of extortion, murder, and kidnapping, is now in jail, awaiting trial. He was infatuated with a lovely Indian actress, Leslie Tripathy. Police speculate that Das irked the gangster by cautioning him to stop harassing Tripathy. If they're right, perhaps Das died for honor. Then again, you could ask why he was hanging out with a violent thug like Acharya in the first place. And was he himself the sort of tough who might thrash a child?

No one (except Budhia himself) will ever know for sure, and there's an outside chance that the boy's scars could have accrued without anyone striking him: in Bhubaneswar's slums, open cook fires are always burning, and rusty nails and broken glass are heaped by the roadside. All that's clear is that nearly every adult in Budhia's life has caused the boy harm.

There is something about kids—their magic innocence, maybe—that can make adults go crazy. Anyone who has ever endured a child-custody battle knows how covetous grown-ups can get. And this is a story about adults going crazy—and about a child trying to remain whole amid the chaos. It's a story about a sort of custody battle, one lacking moral clarity. Biranchi Das wasn't a pure villain; in some ways he shined with devotion.

Back in Puri, he bent to the ground and tied Budhia's shoes. Budhia started to run, at roughly 10 minutes a mile, up a long, slight incline, past roadside shops where vendors sold milky chai for 10 cents a cup and past bald patches of land where long-tailed monkeys crouched by the road, watchful and still.

The police officers surrounded Budhia, their boots scuffing the pavement with a militarized rhythm, and TV cameras craned in at the boy, shooting footage that would later verify that this run was no hoax. Thousands stood at the roadside. Later, everyone in Orissa would speak of how the crowds felicitated Budhia, and that word, carrying hints of fervor and ecstasy, seems to fit. Several times, spectators rushed toward the boy, attempting to garland him with a necklace of orange and red marigolds—the flowers that abound in Indian temples.

Budhia kept going. He crossed a bridge over the River Kushabhadra and passed the fishing village of Chandrabagha. With temperatures climbing into the 90s, Budhia drank only a touch of lemony water. He tired. Then, three miles short of his goal—seven hours, two minutes into his run—Budhia collapsed from exhaustion. He began vomiting and convulsing. Over and over, he bit at the arms of Jyotsna Nayak, the doctor tending to him.

Nayak later told a British filmmaker, "Brain irritation was there. Had I not been there, he certainly would have died." And large questions seemed to hang in the air: Do coaches and parents have the right to conscript children to chase after glory? Who sets the rules? And why are we so transfixed by the bizarre achievements of a 4-year-old boy? Sitting here in the world's most affluent nation, fretting over what type of soy milk our kids are drinking, are we entitled to dictate how the talent of a desperate Indian slum kid ought to be nurtured?

Budhia was thirsty. Nayak gave him water. And before long, the boy bounced back. After all, he'd seen hardship before.

BUDHIA SINGH WAS BORN in Bhubaneswar's Gautam Nagar slum, in a shanty that has since been razed to make way for the railroad. His mother worked, in Indian parlance, as a peon. She did domestic chores, earning $6 a month. Budhia's father, meanwhile, was an alcoholic addicted to ginger—dirt-flecked firewater that women sell from battered metal bowls by the roadside in India. He was unemployed, a beggar who contributed nothing to his family's welfare.

Budhia's parents knew Biranchi Das, who was the president of their slum in Bhubaneswar, the owner of a hotel, and a partner in his family's taxi business. For more than a decade, Das had run an esteemed judo hall, handpicking athletically promising boys and girls from the slums and subjecting them to an almost paramilitary training regimen with twice-daily workouts, strict dietary rules, and classes on combat theory. Seven of his students have become national champions, and more than 1,200 have launched careers with the Central Reserve police force.

I met Das four months before he was killed. He was stout and bearded, rippling with muscles despite a little potbelly, and he exuded the dark, burly beneficence of a Mafia don.

In 2003, he said, Sukanti asked if 1-year-old Budhia could bunk at the judo hall. "She had three daughters, all older than Budhia," Das said, "and already she'd sold the two oldest into servitude, as maids. She told me, 'I can't afford this boy. I can't feed him. Take him.'"

Das said no—Budhia was too young for judo. But about six months later, according to Das, the boy suffered an accident. Riding the crossbar of a neighbor's bicycle, he crashed, fracturing his ankle and shredding the skin on his leg. Untended, the wound festered and got infected. When Sukanti at last took her son to the hospital, doctors advised amputation. Terrified, she returned to Das. This time he said he'd care for the boy. Budhia lived with Das and his wife for six months, until his leg healed.

Then the boy went back to his mother, only to be hit by tragedy. Inside a month, Budhia's father died. Soon after, Das asserted, Sukanti sold her son to a bangle vendor, a man who sold peanuts and gum from his bicycle, with the expectation that, in time, Budhia would work as an assistant. "The vendor didn't take care of Budhia," Das said. "When Budhia visited me after one month, his skin was pale, his clothes were dirty, and he had sores on his body." Das said he bought the boy back for $20. Then one day when Budhia was just 3, the boy cussed. Das punished him, forcing him to run around a dirt oval "until I get back."

Five hours later, Budhia was still running. Soon Das decided that Budhia would become the first Indian runner to win an Olympic medal. He began training the boy, riding on his bicycle as Budhia ran—four miles a day at first, then six, then 10. In time, crowds of adoring fans joined the runs, trotting behind the boy or rolling beside him on bikes.

In October 2005, Das took Budhia, then 3, to his first race—a half-marathon in Delhi. Race officials forbade Budhia to start, but no matter. He was the darling of the 6-K fun run, and the It boy of a postrace gala. British decathlete Daley Thompson tried to score a kiss from Budhia, but Tim Hutchings, international administrator for the London Marathon, fulminated, "For a child of 3 to be training hard is verging on criminal."

By now, a British filmmaker was tracking Budhia's story, making a half-hour TV documentary, and Das was hatching intricate plans. He decreed that, after the Puri run, Budhia would run a marathon in Nayagarh. "After that," he said, "he'll go to Madras, and then there's a race in Cochin, and onto Guwahati. After this we will take him to some events abroad."

He never competed in these races. After his Puri run, Orissa's child welfare department issued a medical report finding him "undernourished, anemic, and under cardiological stress." The agency banned all children from entering distance races before the age of 14. In India, the ruling was largely seen as ridiculous. "How self-indulgent and naive can our liberalism be?" railed *Khaleej Times* columnist Barkha Dutt. "This is a chance for a poor slum child to break down the class divide and travel on the same superhighway to success as everyone else."

Snubbing officials, a public poll named Budhia the second most popular person in Orissa. A steel company hired the boy as a spokesmascot, and a Dubai businessman flew Budhia and his coach to the Emirates for a splashy getaway at an amusement park. Then came the video that nearly deified Budhia. "We hoped the song would clear many misconceptions about the child," said producer Rajesh Kumar Mohanty. "We have tried to compare him with the mythological Lord Krishna."

OVER THE FOLLOWING YEAR, Budhia's prospects seemed to brighten. With his mother's permission, in September 2006, he'd moved to a state-run sports hostel, where he lived and trained with more than 100 other sports hopefuls, most of them teens. He had a new coach named Arun Das (no relation to Biranchi Das), who promised further glory. Then, on a scholarship, he enrolled at the D.A.V. Public School, arguably Bhubaneswar's most prestigious academy. He was treated like a celebrity on his first day. After his classmates, all dressed in uniform plaid pinafore shorts, clambered to kiss him on the cheek, he addressed the entire student body, from a stage, chirping, "I am Budhia Singh. You will all be my friends. I will help you to learn running."

I arrived in Bhubaneswar on a warm day in the winter of 2007. The city is loud 24/7, teeming with a vitality that is both joyful and desperate. From my hotel room, I heard hundreds of garbage-eating crows cawing in a tree, the low throttle of auto rickshaws, and a nightclub downstairs where middle-aged men paid teenage girls to sing for them.

I later moved to a quieter hotel. I also began counting dead dogs I saw squashed on the roads. In one week, I saw eight. Once, when I was riding with an interpreter, he ran over a puppy and never let the conversation falter. "So your brother," he said, "he is staying in New York?"

Crossing the street was life threatening. There were few public bathrooms, so men peed by the roadside; the stink of urine was everywhere. Orissa has the worst child mortality rate in India, and several times young mothers trailed me, tugging at my shirt and begging me to buy food for their infants.

Biranchi Das's judo hall was an oasis, secreted behind high concrete walls on the spacious grounds of the state museum. One day in the coolness just after dawn, recorded chant music echoed over the grounds. Das stood outside the hall, fresh from a six-mile run, dancing in place like a boxer, then vaulting into a handstand. He plucked a little branch off the ground and began using it, as many Indians do, as an improvised toothbrush.

"How's Budhia?" he asked. "What did Budhia say?" I hadn't yet met the boy, but Das continued. "Budhia is a good child," he said. "I miss him. He and I had a dream. It was not fulfilled. That is agony for me. In Japan and Korea, they start training athletes at age 3. If you don't take risks, you don't get results. I am the person who took risks with Budhia, and I got results."

As he spoke, a friend of his stood nearby, radiating his own athletic vigor. Ashwini Das, 55, is a devout yogi and an Art of Living instructor with the regal bearing and prominent clavicle that comes from a lifetime of Ashtanga and belly breaths. A few years ago, he told me, "I became interested in how Biranchi is growing up this Budhia. This child has an inner facility, and Biranchi just explored it."

Biranchi drifted off, and Ashwini and I wandered through the deserted museum grounds. "When Budhia came to him," Ashwini said, "the child had a physical problem, and Biranchi worked for Budhia as no parent can. Look, there are hundreds of millions of kids like Budhia in India—starving, without even a meal—and among all these children, Budhia alone became an inspiration."

He halted and abruptly asked: "What is the nature of the mind?" I had no earthly idea, so I let him answer his own question. "Whatever you resist," he said, "that persists. If you say, 'I want to sleep,' you can't sleep. Meditation means deconcentration—and Budhia achieved this, as few people can. He had an inner quality."

"You mean he was wise?" I asked.

Ashwini looked at me like I was a total idiot. "No," he said. "Budhia is a small child. He knows nothing of the world. I believe that he had a gift inculcated from a past life—a gift beyond imagination. He can run, and Biranchi brought that talent to life. He is the one who put the petrol in the Budhia vehicle."

SUKANTI SINGH FELT OTHERWISE. I met with her one afternoon in a lawyer's office. Budhia's mother looks about 40. Slender and fine-featured, she wore a bindi (a red dot traditionally worn by married women on their foreheads). Her bony brow jutted out of her yellow sari. She was quiet, keeping her eyes downcast as men yelled around her.

"She's illiterate," said the lawyer, Suresh Routray, dismissively waving a hand toward Singh. "She knows nothing."

Singh's boyfriend also spoke over her. "Biranchi Das is a goon," said Pranakrushna Khatua, a convicted bank robber, according to Bhubaneswar police records. "He threatened to kill Sukanti and her three daughters. He told her that if she said anything about the money, she would die."

We were there to discuss the donations and endorsement money that Budhia had received during the 18 or so months he trained under Das. In December 2007, Singh told police that Das had embezzled more than 60 million rupees, about $1.4 million, from the Budhia Singh Trust. Routray, a corpulent man, about 40, with drowsy eyes and a broad mustache, prepared the legal papers. He did so because he's the president of Salia Sahi (the slum Sukanti Singh now lives in) and also a prominent member of Orissa's Communist Party.

Twice, I'd meet Routray in my hotel lobby, to probe him for details on how he arrived at 60 million rupees. His air was breezy and jocular. "Ah, Meester Bill," he said, hailing me with bearish effusion, "Meester Bill! You want the papers? I will get you the papers." He never got me any documents. Biranchi Das said that Routray was showboating to garner publicity for the Communist Party.

Now, in his office, I asked him, "What companies gave Budhia money?"

"Ah, there were so many companies, so many companies," he responded. He named three, each of which, he reckoned, gave $500 or so. Then he repeated himself: "So many companies."

I wanted to hear what Singh thought, and she bitterly lambasted Das. "When they stopped Budhia from competing," she said, speaking to my interpreter, "he couldn't make any more money for Biranchi. So Biranchi started torturing Budhia. There is no other reason."

Singh argued that Das had bullied her into lying to the media. "That story about me selling Budhia," she said, "it wasn't true. I never sold my son. Biranchi just made me say stupid things. I said them because I was depressed."

Singh talked of her husband's death. "He left me without one pie," she said. "My neighbors had to pay for the cremation. When they demolished my house to make way for the railroad, I asked Biranchi for money. I said, 'You have taken all the money that my son earned. You should give me money to rent a house.' He said, 'There is no money left. We spent it on Budhia's training.' He is a liar."

Suddenly Khatua's cell phone rang. Budhia was calling from school. He'd just won a 100-meter race for kindergartners. I could hear his joyous voice coming out of the phone—and it seemed that he'd called to talk to his mother. They were still in touch, after all. Press photos have captured her cradling her slender boy in her own slender arms. She visits Budhia once a week, scraping together 10 rupees for the rickshaw ride.

But this was a big meeting for Sukanti Singh. An unfathomable pile of money was at stake, as she saw it, so she did not get on the phone to say hi. She just sat there stooped over the desk, staring dully ahead as she stewed in disdain for Biranchi Das.

BUDHIA IS STILL FAMOUS in Bhubaneswar. On the streets, he is a one-name hero. "Ah, Budhia!" people will say. "Marathon boy!" "Ah, Budhia, he is a miracle!" Once, when I went to meet him at a D.A.V. Public School picnic, he wasn't present. His minders at the sports hostel forbid him to go out in public without a security guard, and on that day, the guard had a holiday.

I finally met Budhia in his classroom. He sat at a desk in his plaid pinafore and brown V-neck sweater. Budhia was watchful, with the whittled, ropy look of a runner, and he fidgeted—overwhelmed, perhaps, by my looming, pale presence. "This man has come all the way from America to see you," the teacher proclaimed in the singsong universal to kindergarten instructors.

Budhia said nothing; he just looked up at me, skeptically. I'd brought a present for him—a book about children of the world. I'd tried to make the gift speak to his worldview: pasted to the wrapping paper were pictures of Budhia himself, running. He picked open the paper as the teacher translated my questions. "Do you like running?" she asked, vigorously nodding her head. "Yes, you like running. It is very fun, isn't it?"

I looked at Budhia and rolled my eyes. Tentatively, he smiled—and for a while, he seemed amused by me. We went back to the sports hostel, where he sleeps in a large concrete room, and he played a little cricket with me, waving a mop handle as I bowled him a yellow ping-pong ball. At one point, he sprinted into the kitchen and came sprinting back, giddy as he pressed his fist toward my hip. "Want apple?" he said in faltering English, his voice tiny and high as he skittered away.

Soon, though, I was no longer a novelty. Budhia sat down in the corner. I thought that maybe now he'd read the book that I'd given him, but no, very carefully he plucked a piece of paper from out of his pinafore and stared at it, delighted. It was the picture of Budhia himself, running and waving to fans.

"YOU TALKED TO BUDHIA? What did he say?"

I'd expected that Biranchi Das, facing the torture accusations, would shun all my calls and refuse to be interviewed. But in fact he was the most media-friendly person I met in Bhubaneswar. He was polished and genial, and it seemed that impoverished slum dwellers considered his office a small font of hope. One afternoon I found him meeting with a man who needed money for his sister's wedding dowry. Without the money, his sister couldn't marry; her future would be cast into doubt. "Five minutes," Das told me.

The meeting lasted for half an hour, and when the man emerged, he was smiling. Das had promised he would help, personally, in a couple of weeks. "Right now," Das explained to me, "I only have 700 rupees [about $16] in my bank account. I am a poor man. I didn't get rich from Budhia. All the money we got came to 1.32 lakh rupees [about $3,100], and we spent it on Budhia's training."

Yet on another occasion Das hinted that he had profited from Budhia. "I adopted him," he said. "If he makes some money, I deserve some of it, don't I?" Later, Das fed me what seemed an outright lie. "This judo hall," he said, "is the production center for Budhias. Right now I am training four new Budhia runners. They are all between 3 and 5 years old. They are training every day. They are practicing. I have videotapes, but I cannot show you. It is all very secret right now, but when the day comes—when it is time for them to perform—I will tell everybody."

I asked at least five children at the judo hall if they'd seen any preschoolers besides Budhia Singh training as runners. They all looked at me with blank stares. No, they had not seen the new Budhias.

Even when he was joking, Das oozed swagger and bravado. One morning, he smugly summoned me to lie on the judo mat. Then he sicced one of his young behemoths on me as I struggled to break free of the boy's hold. When the farce was over and I lay there, whipped, Das chuckled and tossed me a little tip—a two-rupee coin.

Das's police record was not pretty. After the Child Welfare Committee for Orissa's Khurda District took Budhia out of Das's house, the judo coach allegedly organized a mob of 200 protesters to rally outside the home of Rabi Shankar Misra, the agency's chairman. Misra contends that some protesters burned his effigy, climbed a wall into his property, and surrounded his house for several hours. Misra also accused Das of using Budhia. "He got a free trip to Dubai out of him," Misra told me. "Would he be able to go to Dubai otherwise?" (It was a valid critique, but a few days later Misra himself tried to milk the Budhia story for a free trip. In answering *Runner's World*'s request that he e-mail some legal documents, Misra demurred. "I can give you a presentation on the complex issues," he wrote, "in your office in USA, if invited for this presentation.")

Later, in August 2007, after a street accident in which Das's 7-year-old son was harmlessly clipped by a motorcyclist named Sabeer Ekram, Das allegedly burst into the man's home with 30-odd henchmen. Ekram's mother, M. D. Manju, told police that Das beat her son up. "He pelted us with filthy expletives and threatened to set our house on fire," she told the police.

Still, Das had close ties to the police. One afternoon, he brought me across town to visit his top contact at the Central Reserve police force—deputy inspector G. P. Mastana.

Mastana's building was guarded by several machine-gun-toting officers who wore full khaki uniforms topped by brilliant indigo tricorner hats. Scores of young recruits were training as we arrived, running along in lock-step on a sandy dirt road. We went inside. Mastana's office was grand, with a large desk bearing four black telephones and, above that, a plaque honoring men who'd preceded him as deputies. Mastana, who's a Sikh, was sitting there in a turban, very erect—a bristling, fit 60-year-old.

The mood was a bit stiff, so I tried to break the ice. "Jeez," I said to Mastana, "I wouldn't want to wrestle you." He did not laugh, but after a few minutes he spoke warmly of Budhia. "I admire the boy," he said, "and one time I advised him. I told him he could be a supreme athlete, and I said, 'After that, then you can do something good. You can bring glory to the nation—you can become an officer with us and set an example for others.'"

Das was leaning forward in his chair now, listening with rapt appreciation. The troops scuffed by on the roadway outside, and it seemed almost forgotten that we were talking about a little boy who was still learning to read. "What did Budhia say?" I asked.

Mastana stared me down, somber and earnest. "Budhia said he was willing."

TWO DAYS LATER, I SAW BUDHIA on the track at Kalinga Stadium, but he didn't seem particularly focused on athletic supremacy or national service. He was dribbling a soccer ball as some teenage girls in full soccer regalia made pretend futile attempts to steal the ball. He was laughing.

"Budhia is doing his training," his new coach, Arun Das, told me before detailing the boy's current regimen: seven or eight miles a week, a little stretching, a little hopping and bounding, a little horseplay with the soccer ball and the discus.

Arun Das is a genial and wrinkled man, about 60 and a tad flabby, dressed in a blue nylon track suit. As his older runners muscled their way through a speed workout, he sat on the grass, canted back in a lawn chair, savoring the mild winter sun as he spoke fondly of Budhia. "He's like a son to me," he said before adding with a warm, self-derisive chuckle, "Well, more like a grandson."

I asked if he saw Budhia becoming a champion. He laughed. "Now is not the right time to say. Come back in 12 years and I'll tell you."

"But what kind of times is he running?"

The coach looked skyward for a moment, searching for the numbers. "For the 400," he said, "about two minutes."

Two-flat is good for a little kid; it would put Budhia in about the 85th percentile among 6-year-old American boys. Still, I was surprised. The stories I'd read suggested that, like Biranchi, Arun was driving Budhia toward world-class glory. (One headline read, "Budhia gets new coach, dreams for Olympics.") But now I got an inkling that Arun Das was like no other Budhia caretaker I'd met in all the days I'd spent rattling around Bhubaneswar in auto rickshaws. It seemed he might be playing a gentle trick on the Indian people—administering workouts, proffering photo-ops, and gamely sustaining the illusion that Budhia was on the brink of greatness while simultaneously protecting the boy. He was, it struck me, letting Budhia be a kid in a society where a leisurely childhood is a luxury.

After a few minutes, Budhia trotted toward us to high-five a sprinter standing nearby. I tried to ask him a question, but by the time my words had been translated, he was already running off toward the steeplechase pit for a game of tag with the soccer players. These girls lived with him, and it looked as though they cherished him as a mascot.

"I am playing," he squealed as I stepped toward him with a question. "Just let me play."

I SAW BUDHIA JUST one more time, at his school, on a day his class was doing "magic painting." Again, the teacher came over to his desk to interpret. "Was it hard," I asked, "doing all that running for Biranchi?"

"No, I just did what I was asked."

"Was it stressful?" He shook his head: no.

"Was Biranchi nice to you?"

Now there was an awkward silence and I could hear the high, happy din of the other students larking about, unsupervised.

Budhia stared at the floor, biting his lip.

The question seemed to put him under enormous pressure.

Biranchi Das had helped deliver him to a new and wonderful place in his life. A peon's son destined to caste-bound misery, he was now standing in a cool, pleasant room filled with the nation's elite. He'd transcended social barriers that are more rigid than most Americans can fathom, and he'd performed his own kid-magic. He had survived all the craven adults fighting to control him.

There was something elegant and beautiful about this lean little kid, whose smile, at times, bordered on beatific. Maybe, in time, this magic would prevail. Maybe Budhia would turn out all right. But maybe, too, he was scarred. He seemed brooding and insular now. He kept staring down. He said nothing.

"He is not able to express himself," said the teacher. "The question is difficult."

I stopped my interview. Budhia finished his painting (of a Christmas tree), and then the class streamed outside to do calisthenics in the red, dusty school-yard. There were two parallel lines of kids, and the exercises were supposed to be done in unison. But of course they weren't. Every kid, including Budhia, flubbed the performance. The lines were a melee of children idly scuffing their feet and wiping their noses and scratching their legs. I stood there and thought about how all of these kids would carry their own quirks—and the history and traumas of their earliest childhoods—forward from here, all alone, ultimately, against the challenge of growing up in a world filled with tough questions.

Eventually, the teacher told the kids to sprint to the back of the playground. I watched for Budhia to stand out—to lope ahead like a sad, lone gazelle. But by now every single kid in the crowd was screaming with glee and sputtering and swerving along over the dirt, and I lost him in a swirl of dust.

AN ARMY OF RUN

BY BENJAMIN H. CHEEVER

> *Soldiers, like civilians, run to get fit.*
> *But in wartime, running is also a bonding exercise,*
> *an escape from combat stress, and a connection to home.*
> *You can't go to Iraq to see it for yourself. But we did.*

DECEMBER 2006

RUNNING IS A DELIGHT, and so authority figures disapprove. A doctor waved me in off the road shortly after we moved into the neighborhood 18 years ago to warn that I'd destroy my knees. "Detach your retina," I was told by an editor over lunch. "Compress your spine, shatter your hips." I can't be the only person who has to run this gauntlet. How many times have you been asked about Jim Fixx? Authority figures in uniform are particularly scornful of vigorous exercise. "Trying for a heart attack?" the veterinarian in his blue smock asked me one torrid summer day, when I came in slightly flushed to get the dogs their shots. Uniformed groundskeepers have blown whistles and shooed me off golf courses. A policeman once tried to pull me out of a triathlon after I'd been hit by a car. That's right, after I'd been hit by a car. I remounted and finished the race. The military, I figured, would be the worst. Soldiers come uniformed and are international symbols of authority. I knew they ran in boot camp, but then even policemen are slim during the pupa stage. Which is why I was shocked when a friend, the writer Esmeralda Santiago, said she had two brothers in the service—and both ran. Frank had run as a bodyguard with the Joint Chiefs.

"The Joint Chiefs?" I asked, bewildered. "They run?"

I had figured the higher up the chain of command you went, the more elaborate the uniform and the slower the man inside. Ulysses S. Grant looked as if he'd been shoehorned into his double-breasted getup. As did Bismarck. Churchill favored a roomy one-piece jumpsuit, which failed to disguise his bulk. Even Napoleon, the little corporal, seems to have been about three months pregnant.

I called Esmeralda's brother Frank. General Richard Myers (retired 2005) loved to run, he told me. "The chairman ran as often as he could." Frank and the general ran when the planes stopped in Germany to refuel. The general ran all over the world. Nor, apparently, is this at all unusual for U.S. brass. When he was Army chief of staff, General Dennis J. Reimer (retired 1999) was famous for the thoughts he had while running.

My first contact with the military was in Germany, where I met with soldiers who had been in Iraq and were heading back. I hope I don't lose you here, but I must say at the outset that to run with soldiers at Camp Ray, in Friedberg, was to take all my assumptions about the U.S. Army and have them turned upside down. As much as I'd feared conscription during Vietnam, I had mourned the loss of the democratizing draft and thought it appropriate that an army protecting a democracy include everybody. My father, the writer John Cheever, forged lasting friendships during World War II. He trained with a heavy-weapons battalion in Georgia. Late in his life and signing books, I saw him approached by a man he had known in Georgia. It was immediately clear that my father liked this guy, that the bond formed in the infantry had not been shattered—as many bonds are in this country—by differences in status and economics. The stranger called my father Joey. The name I knew was John.

People go into the Army now because they have to, I had thought; and yet my guide in Germany, Captain Will Bardenwerper, was a Princeton grad. Bardenwerper was working in midtown Manhattan as a financial analyst when the World Trade Center was destroyed. He decided to enlist. My guide's provenance was unusual enough that he was teased about it, but there were also two Rhodes scholars in the 1st Brigade Combat Team of the 1st Armored Division.

"It was a chance to serve my country, a chance to give back, a chance to defend," I heard over and over as I ran with soldiers through the darkened German countryside. This was late in 2005, so the PT (physical training) runs I was invited on—all about six miles—started and ended before the sun came up.

On my first morning in Germany I ran with 1st Lieutenant Brian Braithwaite, who expected to leave soon for Iraq, where he would lead a platoon. The trails in and around Friedberg are exquisitely maintained, which is a lucky thing, because we barreled along in zero visibility. Racing along at my side, Braithwaite explained his responsibilities as the commander of a Bradley fighting vehicle. When the gunner was about to shoot, he, Braithwaite, would also look through the sights and make certain that the target was justified. This raised the terrible question of a commander's responsibility for the misdeeds of others, and I asked if there weren't some men in the platoon who made Braithwaite uneasy. "I love my men," he said.

We were running beside a river, on a mud path, but it was still black night. The lieutenant and I were setting the pace, although this had more to do with Braithwaite's rank and manners than my speed. The soldiers ran in PT uniform—shorts, running shoes, a gray T-shirt under a gray windbreaker, and a striped glow-in-the-dark strap that could be worn around the waist or across the shoulder, bandolier-style. It was much like the many runs I've made in groups in the States. Except when we had to cross a particularly dangerous stretch of road, one man would step out into traffic, raise his arm, and stop the cars. This was not a group of individuals. This was a team, and with authority.

After the run and showers, we all met for breakfast. One man's favorite PT run (maybe "favorite" is the wrong word here) had involved carrying metal road wheels. Taken from Bradleys or tanks, these weigh 30 pounds apiece. In another case they carried jugs of water, but there were fewer jugs than men, so they had to pass off as they moved together as a group, learning each other's strengths and tolerances.

In the infantry the air of respectfulness was present but not forced. Everybody saluted, and I remembered that this gesture may have started when knights wore helmets and used to open their visors to each other in passing. This was done with the right hand, while the left held the reins.

At one point an extremely high-ranking officer came through a crowd I was in, and all the men stood at attention and saluted. This left me feeling embarrassed and out of step. I didn't want to seem disrespectful. "I shouldn't salute?" I asked Bardenwerper.

"No," he said. "You shouldn't salute."

"So what should I do?" I thought of bowing.

"You're a civilian," said Bardenwerper. "We're a democracy. You outrank everybody here."

THE SOLDIERS RUN FOR the same reasons I do.

1) Because they love it.
2) Because it makes them better at the job.
3) For the T-shirt.

When I went to Iraq last summer, I found that many soldiers had fallen in love with the sport only after they'd faced the stress of combat. A run is crucial when a fellow soldier has been killed, Captain Nicole E. Ussery said as I ran with her on the streets of Camp Victory in Baghdad. The officer must metabolize the horror and sorrow to keep them from demoralizing the troops, she explained. "Running allows you to remember who you are."

Camp Victory is huge, more than 60 acres, and adjoins other large camps. Long trails down range are not always available. Soldiers covet FOBs (forward operating bases) with perimeters wide enough that they can get in a good run. Lieutenant Colonel Thomas Graves had a three-mile perimeter last time he was down range. "I even went for a 10-mile run once," he told me. "Felt like I was getting dizzy."

I had met Graves in his office in Germany, which had a T-shirt drying on the closet door and three pairs of identical Nike running shoes on the floor. Now 42, Graves was in the ninth grade living in Germany when he got a copy of Joe Henderson's *Jog, Run, Race*. Graves recalled the book fondly. "It went through my whole family," he said. "My dad was in the military. My mom started running, I started running..."

Graves holds his staff meeting on Wednesday. This is called the commanders' run and is convened at eight minutes per mile. Like General Myers, Graves has run all over the world. "In Iraq, Kuwait, Korea, Qatar, Panama—just about every country in Europe," he said. "Every time I've gone someplace new, I've always used running to get to know the area. My favorite is the first run out. You're not really sure where you're going. New city, new place, different world."

Like their civilian counterparts, soldiers often want to stretch a workout. Six feet tall and weighing about 210 pounds, Bardenwerper was disappointed when we settled on six-plus miles for the morning outings. "Ten," he kept saying. "We could go ten."

I was particularly cheered to learn that in the no-nonsense infantry running was considered essential. All other things being equal, a fitter soldier is a better soldier. If wounded, he or she is more apt to recover quickly and completely. Not to mention—although several people did—how much easier it is to carry a wounded marathoner off the field than it is to carry a wounded fat man. Every soldier has to pass the Army physical fitness test twice a year, and sometimes more frequently. This requires sit-ups, push-ups, and the two-mile run. In order to get 100 points out of 100, the Army wants men ages 17 to 26 to run two miles in 13 minutes. There's a sliding scale for age and sex, with women of that age wanting the same score expected to cover the distance in 15 minutes and 36 seconds.

The soldiers used to run in boots. Now everyone gets running shoes, and the larger PXs have specialists who will match a shoe to the soldier's foot and stride. While the likelihood of finding the exact shoe you want and in your size is as small at a PX as it is at The Athlete's Foot, the prices are great. I saw a pair I'd paid more than $100 for in New York on sale in Baghdad for $30.

WHILE THE MILITARY RUNNING world and the civilian one are quite separate cultures, they do support one another's shared passion. Therefore, many prominent races in the States sponsor simultaneous, or "satellite," races overseas, in Baghdad and Afghanistan. The Honolulu Marathon does this, as does Boston. The mother race will send T-shirts, numbers, and sometimes even timing equipment.

After Germany, I had hoped to go to Iraq for the marathon that the Honolulu race sponsored in December. When the date was changed, I was told the race might be canceled, so abandoned the plan. It wasn't canceled, and I afterward wondered if I hadn't simply chickened out. Therefore I was excited when I learned that the Atlanta Peachtree Road Race 10-K sponsors a satellite event in Baghdad. I wrote organizer Julia Emmons. The 102-pound dynamo, who has turned her July 4th event into the largest 10-K in the world, told me they'd held the Baghdad Peachtree a couple of times already and the story was an old one. This is different, I explained. I wanted to run in Baghdad. She wrote back: "The Atlanta Track Club cannot endorse anyone going into a war zone, thus potentially in harm's way."

I could see her point, but think of it this way: We have about 130,000 military personnel in Iraq. That's a mighty risk. How dramatically is this changed by the introduction of one more journalist, however frightened? The race was just weeks away when my Army contact in Baghdad, Major Todd Breasseale, gave me the green light. Suddenly I could see Emmons's point. Sure, there were 130,000 military personnel in Iraq, but none of them were me. I'd been trying to do this for months, but now it seemed hasty, ill-considered.

My wife—and bless her heart for this—didn't want me to go. Because of the irregularity of military flights into and out of Baghdad, it would take almost a week to get there, and I was going to spend a full week in Iraq. The last days at home passed in a welter of chores, red tape, and anxiety. There were forms I didn't understand, shots I needed. Why did the Army want to know my blood type? Janet walked by my office and found me standing at my desk holding a piece of string that went from the second button on my polo shirt to the top of my belt buckle.

"What are you doing?" she asked.

"Measuring myself for a bulletproof vest."

She warned me not to tell strangers that I was going to Iraq for a 10-K. "They'll know it's a lie, assume you work for the CIA, and kidnap you or kill you."

"I'm writing a book about running," I'd say, when the subject came up in out-of-family conversation. "This will be the biggest race ever held in Iraq," I explained. "July 4th."

"Oh, that's very brave," everybody said, which sounded like code for "Are you out of your mind?" The runners were more direct. "How hot does it get? Is there a T-shirt?"

I took a C-130 from Amman, Jordan, and landed on the military side of Baghdad International Airport, which is mostly outdoors, mostly sandbags and cement abutments. A cheerful Major Breasseale met me there. I was in chinos, a black polo shirt, and my black TravelSmith blazer. The temperature was likely around 120 degrees. Breasseale told me afterward, "I could tell you weren't from around here." We drove down Route Irish, once the most dangerous stretch of road in the world, but apparently now quite safe.

Still, I was glad to pass through the towers and enter Camp Victory. It's set in what had been a vacation complex for Saddam Hussein, his family, and Baath Party loyalists. The palaces—and there are many palaces—are surrounded by lakes, the water brought in from the Tigris River.

The vast complex looks like a health spa, or a sanatorium with all the colors washed out. The buildings and Humvees are brown. The dust—and there's a lot of dust—it's brown also. The roads are gray. The water is gray, as are the giant carp that swim in it. The helicopters are black. I saw leaves on a couple of puny date palms, but aside from the scum in the lakes, almost nothing is the green of life. One morning after a run, I heard machine-gun fire. "The range?" I asked with false bravado.

"No," said the soldier I was with. "It's one of the towers." As he spoke, the high chatter was replaced with the deeper percussion of a much heavier caliber.

"The tower shooting back?" I asked.

"Or another tower," he said, and explained that sometimes the insurgents drive a car toward the towers, firing as they go.

"They can't have much luck," I said.

"Nope," he said. "They don't have much luck."

There's a small dirigible moored over camp, which, with other unmanned aircraft, is constantly spying down on the surroundings. For this reason, the insurgents are afraid to expose themselves long enough to aim their mortars. And so the fire, when it comes at all, is wildly inaccurate. This was told to me repeatedly and seemed a great comfort to the soldiers, although I couldn't quite shake the knowledge that a person could be killed by a mortar, however badly aimed.

The horror of this war was in my face only once. Major Patrick Stich and translator Alex Kurd brought me to the Blackhawk Bazaar, a collection of small shops behind razor wire. Here "fine" watches are sold, pirated editions of movies, old pictures of Saddam, and hookahs as big as cellos.

Coffee brewed in the traditional manner can be purchased by the cup. Stich and Kurd had been given drinks by an extremely welcoming shop owner, a Sudanese, who had refused to let them pay. They were returning to bring this man a goody bag, including fruit, muffins, and blueberry juice. But now the shop was closed. Kurd was told that the proprietor had been murdered by the insurgents for doing business with Americans.

The news made me frantic to go back to Camp Victory. Victory felt safe, although it never felt cozy. Saddam had money, but he did not have taste. The glass beads for the many chandeliers are not glass, but plastic. The hand-painted tiles seem to have been hand-painted by artists with guns pointed at their heads. The main palace is called Al Faw and is named after the place where the Iraqis had a great and bloody victory over Iran. The halls are decorated with sayings from the wise men of history, including, of course, Saddam himself. Breasseale, whose office was inside, describes the building as "the love child of Elvis Presley and Tony Soprano."

The roads around the lakes are often thronged with armed Humvees with signs in English and Arabic warning everybody to stay back 100 meters. Early in the morning and at dusk, the automotive traffic is light, and the running traffic quite heavy. While I was there, the temperature reached 129 degrees. For this reason much of the running is done at dawn or after sunset.

Navy commander Matt Simms codirected the Peachtree satellite race and won it handily in 34:50. He also had won the marathon sponsored by Boston at Camp Adder near Ur in April. He didn't mention this, of course, and I wouldn't have known had the Boston results magazine not arrived at home the day I returned from Iraq.

While the stress of military life makes a run especially delicious, holding a race in a war zone presents its own problems. Just for instance, there's incidental fire. "We have an overhead announcement system called 'the big voice,'" Simms told me. "It'll say 'Uruh, uruh, uruh, uruh,' like that, and you'll say, 'What's it saying?' There's a marathon at an air base at Taji, just north of Baghdad, that they run every year called the Midnight Marathon. In the middle of that race, they had to stop because the big voice came out. You'd better stop and ditch somewhere. Doesn't matter if you're doing a PB.

"We just had a little fun run on a base that's adjacent to this one," Simms continued. "There was activity in the neighborhood adjacent to the base. It sounded like people were discharging weapons. And you never know if they're shooting each other, or if they're shooting in the air, or if the soccer team won. They just about stopped that race, but they let us finish."

It's tough to live in a country where the explosions you hear are not trucks backfiring. And yet the soldiers I ran with seemed to be facing their predicament with grace and—more surprisingly—with humor. I felt honored to be among them.

The soldiers spoke cheerfully about their own risks and mortality, about a friend who had been shot while running—a stray bullet—and who had been shot five or six times altogether. They couldn't decide if they wanted to be with him, because if there were bullets, he'd collect them in his own body, or if they wanted to avoid him, because he was bad luck.

"I never ran before coming into the Army," Captain Ussery told me. "Being a female in the Army, they either think you're squared away or not worth anyone's time. Running is a way to get in shape. When it's time for physical fitness tests or best-lieutenant competitions, I can hold my own.

"Running lets me work out the frustration of fighting a nameless, faceless enemy that doesn't wear a uniform. It's a chance to be alone, to reflect on the day."

IF RUNNING ALONE IS an opportunity to get away from an individual's troubles, then the races held in Baghdad are a sharing of that escape. Even in civilian life there's something absurd about waking in the middle of the night in order to do something devilishly hard, to run a race you won't win and for no money and very little glory.

Talking with Simms on the evening before the race, I heard that General George William Casey Jr., the U.S. commander in Iraq, is a huge supporter of the sport. Simms said that at the last 10-K, "Casey ran just over an hour." Bernard Creque, director of morale, welfare, and recreation, was listening nearby.

"General Casey?" he said. "No, no. He ran it in 30 minutes."

There was laughter, and somebody said, "Promote that man."

But at the end of the interview, when Simms had explained the care that had been taken to make sure that this 10-K was 10-K—and not 9-K or 14-K—he said, "If this race can turn one more person into a runner, then it's all worth it. Because it makes the world a better place."

So at 4:30 a.m. on July 2nd, I climbed into a crowded SUV. (The date was as close to July 4th as they could manage and still catch a Sunday, their day off, although days off are always conditional.) Breasseale's boss was there, Lieutenant Colonel Michelle (Shelly) Martin-Hing. I'd never seen her pull rank at the office, but now any trace of hierarchal preference was absent. Breasseale was wisecracking cheerfully about how slow he'd be. A former marathon-a-year man, he had broken an ankle (rugby), followed by a leg, wrist, and thumb (skiing). Knee trouble was slowing his recovery.

I saw men coming into the start on bicycles with headlights and rifles. The rifles were stacked and guarded. There were lights and there was music, and there were Portosans. Written in black marker above the toilet I used was THERE IS NO SUCH THING AS FRIEDLY [sic] FIRE. THINK OF THAT 101ST. A second toilet poet had drawn an arrow from the word "friedly," and suggested that the first toilet poet learn to spell.

We'd begun to move toward the start when a truck came in from outside the wire and parted the crowd of runners, as if it were a boat and we the sea. The truck was full of stern men in combat gear. Their getups and expressions contrasted sharply with the cheerful, lightly dressed men and women around me.

In the gray light of dawn, Simms and a chaplain got up on a platform. We heard a letter from Stateside Peachtree director Emmons in support of the troops this day and every day. Then we heard a prayer thanking the Almighty for the tremendous good fortune our nation had already experienced, and yearning humbly for more of the same. Then we turned back away from the starting line, stood at attention, and a live band played the national anthem. Some of the men stood with one hand over their hearts, others with their arms down at their sides, fists clenched.

General Casey didn't run that day, but his habit of turning up at these contests was good for me. After Casey, then over 55, had come in ninth in the 50-to-60 age category, race organizers had introduced five-year increments. This gave me—at 58—a much better chance of placing. We ran on pavement around Saddam's ornamental lakes. The event looked and sounded like a lot of 10-Ks held in the States, with runners joking, "I've peaked," or "Is it over yet?" after the first mile. No crowds, though, along the curb, no dogs attached to leashes, or husbands attached to strollers. There were no children holding their hands out to be slapped.

Soldiers, like other runners, are able to channel their competitiveness during a race so that brotherhood comes easily. So when somebody passed me, I said, "Looking good," which is what they said to me when I passed them. "Looking good." Or "Way to go." When I got to the finish table for the 55- to 60-year-olds, the man who gave me the pen said, "You're my first customer," and I was delighted. Turned out nobody had yet finished in the over-50 category either.

"First in my age category," I crowed, as we milled around afterwards. I was a little disappointed by the reaction of my friends. Major Stich, Sergeant Major Paul Stevenson, and Royal Navy Petty Officer Sarah Turner acknowledged my accomplishment, but they didn't exactly jump up and down. I may actually have been jumping up and down.

"First in my age category," I said again and again, as if I might not have been heard or fully understood. When the awards were given, it turned out that Stich had not only won his age category but was also in the top 10 overall, as was the sergeant major, who was running through a bad Achilles. Turner was the fastest woman in her age category. My prize was an Ultimate Direction water bottle with a crimson nipple and a mesh key pocket. It's on my desk at this moment.

Even I agreed that in our little group the hero of the day was Martin-Hing, who took minutes off her personal best and seemed to be teetering on that fulcrum between the regular health-conscious runner and the joyous fanatic. I had heard her say the day before that she'd reached her weight goal.

Of course my success is partly attributable to my antiquity and the dearth of old soldiers. I ran 44:21 and finished 47th out of 767 soldiers. It was the largest race so far in Iraq. I ran to write about it and also for the T-shirt, which is the Peachtree shirt exactly, only with Baghdad Division on the sleeve.

When I was running with Stich the next morning, Simms appeared and slowed to give details of the race. I said I'd noticed that there are Iraqi troops in camp and wondered if any had run. Simms said not yet, but that he's hoping to get some in the next event. Now that does sound like a victory.

Reflecting after the race, Sergeant 1st Class Gene Worthy said, "I think the reason behind the festive atmosphere at the Peachtree is that we had almost 800 people together in one place, in Baghdad. It didn't have anything to do with the bad guys, the good guys. It was 800 people together to go run. I think that's why there was a smile on every face you saw."

MY ASSUMPTION THAT THE ARMY was often a dead end had been dispelled by everybody I spoke with, but had been shattered by Captain Travis Patriquin in Germany. He was dazzling in conversation. He was also an example of an enlisted man who'd been in the Army for years before he decided to go to college and then officers' school. He now speaks several languages and is the civil military officer for his brigade.

Patriquin is eloquent about running. "You see guys in the gym who can do a lot of weight," he told me. "We call them 'all show, no go.' Because if you can move a car once, that's great. But if you can't run somewhere and move the car, and run somewhere again and move the car, you're no good to the military."

The brigade I spent my time with in Germany is commanded by a fit, humorous officer who was reluctant to be interviewed because he thought the men should get the attention. Cornered, though, Colonel Sean B. MacFarland spoke movingly of Dave Wottle, who won the gold at 800 meters in the 1972 Olympics. Wottle, he said, "went from last place to first place for the win mostly in the last 200 meters. The famous 'kick' that won the race for him was an illusion, though.

His 200-meter split times were amazingly consistent: 26.4, 26.9, 26.4, and 26.2. It was a phenomenal display of energy conservation. In the Army we call that 'tactical patience.' It means waiting for the right conditions to commit your reserves. I sometimes use the race as a metaphor to coach junior officers who want everything right away and worry when they see others advancing ahead of them, or who are too quick to commit their tactical reserves in battle. Energy conservation, even splits, or tactical patience all amount to the same principle. It's one of the things running taught me about life."

Next time somebody brings up Jim Fixx and his untimely death at 52, you might want to counter with the elder Johnny A. Kelley, who completed 58 Boston Marathons and died in 2004 at 97. Or take courage from the U.S. infantry. These men are more interested in how they live than in how long. A coward dies a thousand deaths; a hero, only one.

WELCOME TO
MARATHON

BY **STEPHEN RODRICK**

> *Yes, that Marathon. Home of the
> 26.2-mile epic, where beauty—and the truth
> about the race's original route—are both
> in the eye of the beholder.* Opa!

SEPTEMBER 2004

IT'S SUNDAY IN THE Greek town of Marathon and standing room only at St. John the Baptist Church. The Greeks do Communion right—no thin wafer, a hefty chunk of bread that the little ones can teethe on and the old folks substitute for a light breakfast. Afterward, the locals linger on the church steps and smoke unfiltered cigarettes. No one looks like they're going to give their hammies a quick stretch and burn out a quick 10-K.

Which is odd, because I'm in *that* Marathon. The Marathon that made you find Kenya on the map, pump your fist over Frank Shorter's win in Munich, and roll the delightfully alliterative Rosie Ruiz off your tongue. It's the Marathon that had you cursing that damn November sun during the last New York City Marathon as you realized Puffy, Puff Daddy, P. Diddy, or whatever his name is, might be ahead of you. All that training and getting beat by a crappy rapper! Oh, the humanity.

Yes, this sleepy town is the cradle of running, from which flow the Tigris and Euphrates of marathon routes. Two routes—one old, one really old—and without either there would be no entry lotteries, no blackened toenails, and no hideous protein gels. Much like the Bible and American foreign policy, the routes are open to interpretation, with reality not always squaring with the myth. And much like the Bible and American foreign policy, reality doesn't always matter.

According to legend, the original route begins not more than a few wind sprints from St. John's. Back in 490 B.C., the Athenians stomped on the Persians in a battle where they were at least three-touchdown underdogs. The high command sent a poor sap named Pheidippides running from here to Athens, in full armor and undoubtedly low on electrolytes, to tell the city folks. He arrived, gasped "we won," and then kicked the bucket.

Fast forward 2,500 years. It's 1896 and the modern-era Olympics are being hatched in Athens. A suggestion is made that a race be run that mirrors Pheidippides' jaunt. A course is laid out from Athens to Marathon, and that first race is won by a Greek water boy named Spyridon "Spyros" Louis. The modern marathon is born.

Not that you would know it. Here in Marathon, there's no Spyros Louis statue. No T-shirt shops. Not even any limited-edition Gatorade. If this were America—and the locals are quite happy that it is not—there would be an interactive museum, Spyros Louis action figures, and a finish line photo-op where you could stick your head into a cardboard runner so it looked like you won the first marathon.

Maybe there's a lack of hype because the locals know the truth. Or, more correctly, know the lack of truth. Greek historians whisper that while there are records of the Greeks using long-distance runners as messengers, Pheidippides' Athenian run didn't make an appearance in historical accounts until 600 years ago. Translation: Pheidippides' route may be less real than Dorothy's yellow brick road. And, by the way, if Pheidippides or a pal did hightail it to Athens, it almost certainly wasn't on the Olympic route. For one thing, Pheidippides ran, at most, only 20 miles. For another, the Athens Olympic route—the one that modern warriors like Paul Tergat and Paula Radcliffe took on in 2004—is marred by miles of strip malls and well-organized gangs of man-sized wild dogs that nearly devoured my left leg in nearby Rafina. No, Pheidippides' legendary route went straight up through the surrounding steep hills, a run that would cause Khalid Khannouchi's quads to go into full arrest. And the legend of Spyros Louis? Well, more than one Nancy Negativity has suggested he may have taken a shortcut through a shepherd's meadow.

And yet, such conflict serves no one well. So, outdated map in hand, I set out this past spring in search of the two routes that mated and breech-birthed this odd human endeavor known as marathon running. I spent 10 days driving every mile of the official Olympic course, investigating leads about the "real" route, hunting for a Marathon citizen—man, woman, or sheep—who has actually run a marathon, and unraveling strands of myth, heroism, and possible chicanery. But most of all, I discovered an Olympic town that perfectly mirrors the agony and absurdity of running 26 miles for pleasure.

CHURCH SEEMED LIKE A good place to start. For one thing, it's the only place open on a Sunday morning. Okay, it's also a logical spot to atone for my sins of last night—an ill-advised, ouzo-soaked search for Marathon after dark—and get an ecclesiastic take on the upcoming festivities. The Olympics are returning to Greece whether the Greeks are ready or not—and man, they are so not ready.

Sunday services have never been more beautiful. St. John's is filled, in the Greek style, with a kaleidoscope of icons: the Madonna and child, the apostles, and a multitude of saints that my Jesuit education leaves me unable to identify. The pews are like box seats at a new ballpark; all chairs are individual and ornate. Up top, there are literally angels in the architecture, and an explosion of colors created by either God or Crayola. Down below, a husky woman clears the altar. She sternly motions to me that I should uncross my legs, apparently a taboo in Greek churches.

Properly seated and benefiting from a few moments of contemplation, I reverently approach Father Peter, the local pastor. Kindly and bearded, he places a warm hand on my shoulder. Through my translator, I ask him if he's excited about the global attention the Olympics will bring to his flock. The Chamber of Commerce did not vet his answer.

"All the attention to the pagan festivals and pagan gods of the ancient Olympics doesn't sit well with me," says Father Peter. His face goes stern, reminding me of my delinquent altar-boy days. The Greek Orthodox religion is the only show in town, so Father Peter's words carry serious weight. "We're reveling too much in the pagan pastimes," he says. "I don't approve." His eyes lock, Rasputin-like, on mine. I back slowly out of the church. Man, you know it's a tough town when the priest refuses to bless the Olympics.

Seven years ago, it seemed like such a good idea. That's when Greece won the bid for the 2004 Games, making it the smallest country ever to host the modern Summer Olympics. Of course, 2004 was a consolation prize for Athens' failing to get its act together and losing the bid for the '96 Games, the 100th anniversary of its hosting the inaugural games of the modern Olympics. But surely, the IOC organizers theorized, with the seven-year ramp-up, Athens would be ready for 2004. Alas, they didn't consult the Greek artist Yannis Tsarouchis, who once remarked, "Greece is fine as a backdrop, not as a reality."

And the reality is that the Greek work ethic hasn't meshed with Olympic deadlines. Which you might take as an ethnic slur, except that the Greeks embrace it. This is a country that still celebrates a daily siesta from 3 p.m. to 6 p.m. It's considered bad form to use the telephone during those hours; all well and good if you're running a Club Med in the Greek Islands; not so good if you're trying to build Olympic facilities. During my stay, the Greeks cancel plans to build roofs on the Olympic stadium as well as the natatorium. They argue that roofs were always a dealer option. Cynics wonder if the Greeks would declare water and electricity optional next.

Another scotched work project was a light-rail line between Athens and Marathon. This forces me to rent a car in Athens and drive to Marathon in a Hyundai that's ill-prepared for my big fat Greek *Cannonball Run*. There, I meet Maria, my translator. She is beautiful, brilliant, the daughter of a movie star, and, like many Greeks I encounter, believes 9/11 was either ordered by Bush the Younger or was a David Blaine–like mirage. Once we agree not to discuss politics or virtual Armageddons, we get along fabulously.

Perhaps her most endearing quality is that she doesn't smoke, unlike the majority of her nicotine-obsessed nation. There had been multiple signs at baggage claim in the newly opened Karmalis Airport prohibiting smoking. I counted three violators within five minutes, including my customs officer. It reminded me of what a runner who once ran the Athens Marathon observed. "Everywhere I went," he said, "the judges, the people handing me water, little kids, were all smoking." On the way from the airport to the hotel, my taxi driver's Marlboros had filled the cab with so much smoke that I could barely open my eyes long enough to see him or the road. Which was fine, because the ride depicted an urban sprawl of faux classical mansions nestled against tin shacks with satellite dishes. Athens is Tijuana-like in its dismissal of the word *aesthetics*.

Alas, National Route 83, a.k.a. Marathon Avenue, is not paved with gold or good intentions. In spots, it isn't paved at all. Where there's road, backhoes and bulldozers block traffic. As I sit in my Hyundai amid the cacophony of horns, motorcycles, and furious men screaming words I can only assume are not compliments, I drag out the map. I'm supposed to be retracing the Olympic route (albeit in reverse). Clearly, I have taken a wrong turn, ending up on a two-lane road that makes a Costco parking lot look like a Monet painting. I stop at a gas station and ask for directions. The man behind the counter listens, tries to sell me lottery tickets, and breaks into a belly laugh. "Oh you're on the right road," he says in English. "Can you believe it? This is the marathon route." He lets out another belly laugh. "Only in Athens."

A few days later, I pick up an old copy of *The Athens News*, an English language daily, and read of a Greek Olympic official describing Route 83 as a "bordello." While construction promises to expand two lanes to four, no amount of asphalt will beautify a route featuring 17 Shell gas stations, old women selling live chickens out of the back of pickup trucks, and neon signs offering the unique culinary pleasure of "Canadian Pizza."

It's not all the Greeks' fault. Back in 1896, the Olympics featured only 14 countries, no women, and 311 total athletes. So this road, almost all bucolic pasture, was perfect for the 46 runners who ran and the few shepherds who watched the marathon. Unfortunately, 108 years later, the route is unchecked suburban sprawl, Glitter Gulch on acid and day-old feta.

Making matters worse, the fresh blacktop—if it gets laid in time—will still be radiating heat when the men and women marathoners start their respective runs at 6 p.m. To mediate the scorch, organizers were expected to plant hundreds of olive trees for shade. Alas, during my visit, the trees had yet to be planted, and every runner knows a year-old tree provides less shade than a floppy hat. It's as if Major League Baseball decided this year's All-Star game would be held on the site of the old Ebbets Field and ignored that the park was now a high-rise apartment complex. The tragedy is that the Aegean Sea, just a few kilometers to the west, would provide dramatic runner-with-ocean backdrops that would make executives at NBC, which will broadcast these Games, cry real tears of joy.

I PULL INTO MARATHON, unable to find a single sign proclaiming, "Welcome to Marathon, Home to the Original Marathon." A unibrowed taxi driver sits in his cab in the town square. With a gruff point he gestures toward a white marker in the ground that's smaller than gravestones I've seen in pet cemeteries. In Greek, it reads, ON THIS SPOT, THE 1896 MARATHON WAS HELD. IT WAS WON BY SPYROS LOUIS.

Then, it's over to City Hall for a chat with the mayor. Dr. Evangelos Mexis's dual careers dovetail nicely. In the morning, Mexis, a cardiologist, revives people's hearts. In the afternoon, Dr. Mexis tries to revive his town.

"Marathon should be the Vatican for runners," says Mexis, a stylish man in a leather jacket. He politely dismisses a staffer who informs him a contractor wants to do a project off the books. "Runners should make pilgrimages here," he says before letting out a rueful laugh. "Of course, now if there was a pilgrim he wouldn't believe he was in the right place. We don't have a single hotel."

Marathon's mayor pithily captures the challenges confronting his town of 8,000. "We have too much concrete," admits Mexis. Indeed, Marathon, an amalgam of farmers, sheepherders, and retirees fleeing Athens, is a squat city of nondescript two-story buildings, the sporadic crumbling house, and not much else.

Not that Mexis doesn't have dreams. "I would like to sponsor a race between all the diplomats based in Greece," says Mexis, his eyes twinkling. "That way, word would get out all over the world."

We talk for a few minutes about the challenges of selling Marathon as a tourist stop only reachable by the road from hell. After a pause, the mayor edges up in his chair and looks at me and then at Maria. "That's not the route Pheidippides took," he whispers. He points through the walls toward the massive hills that surround his town. "He went up and over."

The mayor then gives a little history lesson on Pheidippides' story. Back in 490 B.C., the Greeks found themselves besieged by the Persians and their boss, Darius the Great. Darius landed 15,000 to 30,000 men just off the coast of Marathon. Freaking out, the Greek high command sent a messenger named Pheidippides on a 150-mile run to Sparta to beg them to send some of their finely trained fighting men. Pheidippides, making the run in full battle dress, traveled to Sparta and back in just three days. To cut a long story short, the Spartans told him they were right in the middle of a big pagan holiday and couldn't possibly get to Marathon for another week.

Without reinforcements, Greek general Miltiades came up with a plan: go on the offensive. Despite being outnumbered, he ordered an attack. The Persians quickly crushed the Athenian center, momentarily believing they had won the battle. Then Miltiades sent in the rest of his men from the two flanks. Surprised, the Persians were routed.

And this is where it gets tricky. While there are ancient accounts of Pheidippides' much more studly Sparta run, there's no record of him running to Athens and dying, as the commonly accepted legend purports. Some historians have suggested the run did occur but was made by another messenger. Furthermore, most scholars agree that the route was likely through the hills. It was more direct and there were actual roads. The 1896 route was adopted so that the race could end in Panathinaiko Stadium, the site of the former Stadia Olympiad, a ruin from the Olympics of ancient times.

The mayor laughs knowingly at the absurdity of trying to gussy up the hideous, historically inaccurate route. "I try and tell people that we should run the real route," says Mexis. "They tell me to keep quiet."

All is not dross, however. The oncoming Olympics have created a bit of a buzz. Finally, Marathon is getting a museum celebrating the town's running heritage. But despite its location on Marathon's main drag, I can't find it. I pop into the hopefully named New Face, a nightclub-cum-coffee bar, for directions.

Inside, a forlorn woman plays video poker. Behind the counter is Angelis Demetrios, the 23-year-old proprietor. He's a beefy man in a black polo shirt who speaks bluntly. "Whoever comes for the Olympics won't come back," says Demetrios. "They will say, 'Wait a minute, we took a wrong turn.'"

He tells me the local economy isn't doing very well. The country's entrance into the European community hasn't been easy for local farmers long dependent on government-set price controls. There was a freak snowstorm a few weeks back that froze much of the olive harvest, as well as other crops. Tourism is hampered because of Greek laws that prohibit construction on sites where there may be archeological ruins. Marathon has 50 no-build zones. "People here are indifferent; they just keep to themselves," says Demetrios. He polishes glasses and smiles. "They don't have big dreams."

With Demetrios's guidance, I find the museum's address on a third pass. I come across two architects with worried expressions. They are standing in front of a roofless house I had mistaken for an abandoned building. Among the weeds is a sign noting it as the future home of a museum consisting of all things Olympic and Marathon. Scheduled opening date is March 2004. Today is March 1.

"We will finish before the Olympics begin," says the lead architect, a middle-aged woman, "or we will be finished."

On the outskirts of town, there's another construction site, but beyond the first row of bulldozers is a running track. This is where the Olympic Marathon will begin. I keep walking and see something. I rub my eyes. Could it be? Yes, finally. Runners!

Okay, there are only four or five kids. But it's a start. They're members of the aptly named Pheidippides Runners Association. I meet Karena Kostas, the mother of three members. Alas, the Kostas family makes up a full quarter of the PRA. "We used to have 110 runners, but we're down to 13," says Kostas. "Parents sign their kids up for basketball; they don't care about the heritage." She shows me the association's training facilities, which consist of some hurdles, free weights, and mats strewn under the stadium's bleachers. "We could use any money or donations," she says. "Can you mention our Web site?"

I tell Karena I'll try. I inquire about Pheidippides' route. She gives me directions to a route starting a few kilometers west of where Mayor Mexis told me to start. Which isn't all that surprising. As Yogi Berra might say, it's hard to pinpoint where something happened when something might not have happened. I also confess to Karena that I have been trying without luck to find a Marathon resident who actually has run a marathon.

Karena crinkles her brow, pulls out her cell phone, and begins dialing. An hour later, I'm sitting in a coffee shop just down the street from New Face. In walks Dimitrios Kassis, a bubbly forty-something man in a Puma sweat suit. Kassis, a Coast Guard clerk, confirms that he had in fact run the Marathon to Athens race. His accounts come with a "kids, don't try this at home" clause.

"I was a soccer player in high school," says Kassis. He pulls out a cigarette, offers me one, and lights up. "So, in 1980, I decided to run the marathon the day before."

I look at him quizzically. The day before?

He smiles triumphantly. "Yes, with no training! And in brand-new shoes!"

You know where this is going. Kassis gives me the gory details. He started well. (Don't they all?) But around the 15-K mark, he noticed his feet were bleeding profusely. He stopped and took off his shoes. His feet were a mess, but Kassis decided to continue. Barefoot. That worked for a few more miles until the pain became unbearable. He contemplated quitting. Then a pal came along. At his urging, he slipped his now-crimson shoes back on. Somehow, he managed to finish in a respectable four-and-a-half hours. That was just the beginning of the adventure.

"I had to take the bus back home," says Kassis, who now runs 10 kilometers a day. "It was crowded and no one would give me a seat. That took an hour." He grimaces at the memory. "Then I got home. My mother came up to me and said, 'Where the hell have you been?' I told her, 'I just ran the marathon.' She looked at me for a second and said, 'Hmmph.' She turned around and left. She didn't even make me soup or lunch."

The shoes, the bleeding, the bus ride, and no soup. Poor Kassis! Then again, he was only following in the footsteps of Spyros Louis, the patron saint of unorthodox marathon training.

KOSTAS KLEFTOYANNIS IS the cultural affairs director in Maroussi, an affluent Athens suburb resplendent with Benetton and Gucci stores. The silver-maned director is an avid runner and also an avid sleeper. "I'd like to run the marathon someday," says Kleftoyannis, who acts on the side. "But they start at eight and I don't like to get up before ten." Having spent a few days on Pheidippides' home turf, I decided it was time to visit Spyros Louis's hometown, in hopes of understanding things better. Plus, Marathon was a bit of a buzz kill.

Kleftoyannis and I meet at the city's storage center. He cracks open the door. Through the weak light, I see the once proud bust of Louis, Maroussi's favorite son. Poor Spyros is now missing his right ear and his nose. There's bird crap on his forehead and a dead cigarette leans against his neck. "It used to be in the town square," says Kleftoyannis. "Some punks vandalized it."

Sensing my disappointment, Kleftoyannis tells me there is someone I should meet. We make the short walk over to the Maroussi Folklore Museum. In a room full of mannequins exhibiting historical Greek wedding garb, I'm introduced to Eirini Louis, the runner's great-granddaughter. She's a shy woman, but agrees to tell me her great-grandfather's story. First, she shows me some pictures, including one of an aged Louis handing an olive branch to Hitler at the 1936 Berlin Games.

"Giving Hitler an olive branch," says Kleftoyannis with ga-ga eyes. "This was before anyone thought he was bad; to know the future, that Hitler was a man of war, is amazing."

Perhaps sensing that Klefty is piling the BS pretty thick, Ms. Louis offers a startling admission. "Some thought he had run through the farms rather than on the route," says Eirini.

Kleftoyannis looks horrified. "Shh!"

Eirini doesn't listen. "I want to tell you that wasn't true," she says with pride. "There were so many reporters watching the course, there was no way Spyros Louis cheated."

The accounts of Louis's 1896 run are only slightly more reliable than those of Pheidippides'. Not that Louis helped much. He was a man of few words. When a reporter asked years later what he remembered about entering Olympic Stadium in the lead, he responded, "Nothing. I was just very hungry." Through the years, various gospels have been passed down: Louis decided to run after he heard folks from another town trashing Marathon; Louis decided to run because one day, while in the military, he forgot his sword and ran home quicker than a horse, inspiring his commanding officer to recommend Louis to try the marathon.

"Those are all wrong," insists Eirini Louis. "He ran for a girl."

According to her, this is how it went: Spyros was a nice guy who delivered water for a living. One day at the Maroussi spring, he spied the beautiful young Eleni Kontu. Alas, Eleni was out of his league. Her parents were rich landowners, and Pops didn't take kindly to Eleni's being courted by the local water boy.

Spyros needed to do something big. Really big. The inaugural Olympics were coming. He remembered an Army officer who had suggested that he try running the 25-mile race, the length for the event at the time. (The 26.2-mile marathon wasn't formalized until the 1908 London Olympics.) He had forgotten all about it until now. The officer pulled some strings and got Louis into the race.

The people of Maroussi raised money and bought him some shoes. The day before the race, Louis said a prayer to the pagan gods for strength. But Zeus didn't hear him. The day was hot and Louis didn't seem to have a chance. Then, running through Pirkemi, Louis spied the beautiful Eleni and her not-too-impressed father. Eleni gave him oranges, Dad a much-needed shot of brandy. Louis kicked it into gear for the last few miles. He won the race by seven minutes. "Needless to say, Eleni's father gave her permission to marry him," says Eirini with a big smile.

Louis was offered many cash inducements after his victory. He turned them all down except a new horse and cart for his business. He and Eleni had three sons. He never raced again. "Why would he?" says Eirini, mirroring the Greek approach to long-distance running. "He got exactly what he wanted."

NEAR THE END OF my Grecian adventure, I get a call from Karena Kostas, who's quite excited. She has found an actual, bona fide Marathon marathon runner—one who actually trained for it.

Boy, had she ever. Kostas Dassis is the guy in your runners' club that you simultaneously envy and hate. He's 63, nearly bald, possesses some wild ear hair, and tries to break all the metacarpals in my right hand when we meet. The man has run 43 marathons. His tidy home, at just about mile marker 6 on the marathon route, features medals, trophies, and photographs of Dassis finishing last year's Athens Classic in just over four hours. He talks like a cranky prophet long ignored.

"I tried coaching kids around here to run marathons," says Dassis. His dutiful wife sits next to him. She lightly touches his forearm when he gets close to blowing a gasket. "The kids here like to gamble, drink, and play cards. When a marathon runner comes to visit, they turn away and don't acknowledge him."

"My husband beats kids half his age," Mrs. Dassis adds.

I ask Kostas if either of his sons run. He shoots me a glare that says the subject is a no-fly zone. Then Dassis painstakingly describes almost every marathon he has run. It seems like the stories actually last the duration of a marathon. "You can't beat the exhilaration of entering the Olympic Stadium," Dassis says. "But the kids just don't listen."

A mention of Pheidippides sends Dassis into paroxysm of ecstasy. "A TV station asked me a few years ago to dress up like Pheidippides," recalls Dassis, lost in reverie. "They were going to film me running into the stadium." He goes quiet and sad. "Then it rained. They said they were going to reschedule." He looks like the waterworks are on the brink of busting. "They never did."

I say my good-byes and mention the debate over Pheidippides' route. Dassis grabs my arm and points toward the mountains as if to say, "He ran through the hills." He gives me directions to yet another supposed starting place on the hill separating Marathon from the Athens suburbs.

Dassis's starting point is different from both the Mayor's and Karena's, but he's such a running zealot I decide to gamble on his. The next day, I put my running shoes on and head for hills. Armed with Dassis's advice and a smattering of hearsay accumulated from townsfolk, I trot up a dirt path that would test the fittest ultra-marathoner. Maria, my translator, follows at a more leisurely pace. After about 15 minutes, my jog slows to a fast walk. I try to channel Pheidippides and the adrenaline he must have felt knowing that his country had been saved from the Evil Empire of their time. That helps for another half mile or so, and then I am in need of oxygen. I pause, my chest heaving. And I'm startled by what I see. I'm near the top of the hill and the olive fields of Marathon lay before me, the Aegean Sea shimmering in the distance. I open and close my eyes, trying to record a mental picture I won't forget.

Spurred on, I kick it back into what passes for high gear. Again, I wonder what Pheidippides must have been thinking as he approached the crest, knowing his beloved Athens awaited on the other side.

And then I stumble upon a field of abandoned televisions.

My Pheidippides role-playing is smashed. Some local genius has decided to use the top of this mountain as his personal dumping ground. I'm disgusted and actually move faster to try and get past the eyesore. And then I stumble on to a garden of spare tires. Tires as far as I could see. Depression sets in. I reconsider all the harsh judgments I made about the Olympic marathon route.

After Maria catches up, we stumble on to a camp where a middle-aged man and a boy are chopping wood. I tentatively approach, crossing a muddy field. The sunburned man's smile shakes away my fear. As he grips my hand, I feel something moist against my sweaty calves. It's a pig, but Bloum Lamai says he is friendly.

I tell him why I'm here. He grins and clasps me on the shoulder as if he's been expecting me. He motions me toward a tin shack across the muddy field. "This isn't Pheidippides' route," he says. "I will show you, but first we have a drink."

He shows us into the two-room dwelling he shares with his wife and their two teenage sons. The floor is dirt and there's no electricity. Beds take up almost all the space, but the place has a simple dignity. On the walls are pictures of flowers and a Christmas tree neatly cut from a magazine. He offers us a glass of wine and a Marlboro. The family came from Albania looking for a better life. After 12 years, he's not sure he has found it, but he's at peace. His biggest dream is that his sons will emigrate to America.

We relax and talk for an hour, comparing notes on the Olympic construction. He hopes to take his boys to a soccer match, their favorite sport, but he is not sure if he can afford it. After I swallow the last of my wine, he pats me on the shoulder and says, "Follow me."

We walk for a mile or so south through a neighbor's field. Suddenly, Lamai stops and says, "Right there." Then he tells me he has to get back to work. He gets paid by the cord. So I wander another hundred yards and find the remnants of a stone path winding through the hills. I'm not sure why, but touching the ancient rocks tells me I've found the route. I trot a few paces and smile, thinking again of Pheidippides putting one sandal in front of the other. Of course, I could be overly optimistic, confused, or just plain wrong. But if I've learned anything in the past 10 days, it's that you won't get anywhere in Greece on logic alone.

CHASING JUSTICE

BY KENNY MOORE

[
*Twenty-five years after running stride for stride with
Ethiopian champion Mamo Wolde in the Olympic marathon,
the author began another, more urgent race: to get his ailing fellow
Olympian out of the prison where he'd languished—
without being charged or tried—for nine years.*
]

JANUARY 2004

THERE'S A STORY all Ethiopia treasures, in which I learned I played a bit part. It's the story of how the country's primal champion, Abebe Bikila, having won the 1960 Rome Olympic Marathon barefoot (symbolically avenging Mussolini's invasion of Ethiopia in the 1930s), and having won the 1964 Tokyo Olympic Marathon in a world record, set out, in the thin air of Mexico City in 1968, to win his third gold medal in a row.

Then 24, green and idolatrous, I ran at Bikila's side in the early miles, through a claustrophobic gantlet of screaming, clutching *Mexicanos locos*. Bikila, protecting his line before a turn, even gave me an elbow. I wanted to tell him that there was no way I'd ever drive him into that crowd, but I knew no Amharic. He had tape above one knee.

Any Ethiopian child can tell you that Bikila was running hurt. After 10 miles, he turned and beckoned to an ebony wraith of a teammate, Mamo Wolde, the 10,000-meter silver medalist and a fellow officer in Emperor Haile Selassie's palace guard. Wolde wove through the pack to Bikila's side. Thirty-four years later, I would learn what they said.

"Lieutenant Wolde."

"Captain Bikila."

"I'm not finishing this race."

"Sorry, sir."

"But Lieutenant, you will win this race."

"Sir, yes sir."

"Don't let me down."

Wolde, thinking some runners were out of sight ahead, took off. None were, but until the tape touched his chest, he couldn't be sure. He took the gold medal in 2:20:27 by a masterful three minutes.

I got blisters. I'd wrapped our trainer's new "breathable" adhesive tape around the balls of my feet, where it came unstuck and rolled up into ridges of fire. I sat down in Chapultapec Park, took off my shoes, and ripped off the tape—and my skin. I got my shoes back on, hobbled until I bled out and went numb, and finished 14th in 2:29:50.

Thus I was in the stadium tunnel when Abebe Bikila emerged from an ambulance. He caught Wolde's eye, came to attention and saluted. Wolde, mission accomplished, crisply returned it. Wolde's victory meant his country hadn't produced a lone prodigy but a succession. Wolde had made the marathon Ethiopia's own.

Wolde went home, had his portrait enshrined among the Olympic rings atop his national stadium, and eventually would inspire Olympic champions Miruts Yifter ("Yifter the Shifter"), Derartu Tulu, Fatuma Roba, Gezahegne Abera, and Haile Gebrselassie. The tale of Captain Bikila's order to the good soldier Wolde became legend in Ethiopia, but I didn't hear about it until April of 2002, from Wolde himself, when he recalled that I was one of the runners he passed to reach Bikila's ear. Why the delay? A simple matter of the champion being made to rot in Ethiopian Central Prison for nine years.

But before we turn to Wolde's great purgation, let's linger with him as long as we can back before the fall, before he was overtaken by the monumental anguish of his nation.

In the Munich Olympic Marathon in 1972, Wolde and I ran almost stride for stride. With five miles to go we were dueling for second, a minute behind Frank Shorter. Wolde was as soft of foot and breath as an Abyssinian cat. The only way I knew he was there was that distinguished widow's peak bobbing at my shoulder. Occasionally our shoes brushed. "Sorry," Wolde said each time.

On a rough path in the English Garden, a cramp shot up the back of my right leg. Wolde watched me slow and grab my hamstring. He ran on. Then he turned and gave me a look I would never forget. His face filled with regret. It was as if he were saying this is all wrong, we were supposed to race together, and the stronger take the silver and the other the bronze. Instead, Belgium's Karel Lismont caught us both and finished second. Wolde took the bronze. I followed in fourth, 30 seconds behind.

Shorter, stunned at his triumph, embraced me. "I thought at least I had bronze," I croaked. "Wolde took my bronze."

Then Wolde and I shook hands, departed the terror-stricken Munich Olympics, and returned to absurdly opposite worlds.

MAMO WOLDE RETURNED to Addis Ababa, was promoted to captain, and promised a nice house. He never got it, because in November of 1974, Emperor Haile Selassie, age 83, was suffocated in his bedchamber, and his 60 top ministers, admirals, and generals were lined up against a prison wall and machine-gunned. For the next 17 years, a fanatic paranoid named Mengistu Haile Mariam changed Ethiopia from a feudal empire to a Marxist dictatorship known as the Dergue (Amharic for "committee"). Revolutionary guards killed tens of thousands suspected of disloyalty. To claim the body of a loved one, a family had to reimburse the government for the bullets used in the execution. More holes meant more revenue, so death squads observed a two-bullet minimum.

Wolde, being Imperial staff, seemed in mortal danger. His Olympic medals and those from many other championships saved him. He was ordered to take a lowly position in a local *kebele*, a sort of neighborhood council that Dergue officials used to spy on, detain, or torture counterrevolutionaries. He married Aymalem Beru, and in 1976 they had a son, Samuel. Aymalem died in 1987, and two years later, Wolde married young, adoring Aberash Semhate. They had two children, Adiss Alem Mamo and Tabor Mamo.

In 1991, the Dergue was overthrown by the forces of the Ethiopian People's Revolutionary Democratic Front. The new government caught 2,000 suspected authors of the Red Terror and created a special prosecutor's office to try them. Wolde was caught up in this sweep and locked up in Ethiopian Central Prison.

Wolde sat for three years without the western world's notice. Then in 1995, Amnesty International reported that he had been imprisoned without even being charged with a crime. Amnesty appealed to the prosecutor to either charge or release him. Ethiopia did neither, refusing even to say what he was suspected of. When the International Olympic Committee (IOC) demanded an explanation, it was told to back off and "await the verdict of the court."

I remember Shorter, a friend and a lawyer, wondering just how well we knew Wolde. I felt we knew enough. A gold medal doesn't guarantee moral integrity, but what is more basic to the Olympics than forsaking violence? Ideals were involved here. The only way to know was to go find out.

An indispensable ally was 1972 Olympic 800-meter bronze medalist Mike Boit, who was then Kenya's sports commissioner. He urged me to come down to Nairobi, where he got me an Ethiopian tourist visa. And so, on a rainy day in August 1995, the photographer Antonin Kratochvil and I landed in Addis Ababa.

First, we called the special prosecutor's office. Spokesman Abraham Tsegaye blandly said Wolde was going to be charged with "taking part in a criminal act, a killing."

I went queasy. I had come all this way on the strength of a backward glance. Suddenly it seemed childishly sentimental.

"Did Mamo Wolde have access to a lawyer?"

"Not now. Not until he is charged."

"If I was detained for three years without charge, I'd sure have a lawyer."

"Well, in your country, every time you shake hands with someone, you need a lawyer. In Ethiopia it's not such a way."

He said he had no authority to let me visit Wolde, and hung up. Kratochvil took a look at my waxen face and asked a question that turned everything around. "Does Mamo have a wife?"

Did he ever. Slender, doe-eyed, and resolute, Aberash Wolde-Semhate, then 24, welcomed us into their mud-and-stick home off a rocky lane, behind a sheet-metal wall. Son Tabor, then three, gave me a brave, cold, trembling little hand-shake. Adiss Alem, Mamo's 5-year-old daughter, showed us his gold and silver medals from Mexico City.

The wood floors were smooth and clean. Frankincense was in the air. Aberash poured us glasses of home-brewed beer and apologized that Wolde was not able to welcome us himself. We looked at a photo album and she sketched his history. He was born in 1932 in Ada, south of Addis Ababa, and was of the Oromo tribe. She had met him when she was 17 after his first wife died. "When I was in school, I ran a little, not seriously," she said. "But I read about them both, our heroes, Abebe Bikila and Mamo."

When asked, Aberash explained that Wolde was being framed. On a night in 1978, Wolde had been ordered by a top official to put on his uniform and go to a nightclub. At the club, Aberash said, he saw a group of officials with a teenage boy, hands tied behind his back, who might have been in a youth group that fought the Dergue. The officials shot the boy, then ordered Wolde to shoot the body again (the ghoulish two-bullet policy). According to Aberash, lots of people saw him purposely miss. At a hearing in 1992, many witnesses testified that Mamo hadn't killed anyone. "Only one accused him," said Aberash. "The official who shot the boy wants to blame Mamo to save himself.

The prosecutors say they have to keep him in detention until they bring charges, but they never do."

Meanwhile, he'd had bronchitis, hearing loss, and liver problems. Prison meals were terrible, but families were allowed to bring in food. Aberash suggested we come along for a visit.

THE APTLY NICKNAMED End of the World Prison was 10 blocks of postapocalyptic depression. Rusty metal walls surrounded cement barns. In the shelter of a crumbling plaster watchtower, guards lounged in thin blue overcoats, their eyes locking instantly on us, the *faranjoch*, the foreigners. We joined perhaps 200 visitors in an open shed. But when we moved with Aberash toward the gate, someone saw Kratochvil's camera and we were encircled by guards yelling that foreigners were never allowed in a prison. It was a national security offense. One guard, a man with a crippled hand, kept shouting we were cunning foreigners and that it was their duty to ignore everything we said and arrest us. We were ordered through the gate and put on a bench in the courtyard as higher authority was summoned. "Now we are detained," said Kratochvil.

We waited six hours, the man with the crippled hand whining ever more hysterically for our heads. They kept asking for our passports, to prove who we were. We'd left them at our hotel. Finally, we were given an escort there, a huge armored vehicle with six guards. You should have seen the face of the Hilton doorman when we all pulled in. I diverted the officers while Kratochvil went to his room and flushed his film of the prison. A Major Neguesse confiscated our passports, and said, ominously, we would talk the next day.

The next morning, we didn't wait. We went to the dreaded Ministry of Internal Affairs and threw ourselves on the mercy of its chief, a Ms. Mahete, a sour, angular Tigrayan woman in a red dress. When our interpreter said I had run against Wolde in the Olympics, Mahete's expression softened. She held up a hand, made a call, and dictated a letter. In a stroke of impossible luck, we had permission to visit Wolde.

At the prison we held up the letter like a cross before a vampire. The gate rolled open. The guards who had terrified us before shrank back against the walls. Major Neguesse begged to be forgiven. We were led down a rocky path toward a two-story building. Guards were coming down a staircase. Among them was a slender man dressed in a green-and-white sweater, and with a distinguished widow's peak. We fought through our guards and embraced on the steps. He was bony but warm, strong, and excited.

"It all comes back," he said. "You had a goatee. Oh, thank you from my family for this! Remember me to the Olympic brothers."

"You are remembered," I said, and poured out the good wishes of the International Olympic Committee, including a standing invitation to run or be grand marshal of the Honolulu Marathon, in Hawaii, where I now live.

Wolde, thunderstruck, said, "These are words from God."

We had maybe eight minutes together. Then he grabbed my forearms. "It restores my soul," he said. "It is something I can feel in my body, that people outside the country remember." They led him back upstairs.

Watching him go, I thought of what a slender thread had brought me there. But this time it was my turn to look back and cry out that this was wrong, this isn't the way things should be happening.

AFTER THE 1995 TRIP, I wrote about Wolde's plight in *Sports Illustrated*. As a result, that Christmas cemented my faith in human nature. Every day the mail brought copies of letters people had sent to the prosecutor, reminding him that justice delayed is justice denied. Schools and churches adopted Wolde in letter-writing campaigns. Athletes United for Peace, headed by Olympic long jumper Dr. Phil Shinnick and former 49ers quarterback Guy Benjamin, flooded the United Nations' Human Rights Commission with appeals, as did the National Council of Churches.

The most unexpectedly galvanized was Bill Toomey, the 1968 Olympic decathlon champion. Toomey has never been accused of taking life too seriously, but something clicked. As president of the Association of U.S. Olympians, Toomey recruited two-time 800-meter Olympic champion Mal Whitfield (who had coached Wolde in Ethiopia) and former assistant commerce secretary Carlos Campbell to urge the U.S. State Department to press for Wolde's release on bail.

Toomey then postponed his honeymoon, went to Switzerland, and hit up IOC president Juan Antonio Samaranch for help. Samaranch made Toomey the IOC point man on the Wolde case, gave him a check to take to Aberash, and wrote a letter appealing for Wolde's freedom and inviting him to be a guest of the IOC at the 1996 Atlanta Olympics.

Toomey ran with it, stopping in Nairobi to pick up 1968 Olympic 1500-meter champion Kip Keino, arguably Africa's greatest sporting ambassador. In May of 1996, they descended upon Addis Ababa. Toomey called to report.

"The minister of justice was almost in tears at the sight of Kip Keino in his office," Toomey said. "And Kip set it up beautifully. He said, 'In three months, 3 billion people are going to watch the Atlanta Olympics. It's the 100th anniversary of the modern marathon, and they're going to see the great contributions Ethiopian runners have made. And then they're going to see the misery of Mamo Wolde.' That had an effect. They said they'd try to let him out for a day or two. I said, 'The Olympics are 16 days.'

"We got 35 minutes with Mamo in prison. What a nice, humble person! Kip was reliving races with Mamo in Europe and Mexico. Everyone there was moved."

Over the next few months, the IOC reaffirmed its invitation to fly Wolde to Atlanta and the reigning Olympic women's 10,000-meter champion, Derartu Tulu, and the rest of the Ethiopian team bravely asked for his release. Wolde began to allow himself to hope. The Olympic offer seemed to resurrect *ekecheiria*, the mythical Greek Olympic truce under which warriors laid down their arms on battlefields and traveled to the sacred contests of Olympia for 1,200 years.

Unfortunately, that cut no ice with Ethiopia's independent prosecutor, Girma Wakjira. "We know Mamo is a hero of the land," he said. "But how would authorities say, 'Okay, Mamo, we shall prosecute the rest of the people but because you are a hero you can go to Atlanta?'" Wakjira said he would prove Wolde was "head of the revolutionary guard in Addis Ababa's Area 16," and involved with the execution of 14 young people in late 1978 or early 1979.

Wolde neared despair. "My lowest point," he would say later, "was when the prosecutor threw all the Olympic appeals in the dump." He was 64, with liver and lung problems, in a country where life expectancy for men was 46. "My days are numbered," he said. "I hope the world will educate my children."

The Atlanta Games took place without him. Ethiopia's Haile Gebrselassie won the 10,000 and Fatuma Roba the women's marathon. And a powerful NBC report showed Wolde racing in Munich and my trek to his home. The last images were of Aberash and the children waiting outside that dismal, decaying prison.

In Atlanta, Billy Mills, the Tokyo Olympic 10,000-meter champion, suggested we sign an Olympic flag for Wolde. He, Toomey, Shorter, Whitfield, Ralph Boston, Willie Davenport, Rafer Johnson, John Naber, Andrea Mead Lawrence, Wyomia Tyus, and I, among many others, covered the white cloth. When Aberash and the U.S. ambassador to Ethiopia, David Shinn, took it to the prison, the wardens were so impressed, they set up a tea party in the yard for the presentation. "It was ecstasy, it was rejoicing," Wolde would recall. "There were 500 other detainees there, many who'd been government dignitaries and university presidents. When Mr. Shinn held up that flag, there was a cheer from them all."

One Sunday after the Olympics, Wolde stretched to take Aberash's hand through the double fence at the prison. He said the only reason he was alive to receive invitations to marathons was her tireless struggle to bring him food and news, and the sight of his kids growing up safe and strong. "I take this oath," he told her. "When I get out of here, and when I get another invitation to go some-where, I won't accept unless you can come too. You are the marathoner here. You are enduring as much as I."

Aberash wet her fingers with her tears and touched his hand. She had often said that visiting the places Mamo had run was her greatest dream. Now it was their sacred promise.

AFTER FIVE YEARS of imprisonment, Wolde was finally indicted in March 1997. He was one of 72 detainees arraigned on charges of "participating in mass killings and torture." Prosecutor Wakjira said, "The trials should take less than three years."

Wolde's attorney, Atanafu Bogale, hired by the IOC, objected that the charges didn't include the place and date of the offense, or what weapons were used, as the law required. It took a year for the prosecutor to respond. In 1998, the court let the vague charges stand.

Then the baton in our Olympian relay was seized by an old friend and Oregon track teammate, the indefatigable Jere Van Dyk. A sub-four-minute miler and Sorbonne graduate, Van Dyk went to Addis Ababa in November 1998 to cover Wolde's trial for the *New York Times*. He struck up a relationship with the special prosecutor and persuaded prison authorities to let him not only interview Wolde, but also photograph him.

"He was small and thin," wrote Van Dyk, "his forehead deeply lined and his eyes watery. He had bronchitis and throughout a 90-minute interview exhibited a deep cough."

When the government's first witnesses testified at the trial, it was front-page news in Addis Ababa. "Complete with a picture of Wolde receiving an award many years ago from Emperor Haile Selassie," Van Dyk wrote to me, "a figure despised by many, most importantly Prime Minister Meles Zenawi and his fellow Tigrayans who are running the government."

Under Bogale's cross-examinations, it became clear that no accuser had actually seen Wolde commit any of the alleged acts. "It was hearsay, hearsay, hearsay," Wolde would later say. "The government case was futile. No one came to testify who had witnessed me do anything wrong."

Before a western judge, that would mean case dismissed. But the prosecutor begged the Ethiopian court for more time to dig up the eyewitnesses he'd promised. Multiple delays were granted. Wolde, then 68, kept wasting away.

Hope drained. It seemed Ethiopia was too unreachable, too destitute, too tribal, too proud, too callous to ever let Mamo Wolde walk free. I said as much to a friend, an Oregon circuit court judge. "Let them save face," he said. "Go for a lesser plea. Go for time served." That became my mantra. Time served.

THE SECRET OF ENDURANCE isn't so much a lesson as an imperative. You obey the dictates of the marathon. You cut your losses and keep on. You go numb, bleed out, and keep on. You fall, get up, and keep on. You go from rock to rock, from tree to tree, and keep on. You take strength in knowing others care about your effort, and keep on.

Wolde kept on. The great, uncrackable marathoner physically outlasted Ethiopia. In January 2002 a judge convicted him of a lesser charge, sentenced him to six years, and released him because he'd already served nine. Time served. That evening he was home with Aberash and his children. "Thank God, I am free at last," he said. "I hold no malice toward anyone."

The news reached me at home in Hawaii on Martin Luther King Day. "Free at last!" I echoed, and celebrated with a dizzy, whooping run. But even as I imagined Mamo finally reunited with Aberash and his family, a fear knifed me. He must be really sick. Maybe they just didn't want him dying in their prison cell.

Not long afterward, a man called and introduced himself as Mengesha Beyene, of the Ethiopian Sports Federation. He wanted to make sure I knew Wolde was free. I told him I desperately wanted to talk with Mamo, and asked if he could help. Beyene not only could, he did, translating during a three-way call with Wolde.

Wolde's first words were, "I feel like we are embracing!"

I said he was a true marathoner.

"Thanks, thanks. Except for the separation from family and the isolation of prison, I haven't felt abandoned. Thanks to the Olympic community."

I asked the big one. "How's your health?"

"Hey," he said, "give me a couple of months to recuperate and I'll race you anywhere you want, any distance you want!"

Wolde said he wanted to stay in Addis "and establish an institute to perpetuate the legacy of Abebe Bikila" (who'd died in 1973). Generations of champions had welcomed him home. Haile Gebrselassie had raised money to help pay off his "prison debts."

"It's reincarnation for me to join my family," Wolde said. "People visit every day and say, 'We recognize you as a great Ethiopian hero.'"

But things were hardly idyllic. "Prices are staggering, and my son is losing his eyesight," he said. "But for now, it's bliss. The children hug me all the time. If I go around the corner to the store, we all have to go together, kids and Aberash and me, all tangled in a group. In the capable hands of my wife, we have made it safely through."

When he hung up, I was weightless. Beyene filled the silence with a few lines from Alfred, Lord Tennyson's *Ulysses*, which he learned in Emperor Haile Selassie's secondary school.

> *... And though*
> *We are not now that strength which in old days*
> *Moved earth and heaven; that which we are, we are;*
> *One equal temper of heroic hearts,*
> *Made weak by time and fate, but strong in will*
> *To strive, to seek, to find, and not to yield.*

I couldn't get Wolde's fire out of my mind. So I called Dr. Jon Cross of the Honolulu Marathon Association and asked whether the old invitation to Mamo still stood. He called back and said, "Get training, buddy! We're not only inviting Mamo and Aberash, but also you, Shorter, and [Karel] Lismont, the top four from Munich 30 years ago, to run here in December."

We all accepted, none of us sure we could actually make the distance. I had a sore tendon. Frank had just had shoulder surgery. He said, "This isn't fair. Mamo has been safe in prison. We free citizens have crippled ourselves."

I imagined how the story might end, with the four of us old Olympians, perhaps in our Munich uniforms, striding barefoot down my Kailua beach, the turquoise sea breaking upon the level white sand. On the dunes, watching, would be Aberash Wolde and Beyene and our choked-up families. Beyene would declaim more Tennyson into the wind:

> *Some work of noble note, may yet be done,*
> *Not unbecoming men that strove with Gods ...*
> *It may be we shall touch the Happy Isles,*
> *And see the great Achilles, whom we knew.*

And every palm tree, every face, every drop splashed up by our feet would glow with perfect clarity as we ran, in the Happy Isles, with the great Achilles, whom we knew.

So I refused to absorb it, in May, when Beyene called to tell me Wolde had died. Jon Cross was equally shocked. "We just talked to him," he said. "When he accepted our invitation, he said his liver condition was flaring up. I said to fax me his prescription and I'd shoot him what he needed. But he never did." Ten days later he was dead.

Thousands wept as an honor guard of Ethiopian Olympic champions escorted his casket three miles from his home through Addis Ababa to St. Joseph's Cemetery. He now lies beside his inspiration and friend, Abebe Bikila, the man who ordered him to win the Olympic gold medal in Mexico City.

I spoke to Aberash Wolde on her twelfth day of mourning, the day in Ethiopian custom when friends call and bring potluck, to assure the bereaved that they're not forgotten. She recalled Mamo's vow not to travel without her. "When Dr. Cross called and invited Mamo to Honolulu in December, he asked if I might come," Aberash said. "And Dr. Cross said I must come. Mamo jubilantly accepted. He was so happy. This was the culmination of our dream. Mamo's liver hurt, but that was completely wiped away by the joy that at last we would keep his promise. And we would do it in Hawaii. It was unimaginable."

Aberash's tears had flowed, she said finally, because she knew that he was dying.

The liver pains had intensified a month before. Mamo had looked a little jaundiced, but he played it down. "My husband lived and died a strong man," she said. She got him to a clinic for a checkup, and the doctor told her it was cancer and Mamo had only weeks left. The clinic did what it could to make him comfortable, then sent him home to be with friends and family. He died peacefully, as befits a marathoner, knowing the rightness of all things physical has an end.

So now it would be Aberash coming in Mamo's place to Honolulu in December. "From here on out," she said, "I duly represent the legend."

ABERASH ARRIVED IN HONOLULU the Friday before the race, escorted by two Olympic marathon champions, Fatuma Roba (Atlanta in 1996) and Gezahegne Abera (Sydney in 2000). We draped her with leis of tuberose and ilima, the latter a flower reserved for royalty in ancient Hawaii. She in turn presented Cross and me each with an airily soft, white, embroidered dashiki,

Ethiopian dress for special occasions. "Christmas," she whispered, "or the coffee ceremony."

Aberash brought out photos showing how fragile Mamo had been—paper and sticks, glue and grit—during the four months before he died.

Thinking we'd be good hosts, we unfolded a map of Oahu. Had she and Mamo had something they especially wanted to do? Aberash began to cry, while we writhed at our ignorant presumption. Recovering, she made it clear that her mission had little to do with mooning over waterfalls.

"Life in Ethiopia," she began, "is very difficult." Neither she nor Mamo has any remaining family, so she is the sole support for Adiss Alem, now 13, and Tabor, 11. Mamo's oldest son, Samuel, 26, can't work because of his vision problems. Their only income is a small stipend from the IOC. The public schools are dead ends, and she couldn't afford to put the children in private education. Famine is once again present in parts of the country. Abera and Roba confirmed all this, and said the assistance other Ethiopian athletes can offer is more emotional than financial.

We adjourned to let Aberash rest. I sought out the other two Munich Olympians. Karel Lismont, who'd claimed "my" bronze, was only 53. He'd finished second in 1972 at age 22 and run in four Olympics in all, taking the bronze in Montreal in 1976, three seconds ahead of Don Kardong of the United States. As Shorter put it, "He's kept more Americans from medals than any other runner." Lismont turned out to be a man of strict pronouncements. He said running 30 minutes three times a week was all men of our age should do, and so didn't enter the Honolulu Marathon.

I had developed a sore hip in training ("See, see!" said Lismont), so didn't run the marathon either. But Shorter did, and beautifully, covering each mile in exactly seven and a half minutes to finish in 3:23. It was his first marathon in seven years. Afterward, the old Olympians were of one equal temper. We wanted to help Aberash.

Things came together over lunch in Kailua the day before she had to leave. Cross reported that the Honolulu Marathon Association was contributing a grant. Shorter and I had taken up collections at runners' gatherings. All told, we presented Aberash with enough for a year of schooling and support for the children.

Beyene translated Aberash's response, not that he needed to, given the relief on her face. "Thank you from my children," she said. "Thank you from my husband, your friend."

Serious matters concluded, the sentimental Cross, who'd never been able to shake the vision of us all striding together on my beach, proposed that we actually do it.

Kailua's sands were windswept and gray as Shorter arranged us in the order we'd finished 30 years before. He was on the high side, then Lismont, then Aberash—a yard ahead, as she was representing our Achilles here—then me, with my toes in the Pacific foam. We walked along tentatively for a while, feeling odd, with Aberash looking back occasionally to see if she was doing what was wished. At last we just clumped together and walked on in each other's arms.

Cross, backpedaling with his camera, shouted and pointed. A rainbow arched down, pouring upon us all the colors of the Olympic rings. Aberash turned and saw it. Her flinch was as electric as Wolde's embrace had been in prison. I looked down. She too has a faint widow's peak.

Her jolt passed through us all, and the circle of 30 years was at last closed. It was so perfect that we hesitated to speak of it. As we drew apart, all the talk was of the future, of safe travel, of hopes for the children, even as we stared up at Mamo's rainbow, strengthening in the sky, signifying that it was all right to go on, that the bond is as strong as ever.

CONTRIBUTORS

BRUCE BARCOTT, a 2009 Guggenheim Fellow, is the author of *The Last Flight of the Scarlet Macaw*. Barcott is an environmental journalist whose articles on humans and wildlife appear in *Runner's World*, *National Geographic*, the *New York Times Magazine*, *Outside*, and other publications. He lives on Bainbridge Island, Washington, with his wife, writer Claire Dederer, and their children.

JOHN BRANT started running in 1972, and began working for *Runner's World* in 1982. He has served the magazine in roles ranging from copy editor to his present position as writer at large. Several of his stories have appeared in *The Best American Sports Writing*. Brant is the author of *Duel in the Sun: Alberto Salazar, Dick Beardsley, and America's Greatest Marathon*. He lives in Portland, Oregon, with his wife, Patricia Gregorio, and two children.

AMBY BURFOOT has been a *Runner's World* editor since 1978. He won the Boston Marathon in 1968, and later that year ran 2:14:29 (fifth place) in the Fukuoka Marathon. He attended high school in Groton, Connecticut, where he was coached by 1957 Boston winner John J. "The Younger" Kelley. In college at Wesleyan University, he roomed with Bill Rodgers and Jeff Galloway. He considers himself a very lucky guy.

CHARLES BUTLER has been an editor at *Runner's World* since 2004. His writing has also appeared in the *New York Times*, *SmartMoney*, and *Fortune*, among others. He lives in Emmaus, Pennsylvania, with his wife and two children.

BENJAMIN H. CHEEVER is a writer at large for *Runner's World* and the author of four novels (*The Plagiarist*, *The Partisan*, *Famous after Death*, and *The Good Nanny*) and two works of nonfiction (*Selling Ben Cheever* and *Strides*). He edited *The Letters of John Cheever*. Most recently, he collaborated with illustrator Tim Grajek on a children's book titled *The First Dog*. He lives in Pleasantville, New York, with his wife, Janet Maslin, film and literary critic for the *New York Times*.

SARA CORBETT has been a contributing writer to the *New York Times Magazine* since 2001 and is a writer at large for *Runner's World*. Her piece about America's best 12-year-old baseball pitcher was included in *The Best American Sports Writing*. She's written for numerous magazines, including *National Geographic*, *Esquire*, *Mother Jones*, and *Elle*. She lives and runs in Portland, Maine. And she still talks on the phone with her friend Clare—about running and not running—pretty much every single day.

BILL DONAHUE has written for the *New Yorker*, the *Atlantic*, *Bicycling*, *Backpacker*, *Men's Journal*, and the *Washington Post Magazine*. A competitive distance runner in college, he is now an avid cyclist and cross-country skier. He lives in Portland, Oregon.

STEVE FRIEDMAN is a writer at large for *Runner's World*, *Bicycling*, and *Backpacker* magazines. His work has appeared in publications such as *Esquire*, *GQ*, *Outside*, the *New York Times*, the *Washington Post*, and *New York* magazine, and been reprinted in *The Best of Outside*, *The Bastard on the Couch*, *Modern Love*, *The Best American Travel Writing*, and *The Best American Sports Writing*. He lives in New York City (http://stevefriedman.net).

CYNTHIA GORNEY, a former reporter for the *Washington Post*, is the author of *Articles of Faith: A Frontline History of the Abortion Wars*, and teaches at UC Berkeley's Graduate School of Journalism. She is a writer at large for *Runner's World* and a contributing writer for *National Geographic* and the *New York Times Magazine*. Her deeply undistinguished running career—two marathons, a few half-marathons and 10-Ks, and a lot of 25-mile weeks—seems to have been stymied, at present, by a trashed left knee.

DON KARDONG, the author of *Thirty Phone Booths to Boston: Tales of a Wayward Runner*, is currently a contributing editor to *Runner's World*. He ran cross-country and track at Stanford University, finishing second behind Steve Prefontaine in the 1971 PAC-8 3-Mile in 13:19.8. He finished fourth in the 1976 Olympic Marathon in Montreal. He is currently the race director of the Lilac Bloomsday Run in Spokane, Washington, where he lives with his wife and two grown daughters.

CHRISTOPHER MCDOUGALL is the author of *Born to Run: A Hidden Tribe, Superathletes, and the Greatest Race the World Has Never Seen*.

KENNY MOORE, a writer at large for *Runner's World*, is the author of *Bowerman and the Men of Oregon* and *Best Efforts*. He was a senior writer for *Sports Illustrated* for 15 years and the co-writer (with Robert Towne) and executive producer of *Without Limits*. He ran for Bill Bowerman at the University of Oregon, and was the National AAU cross-country champion in 1967 and the National AAU marathon champion in 1971. He ran in two Olympic marathons, finishing fourth in Munich in 1972. He splits his time between Hawaii and his native Eugene, Oregon.

JOHN L. PARKER JR. is the author of the novels *Once a Runner* and *Again to Carthage*. He has written for *Runner's World*, *Outside*, and numerous other publications. He was the Southeastern Conference mile champion three times and the United States Track and Field Federation national champion in the steeplechase. He lives in Gainesville, Florida, and Bar Harbor, Maine.

MICHAEL PERRY is the author of the best-selling memoirs *Population: 485*, *Truck: A Love Story*, and *Coop*. In high school he ran a 4:48 mile. Recently he eked out a 5:58. He lives in rural Wisconsin with his small family and some chickens (http://sneezingcow.com).

STEPHEN RODRICK is a contributing editor for *New York Magazine* and a writer at large for *Runner's World*. His writing has been included in *The Best American Sports Writing*, *The Best American Political Writing*, *The Best American Crime Reporting*, and *Wild Stories: The Best of Men's Journal*. With the exception of the two hours he spent circling Athens in a Toyota while lost on the freeway, he considers the two stories in this collection among the favorite stories of his career.

STEVE RUSHIN is the author of a novel, *The Pint Man*, and two nonfiction books, *Road Swing* and *The Caddie Was a Reindeer*. He spent 19 years on the staff of *Sports Illustrated* and was voted National Sportswriter of the Year by his peers. Rushin has run the New York and Chicago marathons (http://steverushin.com).

ROBERT SULLIVAN is a writer at large for *Runner's World* and the author of such books as *The Meadowlands*, *Rats*, *Cross Country*, and *The Thoreau You Don't Know*.